Management of Endometrial Cancer

Mansoor R. Mirza
Editor

Management of Endometrial Cancer

Springer

Editor
Mansoor R. Mirza
Rigshospitalet
Copenhagen University Rigshospitalet
København Ø
Denmark

ISBN 978-3-319-64512-4   ISBN 978-3-319-64513-1   (eBook)
https://doi.org/10.1007/978-3-319-64513-1

© Springer Nature Switzerland AG 2020
This work is subject to copyright. All rights are reserved by the Publisher, whether the whole or part of the material is concerned, specifically the rights of translation, reprinting, reuse of illustrations, recitation, broadcasting, reproduction on microfilms or in any other physical way, and transmission or information storage and retrieval, electronic adaptation, computer software, or by similar or dissimilar methodology now known or hereafter developed.
The use of general descriptive names, registered names, trademarks, service marks, etc. in this publication does not imply, even in the absence of a specific statement, that such names are exempt from the relevant protective laws and regulations and therefore free for general use.
The publisher, the authors, and the editors are safe to assume that the advice and information in this book are believed to be true and accurate at the date of publication. Neither the publisher nor the authors or the editors give a warranty, expressed or implied, with respect to the material contained herein or for any errors or omissions that may have been made. The publisher remains neutral with regard to jurisdictional claims in published maps and institutional affiliations.

This Springer imprint is published by the registered company Springer Nature Switzerland AG
The registered company address is: Gewerbestrasse 11, 6330 Cham, Switzerland

Preface

> In all affairs it's a healthy thing now and then to hang a question mark on the things you have long taken for granted.
>
> *Bertrand Russell (1872–1970)*

Management of endometrial cancer has improved in the past decade. A gynaecologist or an oncologist managing these patients needs to have an update and broad knowledge of all aspects of disease, including epidemiology, tumour biology, diagnostics and deep knowledge of multidisciplinary treatment approaches.

For many decades, treatment of endometrial cancer was based on our beliefs, expert opinions and rather low level of evidence resulting in different treatment approaches depending upon the subspecialty to treat the patient. The level of evidence has improved lately, which was reflected by the first of its kind of consensus report involving all subspecialties.

More high-quality clinical trials are being performed to answer some of the fundamental questions regarding management of this disease, thus improving outcome of our patients. This book tries to capture advances in all fields, and I would like to thank all my colleagues for their great contribution. My special thanks to OvaCure, Ms. Adoracion Pegalajar-Jurado and Ms. Tina Koutouleas for their tremendous organisational support to bring this project to a reality.

I hope that this contribution will help our colleagues in their continuous effort to improve the outcome of our patients.

Copenhagen, Denmark Mansoor R. Mirza

Contents

Part I Classification and Diagnosis of Endometrial Cancer

1. Classification of Endometrial Cancer 3
   Elisabeth Åvall Lundqvist

2. Controversies in Pathology and Advances in Molecular Diagnostics . 7
   Sara Imboden, Denis Nastic, and Joseph W. Carlson

3. Endometrial Cancer Genetic Classification
   and Its Clinical Application 23
   Lorenzo Ceppi, Don S. Dizon, and Michael J. Birrer

4. Advances in Endometrial Cancer Diagnosis 49
   Vincent Vandecaveye

Part II Epidemiology and Risk Factors of Endometrial Cancer

5. Epidemiology, Risk Factors, and Prevention for Endometrial Cancer 61
   Johanna Mäenpää

6. Hormone Interactions in Endometrial Cancer 69
   Areege Kamal, Nicola Tempest, Alison Maclean, Meera Adishesh,
   Jaipal Bhullar, Sofia Makrydima, and Dharani K. Hapangama

7. Hereditary Cancers... 101
   Lorenzo Ceppi, Don S. Dizon, and Michael J. Birrer

Part III International Clinical Guidelines

8. The Need for Level 1 Clinical Evidence in Daily Practice........... 119
   Athina Koutouleas and Mansoor Raza Mirza

9. Summary of Management Guidelines for Endometrial Cancer...... 133
   Ilaria Colombo, Stephanie Lheureux, and Amit M. Oza

Part IV Surgical Management of Endometrial Cancer

10 Surgical Principles of Endometrial Cancer 153
Anne Gauthier, Martin Koskas, and Frederic Amant

11 Surgical Principles in Endometrial Cancer 175
Andrea Mariani and Francesco Multinu

12 The Role of Sentinel Node Dissection 187
Petra Zusterzeel, Annemijn Aarts, Jenneke Kasiu, and Tineke Vergeldt

13 Fertility-Sparing Treatment in Early-Stage Endometrial Cancer 201
Stefano Greggi, Francesca Falcone, and Giuseppe Laurelli

Part V Non-surgical Management of Endometrial Cancer

14 Risk Factors in the Early-Stage Endometrial Cancer 213
Samira Abdel Azim

15 Role of Radiation Therapy 223
Mansoor Raza Mirza

16 Chemotherapy in Endometrial Cancer 231
Domenica Lorusso and Mansoor Raza Mirza

17 Role of Hormonal Therapy in Advanced Stage Endometrial Cancer . 243
Anouk Gaber-Wagener and Christian Marth

18 Targeted Therapy in Management of Endometrial Cancer 249
Yeh Chen Lee, Stephanie Lheureux, Mansoor Raza Mirza, and Amit M. Oza

19 Management of Rare Uterine Malignant Tumors 277
Frederic Amant, Martee Hensley, Patricia Pautier, Michael Friedlander, Satoru Sagae, Keiichi Fujiwara, Dominique Berton Rigaud, Domenica Lorusso, and Isabelle Ray-Coquard

Index 313

Part I

Classification and Diagnosis of Endometrial Cancer

Classification of Endometrial Cancer

Elisabeth Åvall Lundqvist

Endometrial cancer is the most common malignancy of the female genital tract in the more developed regions of the world [1]. Stage of disease, i.e., the extent of tumor spread at the time of presentation, is the most significant prognostic parameter.

The prognosis of endometrial cancer is generally good with a 5-year relative survival around 80% [2], mostly attributable to early detection, i.e., stage I and endometrioid histology. However, survival stage-for-stage is similar to ovarian cancer. Data from Surveillance, Epidemiology, and End Results (SEER) registries report 5-year relative survival rate of 95.8% for stage I, compared to 15.9% for women with stage IV uterine corpus cancer [3].

The main purpose of cancer staging is to help clinicians predict the prognosis for a cancer patient, guide treatment planning, evaluate and compare treatment results, facilitate exchange of information between health professionals, and help in identifying clinical trials that may be appropriate for the patient. Cancer staging systems should be evidence-based and practical, which implies that changes will occur over time based on new knowledge.

The first cancer staging system was published in 1929 under the patronage of the League of Nations, and applied to carcinoma of the cervix uteri [4]. In 1958, the International Federation of Gynecology and Obstetrics, FIGO (Fédération Internationale de Gynécologie et d'Obstétrique), assumed the responsibility for supervising the staging of gynecological cancers as well as the patronage of publishing treatment results (the Annual Report on the Results of Treatment in Gynecological Cancer). The same year, FIGO developed the clinical staging system for carcinoma of the corpus uteri. In 1971, the grade of tumor was added as part of the staging.

E. Åvall Lundqvist (✉)
Department of Oncology and Department of Clinical and Experimental Medicine, Linköping University, Linköping, Sweden
e-mail: elisabeth.avall.lundqvist@liu.se

© Springer Nature Switzerland AG 2020
M. R. Mirza (ed.), *Management of Endometrial Cancer*,
https://doi.org/10.1007/978-3-319-64513-1_1

Table 1.1 FIGO surgical staging for Endometrial Carcinoma (2009)

FIGO stage	
I[a]	Tumor confined to the corpus uteri
IA[a]	No or less than half myometrial invasion
IB[a]	Invasion equal to or more than half of the myometrium
II[a]	Tumor invades cervical stroma, but does not extend beyond the uterus[b]
III[a]	Local and/or regional spread of the tumor
IIIA[a]	Tumor invades the serosa of the corpus uteri and/or adnexae[c]
IIIB[a]	Vaginal and/or parametrial involvement[c]
IIIC[a]	Metastases to pelvic and/or para-aortic lymph nodes[c]
IIIC1[a]	Positive pelvic nodes
IIIC2[a]	Positive para-aortic lymph nodes with or without positive pelvic lymph nodes
IV[a]	Tumor invades bladder and/or bowel mucosa, and/or distant metastases
IVA[a]	Tumor invasion of bladder and/or bowel mucosa
IVB[a]	Distant metastases, including intraabdominal metastases and/or inguinal lymph nodes

[a]Either G1, G2, or G3
[b]Endocervical glandular involvement should be considered only as Stage I and no longer as Stage II
[c]Positive cytology has to be reported separately without changing the stage

Based on the results from several studies of systematic evaluation of surgical–pathological patterns of spread, FIGO decided in 1988 that corpus uteri cancer should be surgically staged [5]. Specifically, lymph node involvement and the depth of myometrial invasion were implemented. A large data collection including over 42,000 patients with surgically staged endometrial cancer was presented in volume 26 of the FIGO Annual Report [6]. The results from the annual report and other supporting publications demonstrated no significant difference in 5-year survival rate between specific substages in stage I, hence these substages were merged in the revised FIGO surgical staging in 2009. The revision also included other changes, i.e., involvement in the endocervical glandular portion of the cervix was allotted to stage I, pelvic and para-aortic lymph node involvement was separated. In addition, isolated peritoneal cytology was eliminated as a criterion to change stage but should be recorded separately [7, 8]. See Table 1.1.

1.1 Rules Related to Staging

The primary site is the corpus uteri. There should be histologic verification of grading and extent of the tumor.

1.1.1 Histopathologic Grades (G)

GX: Grade cannot be assessed.
G1: Well differentiated.

1 Classification of Endometrial Cancer

Table 1.2 FIGO clinical staging for Endometrial Carcinoma (1971)

FIGO stage	
I	The carcinoma is confined to the corpus
IA	The length of the uterine cavity is 8 cm or less
IB	The length of the uterine cavity is more than 8 cm
II	The carcinoma has involved the corpus and the cervix, but has not extended outside the uterus
III	The carcinoma has extended outside the uterus, but not outside the true pelvis
IV	The carcinoma has extended outside the true pelvis or has obviously involved the mucosa of the bladder or rectum. A bullous edema as such does not permit a case to be allotted to stage IV
IVA	Spread of the growth to adjacent organs as urinary bladder, rectum, sigmoid or small bowel
IVB	Spread to distant organs

G2: Moderately differentiated.
G3: Poorly or undifferentiated.

Although endometrial cancer is surgically staged, there will still be a small number of patients who will not undergo primary surgery. In these cases, the clinical staging system adopted by FIGO in 1971 should be applied (see Table 1.2), and the staging system noted. Ideally, distance from serosa surface should be measured. As a minimum, any enlarged or suspicious lymph nodes should be removed in all patients. For high-risk patients (grade 3, deep myometrial invasion, cervical extension, serous or clear cell histology), complete pelvic lymphadenectomy and resection of any enlarged para-aortic nodes is recommended.

Carcinosarcomas should be staged as endometrial carcinoma. A separate staging system, FIGO staging for uterine sarcoma, should be used for leiomyosarcomas, endometrial stromal sarcomas, and adenosarcomas.

References

1. Ferlay J, Soerjomataram I, Dikshit R, Eser S, Mathers C, Rebelo M, et al. Cancer incidence and mortality worldwide: sources, methods and major patterns in GLOBOCAN 2012. Int J Cancer. 2015;136:E359–86.
2. Klint Å, Tryggvadóttir L, Bray F, Gislum M, Hakulinen T, Storm HH, Engholm G. Trends in survival of patients diagnosed with cancer in the female genital organs in the Nordic countries 1964-2003 followed up to end of 2006. Acta Oncol. 2010;49(5):632–43.
3. Siegel R, DeSantis C, Virgo K, Stein K, Mariotto A, Smith T, et al. CA Cancer J Clin. 2012;62:220–41.
4. Odicino F, Pecorelli S, Zigliani L, Creasman WT. History of the FIGO cancer staging system. Int J Gynecol Obstet. 2008;101:205–2010.
5. Shepherd JH. Revised FIGO staging for gynaecological cancer. Br J Obstet Gynaecol. 1989;96(8):889–92.

6. Creasman WT, Odicino F, Maisonneuve P, Quinn MA, Beller U, Benedet JL, et al. Carcinoma of the corpus uteri. FIGO 26th annual report on the results of treatment of gynecological cancer. Int J Gynaecol Obstet. 2006;95(Suppl 1):S105–S43.
7. Pecorelli S, FIGO Committee on Gynecologic Oncology. Revised FIGO staging of the vulva, cervix, and endometrium. Int J Gynecol Obstet. 2009;105:103–4.
8. Creasman W. Revised FIGO staging for carcinoma of the endometrium. Int J Gynecol Obstet. 2009;105:109.

Controversies in Pathology and Advances in Molecular Diagnostics

2

Sara Imboden, Denis Nastic, and Joseph W. Carlson

2.1 Introduction

Pathology is an evolving specialty, and the advancement of knowledge has led to the introduction of new concepts and diagnoses, and the disappearance of others. Just as in clinical medicine, the evolution of the field is rarely due to presence of perfect data. Classification systems evolve and adapt, with the integration of new discoveries. This is particularly true of endometrial cancer, where a number of new molecular factors have been identified in the past few years.

This chapter presents an overview of the histopathological classification of endometrial carcinomas, as defined by the 2014 World Health Organization Classification of Tumors of Female Reproductive Organs [1, 2]. The chapter progresses from a discussion of precursor lesions to the histological carcinoma subtypes and finally to the genomic characterization of endometrial cancer by the Cancer Genome Atlas (TCGA). Where applicable, controversies are discussed under the relevant diagnoses. Finally, at the end of the chapter, a discussion of two simplified molecular classification systems based upon the TCGA is presented; first the ProMisE system, developed at the University of Vancouver and then the PORTEC system, developed at the University of Leiden. These two systems attempt to recapitulate the genomic classification of the TCGA using methods that are readily available in a modern clinical pathology lab.

S. Imboden
Department of Obstetrics and Gynecology, University Hospital of Bern and University of Bern, Bern, Switzerland

D. Nastic · J. W. Carlson (✉)
Department of Oncology-Pathology, Karolinska Institutet, Stockholm, Sweden

Department of Pathology and Cytology, Karolinska University Hospital, Stockholm, Sweden
e-mail: joseph.carlson@ki.se

2.2 Precursor Lesions

The diagnosis of precancers of endometrioid carcinoma has been controversial for a number of years. The hyperplasia classification has been in use for several decades. It is based on defining the complexity of gland architecture (the degree of fusing and branching of glands) as well determining if cytologic atypia is present. This results in a subgrouping with four different histological patterns: simple hyperplasia, complex hyperplasia, simple atypical hyperplasia, and complex atypical hyperplasia. This system has some advantages and it initially promised to be a good predictor of the risk of progression to cancer. However, the hyperplasia system has several weaknesses: throughout the years the criteria for gland complexity and cell atypia have been defined, redefined, and reorganized leading to confusion of pathologists, gynecologists, and oncologists. Additionally, studies have shown poor reproducibility and difficulties with molecular correlation [2].

In the late 1990s the EIN system (Endometrial, changed to "endometrioid" by the WHO, Intraepithelial Neoplasia) has been developed. This system initially used objective morphometric data to assess a "D-score" but later formal morphometry was dropped. The current system only uses routine microscopy. The system is based on assessing three factors: the stroma-to-gland ratio, size of the focus, and nuclear pleomorphism (which is assessed by comparing nuclei in the crowded gland areas to nuclei in the "background"). The system's great advantage is a better reproducibility among pathologists and a relative ease of use in clinical pathology while also showing a close relationship with early molecular events (such as PAX2 inactivation, PTEN, and KRAS mutation). The EIN system was recently endorsed in an opinion paper by the American College of Obstetrics and Gynecology [3]. However, it made several changes to the diagnosis of "atypia," which have been difficult for supporters of the hyperplasia system to accept.

In the latest edition of the WHO 2014 the two systems have been combined into "Atypical hyperplasia/Endometrioid intraepithelial neoplasia (AH/EIN)." The combined system has retained the traditional definition of nuclear atypia while noting that the assessment of atypia can be facilitated by comparing crowded gland cells to adjacent normal gland cells. The EIN classification's increased gland-to-stroma ratio (area of gland exceeds that of stroma) was incorporated fully in the current WHO classification.

It should be noted that the above discussion refers to precancerous lesions of endometrioid carcinoma, which are common. There is, however, a second precursor lesion, named "Serous endometrial intraepithelial carcinoma (SEIC)." SEICs are rare, and are the immediate precursors of invasive serous carcinoma. It is characterized by an underlying p53 mutation. Because SEIC spreads by exfoliation of malignant cells into the uterine cavity, it can be associated with extra-uterine spread even without invasion. Therefore its clinical risk is similar to that of the fully developed carcinoma, and hence is discussed under serous carcinoma (below) [4].

2.3 Endometrioid Carcinoma

Endometrioid carcinomas are the most common epithelial tumors of the endometrium [1, 5]. Microscopically, in their most well-differentiated form, these tumors resemble proliferative phase endometrial mucosa, with columnar cells containing an abundant cytoplasm and oval nuclei (Fig. 2.1a). However, these carcinomas display an architectural complexity that is absent in benign and hyperplastic mucosa. This complexity is seen as either cribriform, solid, villoglandular, or papillary growth [5].

Endometrioid carcinomas are further characterized by the frequent presence of altered cell differentiation (i.e. metaplasia). Note that the term "differentiation" is typically used for changes of cell type in precancers and carcinomas, while the term "metaplasia" is reserved for similar changes in benign endometrial epithelia. Squamous differentiation is common, and so is mucinous, tubal, and secretory (Fig. 2.1b, c). These changes can confirm the diagnosis of endometrioid carcinoma, but can also make the diagnosis challenging, especially when the majority of the tumor is affected.

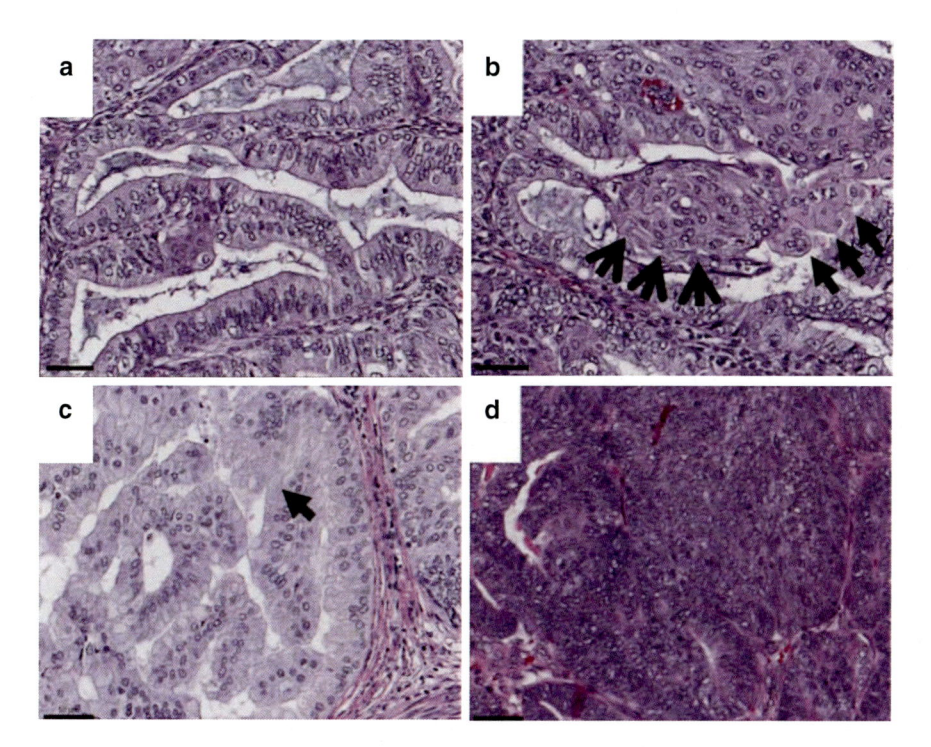

Fig. 2.1 Representative images of endometrioid carcinoma. (**a**) An area of glandular growth, typical of FIGO grade 1 tumors, (**b**) squamous differentiation, both immature (open arrows) and more mature (closed arrows), (**c**) mucinous differentiation with intracytoplasmic mucin (closed arrow), (**d**) an area of solid growth, consistent with a FIGO grade 3 tumor

Grading of endometrioid carcinomas uses the FIGO grading system, presented in Chap. 1 [6]. It has been proposed that this three-grade system be combined into a two-grade system, where grades one and two are combined into a "low-grade" group and grade 3 is synonymous with "high-grade" [7]. Endometrioid FIGO grade 3 tumors are characterized by >50% solid growth, but should show areas of typical endometrioid differentiation, either by demonstrating the correct microscopic appearance of the cells, or by the presence of altered cell differentiation (Fig. 2.1d).

The molecular aberrations identified in endometrioid carcinomas vary with the grade of the tumor. Low-grade tumors are characterized by frequent mutation or inactivation of PTEN (>50%), PIK3CA, PIK3R1, and ARID1A [1]. FIGO grade 3 tumors can show mutation or inactivation of TP53. The presence of a TP53 mutation is sufficiently associated with poor prognosis and aggressive behavior that it should essentially exclude a FIGO grade 1–2 endometrioid carcinoma [8, 9].

Controversial areas within the diagnosis of endometrioid carcinoma include the distinction of FIGO 3 tumors from serous carcinomas, the correct identification of lymphovascular space invasion (LVSI), and the clinical significance of the microcystic, elongated, and fragmented (MELF) growth pattern. Within each of these there are variations in diagnosis between labs. The distinction of high-grade tumors from each other is one area where molecular methods, discussed below, may have significant impact. The presence of LVSI is used in several risk stratification models, including the European joint guidelines for risk stratification [10].

LVSI assessment can be quite difficult, and endometrioid tumors often show "retraction artifacts" in hysterectomy specimens which can mimic true LVSI. Immunohistochemical markers for endothelial cells (CD31, CD34, ERG) and Elastin-stains for Elastin fibers in vessel walls often aid the assessment.

The MELF-pattern has been linked to increased risk of deep myometrial invasion, LVSI, and above all lymph node metastasis [11]. In broad terms it should be a straightforward diagnosis and is usually found unexpectedly in preoperatively low-risk patients. The morphology is of a low-grade endometrioid cancer with distinct widely scattered microcystic glands that deeply invade the myometrium without a desmoplastic reaction. At the deep invasive front there are usually only a few elongated glands and LVSI. Problems arise when trying to assess this morphologic pattern in "nonclassical" cases; the most common problem being that only a part of the tumor shows the MELF-pattern morphology. It is therefore difficult to clearly define how extensive the MELF patterns should be to define a cancer as MELF. It also invites a highly subjective assessment (and therefore low reproducibility) as clear and objective definitions for MELF are missing.

2.4 Serous Carcinoma

Serous carcinomas are typically seen in association with endometrial polyps and an atrophic endometrial mucosa. Of note, these carcinomas can grow by replacing the endometrial epithelium, leading to an appearance that has been called "serous endometrial intraepithelial carcinoma" (the preferred term) or, alternatively, "serous carcinoma in-situ" or "early serous carcinoma" [1]. Whatever the term, it is vitally important that treating surgeons and oncologists realize that serous carcinomas spread by exfoliation of cells directly into the uterine cavity and, via the fallopian tubes, to the peritoneal cavity and omentum. Thus, even in the absence of invasion, SEIC has a risk of metastasis to extra-uterine sites [12].

Serous carcinomas are rare in the endometrium, in contrast to the ovary. These tumors resemble high-grade serous carcinomas of the ovary, with high-grade nuclear atypia, a brisk mitotic rate, and single-cell necrosis (see Fig. 2.2a, b) [8, 13] Additionally, just like ovarian high-grade serous carcinomas, these tumors show a wide variety of growth patterns, such as solid, cribriform, and gland-like, in addition to the classic papillary and micropapillary growth. Micropapillary growth is commonly seen in serous carcinomas but is not required for the diagnosis. Thus, the name "seropapillary carcinoma" should be avoided.

One characteristic feature of serous carcinomas is the near ubiquitous presence of a deletion or mutation of the TP53 gene. This mutation leads to a characteristic immunohistochemical pattern, with approximately 90% of tumors showing strong nuclear positivity in over 80% of tumor cells (Fig. 2.2c) [14]. The remaining 10% can show a completely negative staining result, which has been called the "null

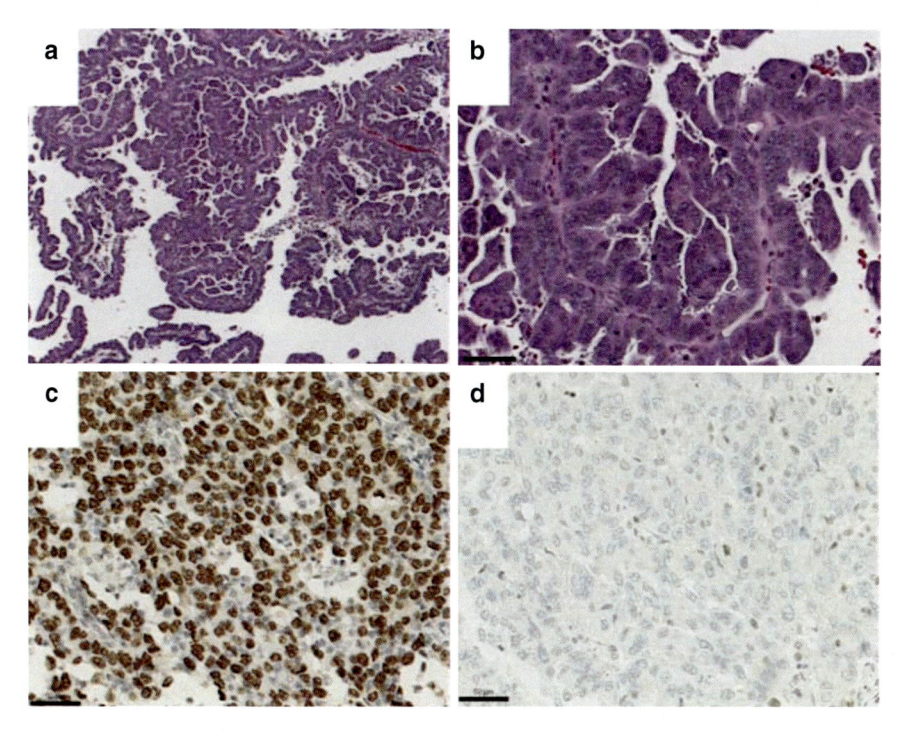

Fig. 2.2 Representative images of serous carcinoma. (**a**) Low-power and (**b**) high-power images of the prototypical papillary growth pattern. (**c**) p53 immunohistochemistry consistent with a TP53 gene mutation. (**d**) The so-called null-pattern staining, which is also consistent with a TP53 mutation

staining pattern" (Fig. 2.2d). The sensitivity and specificity of immunohistochemistry is high but not 100%, and so in discrepant cases consensus histology, or even TP53 sequencing, may be necessary. Serous carcinomas are not graded, as in the endometrium they are all high-grade.

Beyond the near ubiquity of TP53 mutations, serous carcinomas can show mutations in PIK3CA, FBXW7, and PPP2R1A [1]. There is some data indicating that germline BRCA1/2 mutations are associated with the development of endometrial serous carcinomas [15].

2.5 Clear Cell Carcinoma

Clear cell carcinomas are among the rarest of subtypes, making up roughly 2% of endometrial carcinomas [1, 2, 16]. Microscopically, these tumors consist of round to polygonal tumor cells with an abundant clear to granular cytoplasm and a typically central round to polygonal nucleus. The tumor cells contain abundant glycogen, which can be demonstrated using special stains. The characteristic feature of these tumors is the presence of papillary, tubulocystic, and solid growth patterns and the presence of myxoid or hyalinized stroma (Fig. 2.3a, b). Hobnail cells are the most common cell seen [16].

Immunohistochemistry can be useful in the diagnosis of these tumors, where they are characteristically ER and PR negative, and can show expression of Napsin A [17]. Approximately 30% of cases can show a mutation in p53, as detected by immunohistochemistry [18].

Molecular studies have demonstrated a variety of mutations in these tumors, such as mutations in PTEN, TP53, ARID1A, and PIK3CA [19].

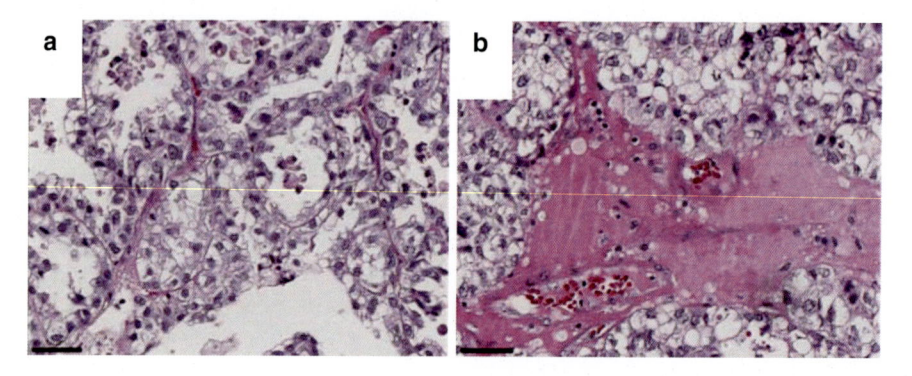

Fig. 2.3 Clear cell carcinoma. (**a**) Low-power and (**b**) high-power images of clear cell carcinoma

2.6 Undifferentiated and Dedifferentiated Carcinoma

There is increasing recognition of undifferentiated carcinomas as a distinct tumor type, separate from other high-grade carcinomas, such as FIGO 3 endometrioid tumors and carcinosarcomas. In the pure form, where no other tumor component is seen, they are called undifferentiated carcinomas. In a dedifferentiated carcinoma, the undifferentiated component is seen in combination with a FIGO1-2 endometrioid carcinoma. The identification of dedifferentiated carcinomas implies that biologically the tumor represents a dedifferentiation, or transformation, of the lower-grade endometrioid tumor to the high-grade undifferentiated component.

Microscopically these tumors are made of solid sheets of high-grade tumor cells showing no particular differentiation. In practice, this means a lack of endometrioid or serous type growth patterns, a lack of variant differentiation (e.g. squamous differentiation). The tumor cells are typically highly dyscohesive and thus can resemble a high-grade lymphoma (Fig. 2.4a). These tumors typically show a reduction in staining with epithelial markers such as keratin, but epithelial membrane antigen is typically retained.

Molecularly these tumors appear to be associated with mutation of members of the SWI/SNF family of genes, as well as loss of functional mismatch repair, as demonstrated by immunohistochemistry for the proteins MLH1, PMS2, MSH2, and MSH6.

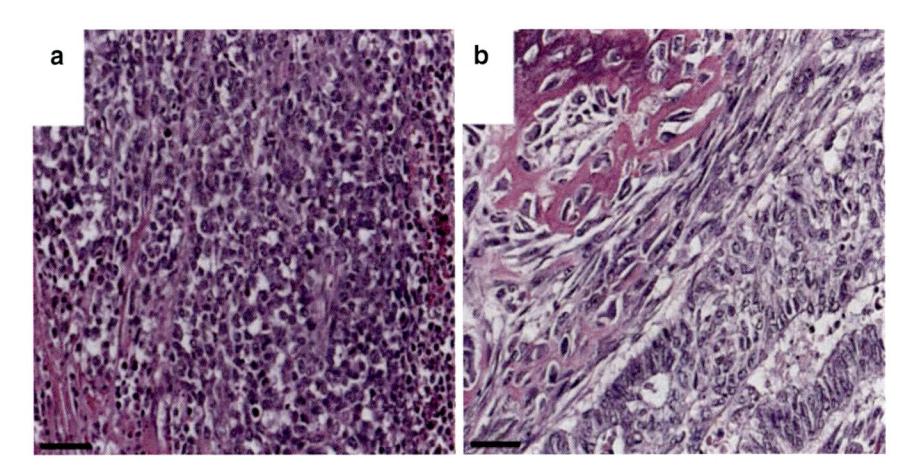

Fig. 2.4 (**a**) Undifferentiated carcinoma showing solid growth of dyscohesive cells lacking in differentiation. (**b**) Carcinosarcoma showing high-grade mesenchymal (upper left) and epithelial (lower right) components

2.7 Mixed Carcinoma

Mixed carcinomas are defined in the WHO 2014 as a tumor composed of a mixture of two tumor types, where at least one of them must be a "Type 2" tumor. The two types must be readily recognizable in routine hematoxylin- and eosin-stained sections. The minimum percentage of the secondary component has been arbitrarily set to 5%, and the behavior of the tumor clinically is expected to follow the most high-grade component. Indeed, research has shown that as little as 5% serous carcinoma can adversely affect outcome [20]. Immunohistochemistry can be used to further support a diagnosis of a mixed carcinoma.

2.8 Neuroendocrine Tumors

Neuroendocrine tumors range from low-grade neuroendocrine tumor (carcinoid tumor) to high-grade neuroendocrine carcinoma (small cell and large cell neuroendocrine carcinoma). These tumors share a characteristic neuroendocrine morphology, and the neuroendocrine differentiation should be confirmed using immunohistochemistry.

Low-grade neuroendocrine tumors of the endometrium are extremely rare; they have been described only in a few case reports. Clearly a metastasis from a low-grade neuroendocrine tumor outside the uterus needs to be excluded before a primary endometrial tumor can be considered. This exclusion must be done with careful clinical and radiological correlation. Microscopically, low-grade neuroendocrine tumors show a variety of growth patterns and a characteristic "salt and pepper" chromatin of the nuclei.

High-grade neuroendocrine tumors can be divided into small cell and large cell types. Small cell neuroendocrine carcinomas resemble the tumor of the same name seen in the lung, with poorly cohesive cells with minimal cytoplasm, nuclear molding, high mitotic rate, karyorrhexis, and the common presence of "crush" artifact. Large cell neuroendocrine carcinomas should only be diagnosed if they show the characteristic growth patterns of well-demarcated nests, trabeculae, and cords, with peripheral palisading. Immunohistochemistry with chromogranin, synaptophysin and CD56, can be used to confirm neuroendocrine differentiation.

2.9 Carcinosarcoma

These tumors are defined as biphasic tumors consisting of high-grade carcinomatous (i.e. epithelial) and sarcomatous (i.e. mesenchymal) components. They were previously called "Malignant mixed Müllerian tumor," and this term, as well as its abbreviation MMMT, is still commonly in use.

Microscopically there is typically an intimate mixture of the two components (Fig. 2.4b). The carcinomatous component is usually either endometrioid or serous. The sarcomatous component is typically high-grade and nonspecific (i.e. showing no particular diagnostic features of a more specific sarcoma type); however, tumors can show rhabdomyosarcoma, chondrosarcoma, and even osteosarcoma differentiation. Regardless of the type of sarcomatous differentiation it is believed that the origin of these tumors is from the carcinoma, which is why they have been included in this section. Immunohistochemistry is not helpful in the diagnosis and the immunophenotype can be more confusing than helpful.

The Tumor Cancer Genome Atlas recently sequenced 57 untreated patients with carcinosarcoma. The tumors had extensive copy-number alterations and highly recurrent somatic mutations. Frequent mutations were seen in TP53, PTEN, PIK3CA, PPP2R1A, FBXW7, and KRAS, also often found in endometrioid and serous carcinomas [21].

2.10 The Cancer Genome Atlas (TCGA) Endometrial Carcinoma Analysis

In 2013 the TCGA completed its integrated genomic characterization of 373 endometrial cancers, including low- and high-grade endometrioid and serous tumors [22]. Tumors were studied by a comprehensive series of methods, including somatic copy-number alterations, exome sequencing, mRNA expression, protein expression, microRNA expression, and DNA methylation. Given the wealth of data, and the number of different methods applied, a custom-built clustering algorithm called "SuperCluster" was developed to derive overall subtypes across all methods. The SuperCluster data indicates the limitations of current diagnostic methods. Within tumors diagnosed "endometrioid" (based on routine light microscopy) are multiple molecular subtypes. Four molecular subtypes were identified, including ultramutated "POLE," hypermutated "MSI," copy-number low "endometrioid-like," and copy-number high "serous-like," as described in (Table 2.1).

Ultramutated "POLE" Group One of the most fascinating finding of the TCGA classification was the identification of an ultramutated tumor type with an extremely favorable prognosis. These tumors show high mutation rates (232×10^{-6} mutation per Mb) and an increased C to A transversion frequency. All of these tumors show mutations in the exonuclease domain of POLE, the catalytic subunit of polymerase epsilon, which is involved in nuclear DNA replication and repair. Mutation rates seen in these tumors exceed those found in any other tumor lineage.

Prognosis of these tumors appears to be extremely favorable [22, 24–27]. The TCGA showed a progression-free survival of 100%. Subsequent studies have confirmed this finding. A European study using the PORTEC-1 and -2 trial cohorts ($n = 788$) identified 48 POLE tumors (6.1%) [25]. There was a strong association of POLE mutation status with high tumor grade; however, none of the patients with high-grade POLE tumors experienced progression or death. These results have been confirmed in a number of subsequent studies. The conclusion of these studies is that POLE tumors of all grades display excellent prognosis, independent of other known prognostic factors. In vitro studies showed that POLE mutated cells had resistance toward cisplatin, suggesting that the good outcome is not secondary to the response

Table 2.1 Summary of the molecular, pathological, and clinical characteristics of the TCGA genomic subtypes [22, 23]

Subgroup	Molecular character	Pathological and clinical character
POLE mutated (7%)	Missense mutation (C → A transversions) in POLE exonuclease domain (catalytic subunit involved in DNA replication and repair) leading to very high mutation rates (ultramutated) Typical mutations: PTEN, PK3R1, PIK3CA, FBXW7, KRAS	Most stage I, endometrioid, also grade 3 tumors High neoantigen loads and number of TILs, overexpression of PD-1 and PD-L1, possibly eligible for checkpoint inhibitors Excellent progression-free survival
Microsatellite instability (MSI) (28%)	MSI mutated, leading to impaired mismatch repair (proofreading in DNA replication), leading to high mutation rates (hypermutated) Alterations of the TK/RAS/β-catenin pathway (70%) and IK3CA/PIK3R1-PTEN pathway (95%)	This group can correlate with Lynch syndrome, allowing preventive strategies for colorectal cancer. Possible targeted therapy options include the mTOR pathway or immunotherapy with checkpoint inhibitors (pembrolizumab (PD-1 inhibitor)
Copy-number low (39%)	16 different genes with frequent alterations in the PI3K pathway (92% of tumors), alterations in the RTK/RAS/β-catenin pathway (83%), and somatic mutations in *CTNNB1*	This group represents most of the grades 1 and 2 endometrioid cancers and has an intermediate prognosis
Copy-number high, serous like (26%)	High degree of somatic copy-number alterations (duplications of segments of the genome) with frequent *p53* mutations (90%), amplifications of the *MYC* and *ERBB2* oncogenes	In this group, 25% were endometrioid high-grade tumors, all showing poor prognosis. This group may profit from treatments closer to the treatments of other serous cancers

TILS tumor infiltrating lymphocytes

to chemotherapy [23, 28]. The ultra-mutated status of these tumors produces a strong immunogenic reaction, this is seen in intra- and peritumoral lymphocyte infiltration, expression of PD-1 and PD-L1, as also additional T cell markers thus being a possible target for checkpoint inhibitors [29–32].

Hypermutated "MSI" Group These tumors show an intermediate mutation frequency (18×10^{-6} mutations per Mb) and were associated with MLH1 promoter methylation. These tumors showed microsatellite instability, few somatic copy-number alterations, and frequent nonsynonymous KRAS mutations.

Copy-Number Low "Endometrioid-Like" Group These tumors have a low mutation rate (2.9×10^{-6} mutations per Mb). This group consists primarily of microsatellite stable endometrioid cancers. These tumors showed an unusually high frequency of CTNNB1 mutations (52%).

Copy-Number High "Serous-Like" Group These tumors also have a low mutation rate (2.3×10^{-6} mutation per Mb), but they have extensive somatic copy-number alterations. These tumors had a significantly worse progression-free survival than the endometrioid groups. Of note, 25% of cases diagnosed by light microscopy as "high-grade endometrioid" cancer had a genomic profile matching the serous-like group. Several potential therapeutic copy-number alterations were detected, including 15q26.2 (amplification in IGF1R) and ERBB2, FGFR1 and FGFR3, and LRP1B deletion. A subset of serous-like endometrial cancers may in fact be derived from the fallopian tube [33]. Tubal serous carcinomas are treated differently than uterine, but this distinction cannot be made without molecular testing. These similarities were seen in the TCGA analysis, where uterine serous cancers show demonstrated similarities to both ovarian serous cancers basal-like breast carcinoma, including high frequencies of TP53 and PTEN mutations. Differences included the higher frequency of PIK3CA, FBXW7 and PPP2R1A1 in uterine serous carcinomas.

2.11 ProMisE (*Proactive Molecular Risk* Classifier for *Endometrial* Cancer)

Researchers at the University of British Columbia have developed and studied a classification system, with the goal of recapitulating the TCGA genomic classifier, but using readily available methods such as immunohistochemistry and gene sequencing [34, 35]. Here markers such as POLE mutation, p53 IHC and TP53 mutation, PTEN, MMR IHC (MLH1, MSH2, MSH6, and PMS2), and FISH for three specific loci (FGFR (4p16.3), SOX17 (8q11.23), and MYC (8q24.12) to determine the copy-number groups, were tested. The result is a molecular classifier called ProMisE, which divides patients with endometrial cancer into MMR abnormal, POLE-mutated, and p53 abnormal or wild-type (Fig. 2.5). These groups correlate with the TCGA subgroups concerning outcomes, and could be a base for developing clinical studies on treatment (Table 2.2).

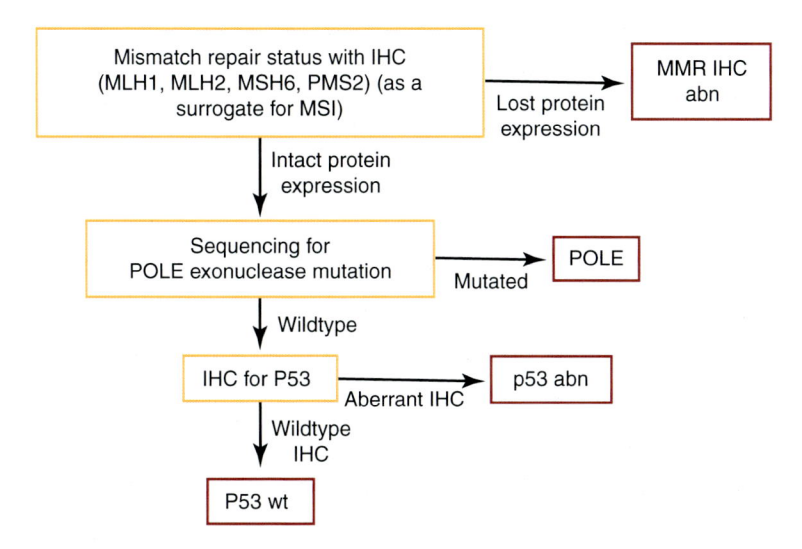

Fig. 2.5 A schematic diagram showing the application of the ProMisE, molecular subtyping

Table 2.2 Summary of proposed molecular risk stratification systems

	Group 1	Group 2	Group 3	Group 4
TCGA $N = 373$	POLE • Ultramutated >232 × 10^{-6} per Mb • POLE mutation • 7%	MSI • Hypermutated >18 × 10^{-6} per Mb • MSI mutation • MLH1 promoter Methylation • 28%	Copy-Nr high • Serous like • Extensive SCNA • Low mutation rate • 39%	Copy-Nr low • MSS • Low copy Nr • Low mutation rate • Endometrioid • 26%
ProMisE $N = 152$	MSI • MMR IHC (MLH1, MLH2, MSH6, PMS2) • 29%	POLE • POLE mutation in (Exon 9–14) • PTEN (not in all) • MSS • 8%	P53 abnormal • p53 IHC 0 or 2+ or TP 53 sequencing • 18%	P53 wild-type • MSS • No POLE mutation • p53 (IHC 1+) • 45%
PORTEC $N = 836$ early stage $N = 116$ High risk	P53 • IHC p53 pos (>50% strong nuclear staining or >50% tumor cell positivity) if unclear TP53 sequenced • 9%/33%[a]	POLE • POLE mutation in exons 9 or 13 • 6%/12%[a]	MSI • MMR IHC (MLH1, MLH2, MSH6, PMS2) • MLH1 hypermethylation • 26%/17%[a]	NSMP • P53 wt, no POLE mutations, MMR stained • 59%/38%[a] • LVSI, L1CAM, p53 remain independent prognostic factors

Original TCGA genomic subtypes ([22]; ProMisE [35] and PORTEC [36]
NSMP No specific molecular profile, *MSS* microsatellite stable, *MSI* microsatellite unstable, *MMR* Mismatch repair, *MLH1* MutL homolog 1, *SCNA* somatic copy-number alterations, *POLE* Polymerase Epsilon, *IHC* Immunohistochemistry, *LVSI* lymphovascular space invasion, *L1CAM* L1-cell adhesion molecule
[a]In the early-stage cohort/in high-risk cohort

2.12 PORTEC

Researchers at the Leiden University Medical Center have developed and tested a molecular classification, using some additional methods when compared to ProMisE [36, 37]. This classification uses microsatellite instability testing, sequencing for hotspot mutations in 14 genes (including POLE), and immunohistochemistry for a number of biomarkers (Table 2.2). The sub-analysis for early-stage endometrial cancer gave an indication that applying the MSI, POLE and p53 analyses, and also stratifying into favorable and nonfavorable by using other markers such as L1CAM, LVSI, CTNNB1 [36]. The use of these markers can help to identify subgroups eligible to targeted treatment. However, in the same cohort, the identification of p53, POLE mutations, and MSI status alone lead to an identification of four subgroups similar to those proposed by the TCGA. The clinical utility of these groups will be assessed in the prospective PORTEC-4 study.

2.13 Outlook and Future Directions

The validation of the proposed molecular classification systems is an important next step to proving their sustainability and applicability to different cohorts in clinically different settings. Prospective studies will be necessary to evaluate adaptations of adjuvant treatment in different subgroups. The evolution towards combining known pathological risk factors with newer molecular markers is a large step towards personalized medicine, with associated improvements in treatment selection.

References

1. Kurman RJ, Carcangiu ML, Herrington CS, Roung RH, IARC. WHO classification of tumours of female reproductive organs. Lyon: IARC Press; 2014.
2. Zaino RJ, Kauderer J, Trimble CL, Silverberg SG, Curtin JP, Lim PC, Gallup DG, Mackey D. Reproducibility of the diagnosis of atypical endometrial hyperplasia: a gynecologic oncology group study. Cancer. 2006;106(4):804–11. https://doi.org/10.1002/cncr.21649.
3. ACOG. Endometrial Intraepithelial Neoplasia Committee Opinion No. 631. 2015.
4. Owings RA, Quick CM. Endometrial intraepithelial neoplasia. Arch Pathol Lab Med. 2014;138(4):484–91. https://doi.org/10.5858/arpa.2012-0709-RA.
5. Malpica A. How to approach the many faces of endometrioid carcinoma. Mod Pathol. 2016;29(S1):S29–44. https://doi.org/10.1038/modpathol.2015.142.
6. FIGO. Announcements. Gynecol Oncol. 1989;35(1):125–7. https://doi.org/10.1016/0090-8258(89)90027-9.
7. Alkushi A, Abdul-Rahman ZH, Lim P, Schulzer M, Coldman A, Kalloger SE, Miller D, Gilks CB. Description of a novel system for grading of endometrial carcinoma and comparison with existing grading systems. Am J Surg Pathol. 2005;29(3):295–304. https://doi.org/10.1097/01.pas.0000152129.81363.d2.
8. Gatius S, Matias-guiu X. Practical issues in the diagnosis of serous carcinoma of the endometrium. Mod Pathol. 2016;29(S1):S45–58. https://doi.org/10.1038/modpathol.2015.141.
9. Soslow RA. Endometrial carcinomas with ambiguous features. Semin Diagn Pathol. 2010;27:261–73. https://doi.org/10.1053/j.semdp.2010.09.003.

10. Colombo N, Creutzberg C, Amant F, Bosse T, González-Martín A, Ledermann J, Marth C, et al. ESMO-ESGO-ESTRO consensus conference on endometrial cancer: diagnosis, treatment and follow-up. Ann Oncol. 2016;27(1):16–41. https://doi.org/10.1093/annonc/mdv484.
11. Cole AJ, Quick CM. Patterns of myoinvasion in endometrial adenocarcinoma: recognition and implications. Adv Anat Pathol. 2013;20(3):141–7. https://doi.org/10.1097/PAP.0b013e31828d17cc.
12. Hui P, Kelly M, O'Malley DM, Tavassoli F, Schwartz PE. Minimal uterine serous carcinoma: a clinicopathological study of 40 cases. Mod Pathol. 2005;18(1):75–82. https://doi.org/10.1038/modpathol.3800271.
13. Sherman ME, Bitterman P, Rosenshein NB, Delgado G, Kurman RJ. Uterine serous carcinoma. A morphologically diverse neoplasm with unifying clinicopathologic features. Am J Surg Pathol. 1992;16(6):600–10.
14. Köbel M, Piskorz AM, Lee S, Lui S, LePage C, Marass F, Rosenfeld N, Mes Masson A-M, Brenton JD. Optimized p53 immunohistochemistry is an accurate predictor of TP53 mutation in ovarian carcinoma. J Pathol Clin Res. 2016;2(4):247–58. https://doi.org/10.1002/cjp2.53.
15. Lavie O, Ben-Arie A, Segev Y, Faro J, Barak F, Haya N, Auslender R, Gemer O. BRCA germline mutations in women with uterine serous carcinoma--still a debate. Int J Gynecol Cancer. 2010;20(9):1531–4. https://doi.org/10.1111/IGC.0b013e3181cd242f.
16. Fadare O, Zheng W, Crispens M a, Jones HWI, Khabele D, Gwin K, Liang SX, et al. Morphologic and other clinicopathologic features of endometrial clear cell carcinoma: a comprehensive analysis of 50 rigorously classified cases. Am J Cancer Res. 2013;3(1):70–95.
17. Fadare O, Desouki MM, Gwin K, Hanley KZ, Jarboe EA, Liang SX, Quick CM, Zheng W, Parkash V, Hecht JL. Frequent expression of napsin A in clear cell carcinoma of the endometrium: potential diagnostic utility. Am J Surg Pathol. 2014;38(2):189–96. https://doi.org/10.1097/PAS.0000000000000085.
18. Fadare O, Gwin K, Desouki MM, Crispens MA, Jones HW, Khabele D, Liang SX, et al. The clinicopathologic significance of p53 and BAF-250a (ARID1A) expression in clear cell carcinoma of the Endometrium. Mod Pathol. 2013;26(8):1101–10. https://doi.org/10.1038/modpathol.2013.35.
19. Hoang LN, Mcconechy MK, Meng B, Mcintyre JB, Ewanowich C, Gilks CB, Huntsman DG, Köbel M, Lee CH. Targeted mutation analysis of endometrial clear cell carcinoma. Histopathology. 2015;66(5):664–74. https://doi.org/10.1111/his.12581.
20. Quddus M, Ruhul CJS, Zhang C, Dwayne Lawrence W. Minor serous and clear cell components adversely affect prognosis in mixed-type endometrial carcinomas: a clinicopathologic study of 36 stage-I cases. Reprod Sci. 2010;17(7):673–8. https://doi.org/10.1177/1933719110368433.
21. Cherniack AD, Shen H, Walter V, Stewart C, Murray BA, Bowlby R, Hu X, et al. Integrated molecular characterization of uterine carcinosarcoma. Cancer Cell. 2017;31(3):411–23. https://doi.org/10.1016/j.ccell.2017.02.010.
22. Network, Cancer Genome Atlas Reserach. Integrated genomic characterization of endometrial carcinoma. Nature. 2013;497(53):67–73. https://doi.org/10.1038/nature12113.
23. Bellone S, Bignotti E, Lonardi S, Ferrari F, Centritto F, Masserdotti A, Pettinella F, et al. Polymerase ε (POLE) ultra-mutation in uterine tumors correlates with T lymphocyte infiltration and increased resistance to platinum-based chemotherapy in vitro. Gynecol Oncol. 2017;144(1):146–52. https://doi.org/10.1016/j.ygyno.2016.11.023.
24. Billingsley CC, Cohn DE, Mutch DG, Stephens JA, Suarez AA, Goodfellow PJ. Polymerase?? (POLE) mutations in endometrial cancer: clinical outcomes and implications for lynch syndrome testing. Cancer. 2015;121(3):386–94. https://doi.org/10.1002/cncr.29046.
25. Church DN, Briggs SEW, Palles C, Enric Domingo SJ, Kearsey JM, Grimes MG, et al. DNA polymerase {varepsilon} and δ exonuclease domain mutations in endometrial cancer. Hum Mol Genet. 2013;22(14):2820–8. https://doi.org/10.1093/hmg/ddt131.
26. Hussein YR, Britta Weigelt DA, Levine JKS, Dao LN, Balzer BL, Liles G, et al. Clinicopathological analysis of endometrial carcinomas harboring somatic POLE exonuclease domain mutations. Mod Pathol. 2015;28(4):505–14. https://doi.org/10.1038/modpathol.2014.143.

27. Meng B, Hoang LN, McIntyre JB, Duggan MA, Nelson GS, Lee CH, Köbel M. POLE exonuclease domain mutation predicts long progression-free survival in grade 3 endometrioid carcinoma of the endometrium. Gynecol Oncol. 2014;134(1):15–9. https://doi.org/10.1016/j.ygyno.2014.05.006.
28. Santin AD, Bellone S, Buza N, Choi J, Schwartz PE, Schlessinger J, Lifton RP. Regression of chemotherapy-resistant polymerase ε (POLE) ultra-mutated and MSH6 hyper-mutated endometrial tumors with nivolumab. Clin Cancer Res. 2016;22(23):5682–7.
29. Bellone S, Centritto F, Black J, Schwab C, English D, Cocco E, Lopez S, et al. Polymerase?? (POLE) ultra-mutated tumors induce robust tumor-specific CD4 + T cell responses in endometrial cancer patients. Gynecol Oncol. 2015;138(1):11–7. https://doi.org/10.1016/j.ygyno.2015.04.027.
30. Eggink FA, Van Gool IC, Leary A, Pollock PM, Crosbie EJ, Mileshkin L, Jordanova ES, et al. Immunological profiling of molecularly classified high-risk endometrial cancers identifies POLE -mutant and microsatellite unstable carcinomas as candidates for checkpoint inhibition. OncoImmunology. 2017;6(2):e1264565. https://doi.org/10.1080/2162402X.2016.1264565.
31. Van Gool IC, Eggink FA, Freeman-Mills L, Stelloo E, Marchi E, De Bruyn M, Palles C, et al. POLE proofreading mutations elicit an antitumor immune response in endometrial cancer. Clin Cancer Res. 2015;21(14):3347–55. https://doi.org/10.1158/1078-0432.CCR-15-0057.
32. Mehnert JM, Panda A, Zhong H, Hirshfield K, Damare S, Lane K, Sokol L, et al. Immune activation and response to pembrolizumab in POLE-mutant endometrial cancer. J Clin Investig. 2016;126(6):2334–40. https://doi.org/10.1172/JCI84940.
33. Jarboe E, Folkins A, Nucci MR, Kindelberger D, Drapkin R, Miron A, Lee Y, Crum CP. Serous carcinogenesis in the fallopian tube. Int J Gynecol Pathol. 2008;27(1):1–9. https://doi.org/10.1097/pgp.0b013e31814b191f.
34. Talhouk A, McAlpine JN. New classification of endometrial cancers: The development and potential applications of genomic-based classification in research and clinical care. Gynecol Oncol Res Pract. 2016;3(1):14. https://doi.org/10.1186/s40661-016-0035-4.
35. Talhouk A, McConechy MK, Leung S, Li-Chang HH, Kwon JS, Melnyk N, Yang W, et al. A clinically applicable molecular-based classification for endometrial cancers. Br J Cancer. 2015;113(2):299–310. https://doi.org/10.1038/bjc.2015.190.
36. Stelloo E, Nout RAA, Osse EMM, rgenliemk-Schulz IJJ, Jobsen JJJ, Lutgens LCC, van der Steen-Banasik EMM, et al. Improved risk assessment by integrating molecular and clinicopathological factors in early-stage endometrial cancer - combined analysis of PORTEC cohorts. Clin Cancer Res. 2016;22(16):4215. https://doi.org/10.1158/1078-0432.CCR-15-2878.
37. Stelloo E, Bosse T, Nout RA, MacKay HJ, Church DN, Nijman HW, Leary A, et al. Refining prognosis and identifying targetable pathways for high-risk endometrial cancer; a TransPORTEC initiative. Mod Pathol. 2015;28(6):836–44. https://doi.org/10.1038/modpathol.2015.43.

Endometrial Cancer Genetic Classification and Its Clinical Application

3

Lorenzo Ceppi, Don S. Dizon, and Michael J. Birrer

3.1 Introduction

Each year, epithelial endometrial cancer (EC) incidence accounts for 7% of all cancers in women worldwide, representing the fourth most common malignancy arising in women. In the United States alone, over 54,000 new cases are expected and over 10,170 women will die of this disease in 2015 [1].

This disease consists of multiple variants, where the most relevant are the endometrioid and serous EC histotypes. Despite several classifications that divide EC into different histotypes or clinical types, a better understanding of the different genomic events harbored in uterine cancer allowed the scientific community to gain a deeper knowledge of the differences among this disease. This knowledge is driving the actual amount of precision medicine research in EC.

L. Ceppi
Center for Cancer Research, The Gillette Center for Gynecologic Oncology,
Massachusetts General Hospital, Harvard Medical School, Boston, MA, USA

Department of Medicine and Surgery, Milano-Bicocca University,
ASST-Monza, Desio Hospital, Monza and Brianza, Italy

D. S. Dizon
Center for Cancer Research, The Gillette Center for Gynecologic Oncology,
Massachusetts General Hospital, Harvard Medical School, Boston, MA, USA

M. J. Birrer (✉)
Center for Cancer Research, The Gillette Center for Gynecologic Oncology,
Massachusetts General Hospital, Harvard Medical School, Boston, MA, USA

O'Neal Cancer Center, Birmingham, AL, USA
e-mail: mbirrer@uab.edu

3.2 Clinical/Epidemiological Classification (Type I–II EC)

The World Health Organization (WHO) pathologic classification divides EC histotypes in endometrioid and serous adenocarcinoma. In addition rarer histotypes include others, such as clear cell, mucinous adenocarcinoma, mixed cell, metaplastic (carcinosarcoma), squamous cell, transitional cell, small cell, and undifferentiated carcinoma [2].

A two-tier category was established by Bokhman [3] to discriminate EC into two types (type I and type II), which acknowledged the divergent clinical, pathological, and molecular features that separate them, as discussed below [4].

Type I EC is characterized by estrogenic stimulation, such as the elevated estrogenic state in obese women and postmenopausal women taking hormone replacement therapy. It builds on a theory that unopposed estrogenic stimulation environment may promote carcinogenesis, which is supported by data that demonstrates high estrogen serum levels in type I EC patients [5]. Type I tumors are characterized by endometrial hyperplasia, where atypical hyperplasia (AEH) could constitute the precursor lesion for EC. Findings demonstrated that PTEN alteration, an important cell cycle tumor suppressor that regulates cell growth and survival, is already present in AEH, representing a plausible early mutational hallmark for type I EC [6]. It is by far the most common EC histotype, representing 85% of all new diagnoses [7], and usually the prototype of type I is low-grade (grade 1–2), low-stage endometrioid histotype endometrial cancer (EEC), with good prognosis.

Type II EC is clinically characterized by diagnosed at older age, no association with estrogen stimulation, and it commonly arises in a background of atrophic endometrium. Compared to Type I tumors, they are often more aggressive behavior and tend to be diagnosed at a higher stage. Although not as common as Type I EC, it substantially contributes to overall EC mortality [8]. Uterine serous carcinoma (USC) is the prototype of type II carcinoma, and genomically, it is associated with a high frequency of TP53 mutations [9]. A number of studies suggest that TP53 mutations may occur as early events [10].

Although this classification is commonly accepted in the scientific community and represents a basic understanding of EC behavior, an ongoing debate centers on whether it is sufficiently comprehensive to explain the heterogeneity of EC [11]. For example, high-grade endometrioid EC, representing up to 19% of EC, may be included as either Type I or Type II categories, since it is associated with an aggressive behavior is poorly correlated with obesity, and has no association with hyperplasia [12]. Moreover, a small subset of serous EC has indolent behavior (2%), without evidence o myometrial invasion, representing a rare subgroup of USC [13]. Lastly, clear cell and rare histotypes are not taken into account in this classification and should be considered separately [14].

To complicate the classification even more, there are known morphologic overlaps between type I/II EC which results in poor interobserver reproducibility among pathologists [15]. At this time there are no prognostic tools such as IHC markers to help distinguish such cases. In that sense, a deeper knowledge of the molecular level of EC cancer is paving the way of further understanding and classification.

3.3 Genetic Correlation to Tumor Types

The vast majority of EC is caused by sporadic mutations and gene alterations. In addition to clinical and epidemiological features, there are distinct genomic alterations that distinguish Type I and II EC [16], which are discussed below.

3.3.1 Candidate Genes and Pathways

Many studies describe several deregulated pathways in EC [17] (refer to Table 3.1).

1. *PI3K-AKT-mTOR* pathway is one of the most studied downstream regulators of cell growth and survival [18, 19]. Briefly, membrane growth factor receptors activate PI3K, which phosporylates PIP3 (phosphatidylinositol 3,4,5 phosphate), under PTEN negative control. This leads to activation of intracellular transcription regulators such as *AKT* and *mTOR* (mammalian target of rapamycin) complex, composed of mTORC1 and 2, and subsequently to transcription factors, such as S6K-1 (ribosomal S6 kinase 1) and 4E-BP1, affecting cell proliferation.

Table 3.1 Prevalence of mutations between Endometrioid and Serous Histotypes

Alteration	Prevalence in EEC (%)	Prevalence in USC (%)
Aneuploidy	10–50	70–95
Microsatellite instability	20–23	15
AKT1 mutation	2–3	13
ARID1A mutation	40	18
BRAF mutation	0–23	11
CDKN2A mutation	10–30	44
CTNNB1 mutation	2–45	0
FBXW7 mutation	2–16	0
FGFR2 mutation	5–16	2–3
KRAS2 mutation	8–43	3
PIK3CA mutation	36–52	33
PIK3R1 mutation	21–43	12
PIK3CA amplification	2–14	46
PPP2R1A	21–43	12
PTEN mutation/loss of function	57–78	13–19
TP53 mutation	5–20	53–90
Nuclear accumulation of β-catenin	18–47	0
E-cadherin loss	5–53	62–88
p16 positive expression	5–38	63–100
CCNE1 amplification	5	42
HER2 overexpression	3–10	32
HER2 amplification	1–63	17–42
Claudin-3 positive expression	38	74
Claudin-4 positive expression	9	63

EEC endometrioid endometrial cancer, *USC* papillary serous endometrial cancer

Among membrane growth factors, several are described to be related to cancer development in EC. *ERBB2* gene amplification and its product HER2 overexpression, *EGFR* gene amplification, and *FGFR2* gene mutation can be activators of PI3K pathway [20–22]. *PTEN* gene is a tumor suppressor protein that negatively regulates this pathway, and it is found mutated in up to 80% of EC. *PIK3CA* gene, which encodes the catalytic subunit of PI3K, p110α and *PIK3R1*, which encodes the regulatory subunit of PI3K, p85α, are globally mutated in about 43% in EC.

2. RAS-RAF-MEK-ERK pathway mediators are importantly deregulated in several cancers, and also present in EC. This deregulation can also cross talk and activate the PI3K-AKT-mTOR pathway, *KRAS* is the main target of mutation in EC [23].
3. *WNT-βcatenin* signaling pathway regulates gene transcription and development. Its alteration is through loss of *E-cadherin* expression and subsequent *βcatenin* nuclear accumulation, is present in up to 50% of endometrioid, and up to 80% of serous EC [24]; *CTNNB1* (β-catenin) gain-of-function mutations are also present in around 25% of endometrioid EC, rarely present in their serous counterparts [25].
4. *Microsatellite instability* (MSI), alteration of repetitive nucleotide sequence lengths is an event that scars the DNA in multiple regions. It occurs due to mismatch repair system deficiency (MLH1, MSH2, MSH6, PMS2) and MLH1 promoter hypermethylation [26]. This condition is the distinguishing trait in Lynch Syndrome, but it is also present in sporadic EC.
5. *TP53* master regulator gene suppression due to mutation, is present in the majority of USC, though in a smaller portion of EEC.
6. *ARID1A* tumor suppressor and the encoded protein product *BAF250a* are a part of chromatin remodeling complex (SNF/SWI) that regulates transcriptional activation of chromatin-repressed genes. Its mutation and loss of expression lead to a common deregulation in EEC [27].
7. *PPP2R1A* encodes the α-isoform of the scaffolding subunit of the PP2A enzyme, a putative tumor suppressor complex. This hypothesis has been confirmed by the evidence of its activity loss due to gene mutations as a pro-oncogenic event in hematologic and solid tumor growth, like endometrial and ovarian cancer [28, 29], leading to unregulated kinase activity, disease maintenance, transformation, and tumor cell survival.

3.3.2 Endometrioid Endometrial Adenocarcinoma

Numerous studies have been done and show that endometrioid carcinomas (EEC) are chromosomally stable, preserving the diploidic gene number [30]. However, a certain level of genetic instability can be ascribed to mismatch repair-related genes, PTEN loss of function [31], adenomatous polyposis coli protein [32], RAS-associated domain family member protein 1 (RASSF1A) [33] and E-cadherin [34]. Also MSI, due to MLH1 promoter hypermethylation occurs in up to a third of sporadic EEC [35], it is instead rare in USC.

The most frequently altered genes in EEC are PTEN (present in 57–78%), PIK3CA (36–52%), and PIK3R1 (21–43%) [18, 36–38]. These findings highlight the importance of the PI3K-AKT-mTOR pathway in this disease. KRAS gene (18% of cases) or promoter hypermethylation (62–74%) [39] is also a common event in EEC, less common in USC (3%). FGFR2 receptor mutation is present in up to 16% of EEC and, interestingly, FGF and KRAS pathway mutations are mutually exclusive, indicating differences in their phenotype correlate [40].

As mentioned, CTNNB1 mutation (2–45%) [24, 41] and β-catenin stabilization are responsible for the WNT signaling pathway alteration. WNT- and RAS-dependent pathway alteration seem to drive tumor growth in a mutually exclusive fashion, giving insights on pathway redundancy [40].

ARID1A is found mutated in 40% of low-grade endometrioid endometrial cancers, but this mutation is also related to up to 39% of high-grade endometrioid EC and 16% of endometrial hyperplasias [42, 43]. Further, it is found mutated in 18% of USC.

3.3.3 Uterine Serous Carcinoma

Since first pathologic [35] and genomic profiling studies and confirmed from recent genome wide analyses [44, 45], robust evidences demonstrate a recurrent mutated status in TP53 gene in up to 90% of cases, which broadly affects the chromosomal and DNA copy number stability. Animal models with P53 knock down demonstrated that a serous-like EC could arise [46]. A portion of 12% EEC harbors the same alteration in TP53 gene, mostly linked to high-grade tumors.

Other frequent mutations are present in PIK3CA, PIK3RI, and PTEN belonging to PI3K-AKT-mTOR pathway, 35%, 8%, 13%, respectively [18, 47]. Alterations in gene expression are affecting transcripts such as cyclin E and p16, HER2 expression, loss of BAF250A production, altered amounts of the cell adhesion proteins claudin-3, claudin-4, L1CAM (L1 cell adhesion molecule), EpCAM (epithelial cell adhesion molecule), and E-cadherin [43]. Interestingly, PPP2R1A mutation is found in 40% of USC and 5% of EEC [48].

Comparing these composite findings, it is clear that the clinical–epidemiological two-tier classification does not allow describing all the different overlapping features: USC tumors are not entirely TP53 or PPP2R1A carriers, as well as EEC cannot be related uniquely to PTEN, KRAS, CTNNB1, or PIK3CA mutations.

3.3.4 Hormonal Receptors Expression

Endometrial tissue is known to be a hormone-dependent tissue, and the driving component of estrogen/progesterone interaction alteration in EC is one of the mostly studied proliferation promoter. Unopposed estrogen stimulation is demonstrated to promote neoplastic transformation in endometrial tissue [49, 50]. Lebeau showed that amplification of ESR1 gene, encoding for ERα receptor, is a common event in EC. This phenomenon may result in a beneficial effect from anti-estrogenic therapy [51]. Expression of ERα is decreased in poorly differentiated tumors and high-stage disease, and this event is related to poor outcome. However, the disruption of ERα expression is not related to ESR1 mutations.

Moreover, lessons learned from basic researches in breast cancer show mechanisms of endocrine therapy resistance through aberrant activation of the PI3K–AKT–mTOR signaling pathway. These evidences support a close interaction between the mTOR pathway and ER signaling: mTORC1 substrate, S6 kinase 1, is capable of phosphorylation of the function domain of ER, which is responsible for ligand-independent receptor activation [52]. This interaction and its complementary inhibition was demonstrated effective in preclinical models [53]. Eventually, aromatase and mTOR complementary blockade showed successful clinical application in breast cancer [54].

Progesterone receptors are also found to play a role in EC carcinogenesis. For example, PR-A disrupted expression correlates with a worse prognosis in high grade EC [55] and it is an independent prognostic factor for disease-free survival in patients with EEC [56]. Evidences of tumor response are well known, last trials showed a combined effect of progestin and antiestrogenic therapy in up to 27% [57]. Personalized treatment may also consider the regulation of this downstream activator as a regulating target.

3.4 Molecular Classification of EC-TCGA

An integrated genomic analysis of primary diagnosis EC was reported in 2013 among The Cancer Genome Atlas project, providing a multilevel profile of EC of endometrioid, serous, and mixed histology [58].

This project provided a comprehensive description of mutation rates, copy number alterations frequency, microsatellite instability status, and RNA expression based on different platforms such as genome-wide copy number analysis, whole-exome sequencing, whole-transcriptome sequencing, expression profiling, reverse-phase protein array, methylation profiling, and MSI assessment. Complete profiles were obtained from 232 patients' samples; the entire cohort comprises 373 clinically annotated cases.

In summary, serous histology tumors and 25% of the high-grade endometrioid tumors have extensive copy number alterations, few DNA methylation changes, low estrogen receptor/progesterone receptor levels, and frequent TP53 mutations. Conversely, endometrioid tumors had few copy number alterations or TP53 mutations, but frequent mutations in PTEN, CTNNB1, PIK3CA, ARID1A, and KRAS and novel mutations in the SWI/SNF chromatin remodeling complex gene ARID5B.

Higher mutation frequencies than previous reports were found in TCGA dataset; this may be due to more comprehensive sequencing methods. A selected mutational status is reported in Tables 3.1 and 3.2, Le Gallo and Bell extensively summarized it in a recent review [59].

TCGA project provided four subtypes classification based on the multilevel analysis that also showed different outcomes in progression-free survival (PFS) outcome. The established four subgroups are named "*POLE* ultramutated," "Hypermutated/microsatellite-unstable," "copy number low/microsatellite-stable,"

3 Endometrial Cancer Genetic Classification and Its Clinical Application

Table 3.2 Mutational status among TCGA subgroups, adapted from cBioPortal (http://www.cbioportal.org/public-portal/)

Gene Name	POLE ultramutated ($n = 17$)	Hypermutated/ MS unstable ($n = 65$)	Copy number low/ MS stable ($n = 90$)	Copy number high/ serous-like ($n = 60$)	Total of four subgroups ($n = 232$)
PTEN (%)	94	88	77	10	64
ARID1A (%)	76	37	42	5	34
PIK3CA (%)	71	54	53	47	53
PIK3R1 (%)	65	40	33	13	32
CTNNB1 (%)	41	20	52	3	30
TP53 (%)	35	8	1	92	29
KRAS (%)	53	35	16	3	21
CSMD3 (%)	94	22	10	10	19
CTCF (%)	41	23	21	0	18
ZFH3 (%)	82	31	2	7	17
FBXW7 (%)	82	9	6	22	16
TAF1 (%)	82	25	1	5	15
FAT3 (%)	76	31	1	0	15
CHD4 (%)	65	6	12	13	15
USH2A (%)	76	18	4	5	14
FGFR2 (%)	29	14	13	5	14
MKI67 (%)	94	18	2	0	13
KMT2B (%)	65	22	4	0	13
RPL22 (%)	29	37	0	0	13
SPTA1 (%)	76	14	6	0	12
BCOR (%)	65	17	7	0	12
GIGYF2 (%)	59	20	0	7	12
ARID1B (%)	47	23	6	0	12
POLE (%)	100	8	3	2	11
FAM135B (%)	76	11	4	2	11
COL1 1A1 (%)	71	9	2	8	11

(continued)

Table 3.2 (continued)

Gene	POLE ultramutated	Hypermutated/ MS unstable	Copy number low/ MS stable	Copy number high/ serous-like	Total of four subgroups
PPP2R1A (%)	29	9	1	22	11
USP9X (%)	59	17	1	2	10
CSDE1 (%)	59	15	1	0	9
ATR (%)	65	9	0	2	8
SIN3A (%)	35	14	4	0	8
CDH19 (%)	59	5	1	5	7
LIMCH1 (%)	53	12	0	0	7
SLC9C2 (%)	53	5	2	3	7
SGK1 (%)	35	3	6	2	6
INPP4A (%)	29	9	2	0	6
CCND1 (%)	18	12	4	0	6
RBMX (%)	24	12	0	0	5
MECOM (%)	24	5	4	0	5
ESR1 (%)	24	2	6	2	5
NFE2L2 (%)	12	11	3	0	5
ZNF770 (%)	41	5	0	0	4
PNN (%)	35	6	0	0	4
AMY2B (%)	29	8	0	0	4
METTL14 (%)	24	5	3	0	4
TNFAIP6 (%)	29	2	1	0	3
HOXA7 (%)	18	6	0	0	3
HPD (%)	12	6	0	0	3
MIR1277 (%)	12	6	0	0	3

3 Endometrial Cancer Genetic Classification and Its Clinical Application

Table 3.3 Distribution of histologies through TCGA groups

Gene	POLE ultramutated (%)	Hypermutated/MS unstable (%)	Copy number low/ MS stable (%)	Copy number high/ serous-like (%)	Total (%)
Low-grade endometrioid	6.4	28.6	60.0	5.0	100.0
High-grade endometrioid	17.4	54.3	8.7	19.6	100.0
Serous	0.0	0.0	2.3	97.7	100.0
Mixed	0.0	0.0	25.0	75.0	100.0

"copy number high (serous-like)" (Table 3.3). Figure 3.1 is a comprehensive mutational and copy number variation representation of the four subgroups.

1. *POLE ultramutated group* is named due to the prevalent highest mutation rate (232×10^{-6} mutations/Mb; 867–9714 mutations/tumor) and consists of 7% of the entire dataset. It is characterized by an increased Cytosin→Adenosin transversion frequency, with mutations in the exonuclease domain of POLE. POLE is a catalytic subunit of DNA polymerase-ε involved in nuclear DNA replication and repair and its mutation brings numerous genomic alterations. Most frequent mutations occur in PTEN (94%), PIK3R1 (65%), PIK3CA (71%), FBXW7 (82%), KRAS (53%), and POLE (100%). Those patients are composed by 6.4% of low-grade endometrioid EC, 17.4% of high-grade endometrioid ECs, and any of non-endometrioid histology tumors. Interestingly this small subset of patients showed a better outcome in progression-free survival analysis.

2. *Hypermutated/microsatellite-unstable group* is characterized by high level of MSI and low MLH1 mRNA expression due to MLH1 promoter methylation. Among the TCGA dataset, 28.6% of low-grade endometrioid carcinomas and 54.3% of high-grade endometrioid carcinomas are grouped here. The methylation pattern in this subgroup is importantly enriched also throughout the entire genome. Several mutations are recurrent in this subgroup: PTEN (88%), PIK3CA (54%), PIK3R1 (42%), ARID1A (37%), RPL22 (37%), KRAS (35%), CTNNB1 (20%), ATR (18%), FGFR2 (14%), and CCND1 (12%). Novel EC mutations are reported as recurrent events: ARID5B (23%), CSDE1 (15%), CTCF (23%), GIGYF2 (17%), HIST1H2BD (8%), LIMCH1 (12%), MIR1277 (6%), NKAP (11%), RBMX (12%), TNFAIP (68%), and ZFHX3 (31%).

3. *Copy number low/microsatellite-stable group* gathers 60.0% of low-grade EC, 8.7% of high-grade EC, 2.3% of serous carcinomas, and 25% of mixed-histology carcinomas. Known mutations are found in some genes: PTEN (77%), PIK3CA (53%), CTNNB1 (52%), ARID1A (42%), PIK3R1 (33%), KRAS (16%), FGFR2 (13%), CHD4 (12%), and SPOP (10%). Other altered genes, not previously described are: BCOR (7%), CSMD3 (10%), CTCF (21%), MECOM (4%),

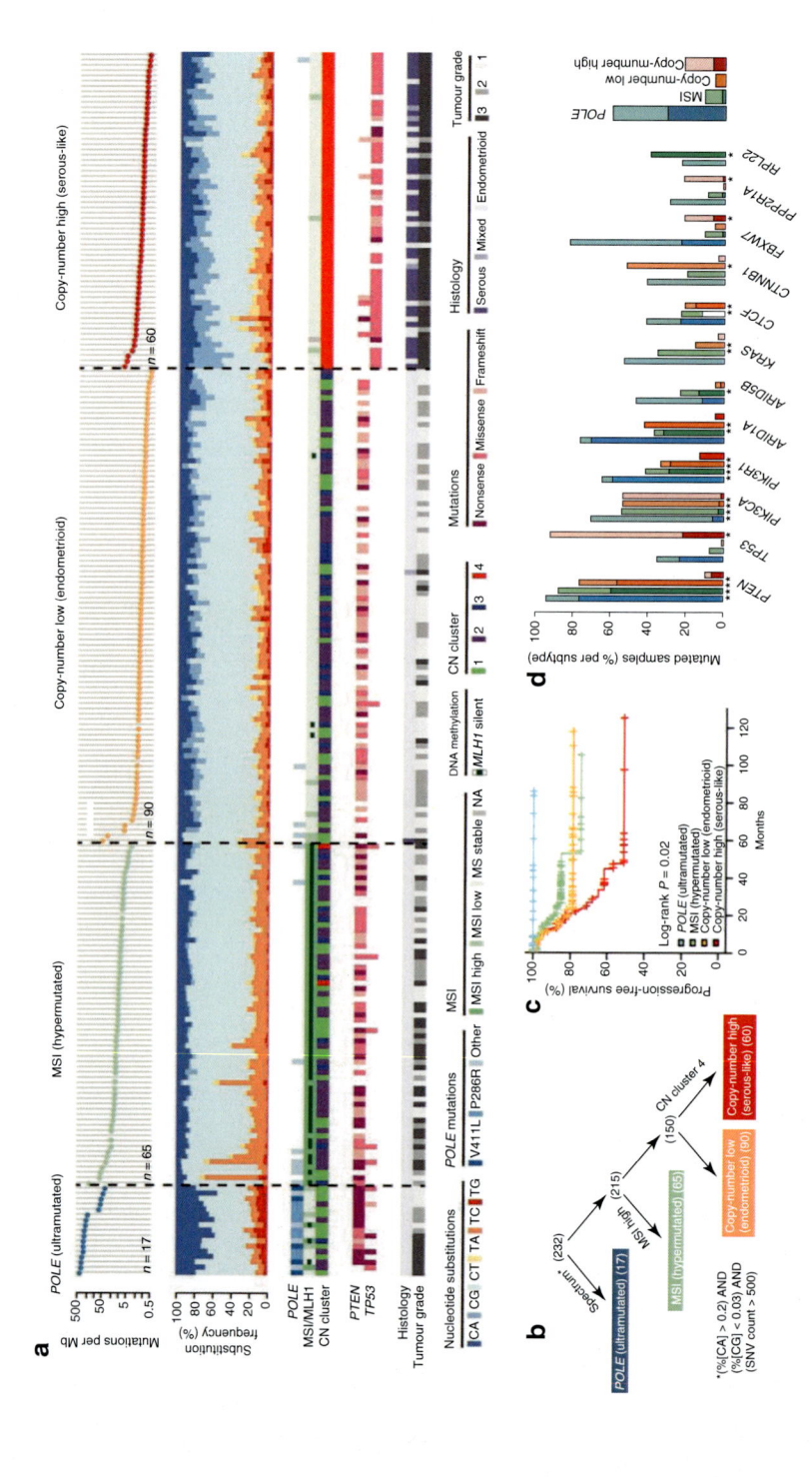

Fig. 3.1 Mutation and copy number alteration spectra across endometrial carcinomas, from the Cancer Genome Atlas Research Network, 2013

METTL14 (3%), SGK1 (7%), and SOX17 (8%). Based on this mutational landscape, among the first three subtypes, PI3K-AKT-mTOR, KRAS, and FGFR2 pathways carry one-third of the driving mutations.
4. *Copy number high (serous-like) group* represents 5.0% of low-grade endometrioid EC, 19.6% of high-grade endometrioid EC, 97.7% of serous carcinomas, and 75% of mixed-histology carcinomas.

Most significantly mutated genes in this subset are confirmed to be as TP53 (92%), and PPP2R1A (22%). Novel mutations were discovered, such as FBXW7 (22%) and CHD4 (13%). The analysis confirmed that the PI3K-AKT-mTOR pathway is less involved in this subtype, with mutation frequencies for PIK3CA (47%), PIK3R1 (13%), and PTEN (10%).

Due to the highest copy number variation harbored in this subgroup, it is appropriate to describe which regions carry some importantly amplified genes. In up to 25% of the cases, significantly recurrent focal amplifications are present on the oncogenes MYC (8q24.12), ERBB2 (17q12), and CCNE1 (19q12). Few novel amplifications are also discovered in genes loci FGFR3 (4p16.3) and SOX17 (8q11.23). This finding is consistent with previously mentioned analyses [16, 17]. In addition PIK3CA, FBXW7, CHD4, and MBD3 are also present in amplified regions.

TCGA also provides a clustering based on mRNA, to highlight different expression patterns. Patients are grouped depending on the importantly hallmark features expressed in their cancers: "mitotic, hormonal, and immunoreactive."

Examples of cross clustering between subgroups is the following: 85% of tumors in the subgroup 4 (copy number–high, serous-like) are also clustering in a "mitotic subgroup," where altered expression is shown related to G1/S checkpoint regulation, growth hormone signaling, Her-2 signaling in breast cancer, endothelin-1 signaling, cyclins and cell cycle regulation.

3.4.1 Microarray mRNA Expression from TCGA and Its Independent Validation for Endometrioid EC

An interesting publication independently analyzed the mRNA microarray data of TCGA, focusing on EEC only [60]. An integrated analysis performed on 271 endometrioid EC ended up with an alternative grouping that may exploit the heterogeneity of EEC. After that a validation in an independent dataset was performed on 184 EEC cases from MD Anderson Cancer Center, TX. In summary the four clusters identified different prognostic expression profiles, where the most translatable finding is the correlation of CTNNB1 mutation and Wnt/B catenin activation to a subset of low-grade EEC with poor outcome. This activation may further be explored in models to identify possible targetable molecules.

3.4.2 Comparison to Ovarian and Breast Cancers

In addition, TCGA provides a thorough multilevel comparison between copy number high (serous-like) EC group, high-grade serous ovarian cancer [61] and basal-like breast carcinoma [62]. The level of similarity is based on focal somatic copy number alterations, transcriptomic supervised analysis and methylation patterns. Mutations frequencies encompass TP53 mutations in 91% in serous EC, 96% in high-grade serous ovarian cancer and 84% in basal-like breast cancer, whereas few PTEN mutations are found (2, 1 and 1%, respectively). In addition, no frequent mutations as in serous-like EC such as FBXW7, PPP2R1A, and PIK3CA were found in ovarian and breast similar type.

3.4.3 High-Grade Endometrial Cancers

About 20% of high-grade (grade 3) endometrioid EC are "serous-like" at the molecular level. As noted in the TCGA study, the distinction between the histologic and molecular classification of these cases has important clinical implications—suggesting that patients who have grade 3 EECs with a "serous-like" genomic profile might be better treated with regimens that are used for USC. The implementation of the proposed molecular classification might enhance standard pathologic classification and might tailor adjuvant therapies.

It is important to state possible confounding factors in multilevel genomic analyses such as transient mutation accumulations in non-oncogenic genes, as TCGA users cannot omit in data analysis interpretation. A multi-institutional revision analysis project [63] related to TCGA network comprehensively reviewed the mutational results throughout all the different cancer types and revealed an amount of not plausible findings. Mutations encoding olfactory receptors or muscle proteins suggest extensive false-positive findings that may overshadow true driver events.

3.5 Clinical Applications: Therapeutic Targets in Development

So far EC treatment is based on comprehensive staging surgery and adjuvant chemo-radiotherapy based on risk factors for early stage of the disease, surgery combined with first line chemo-radiotherapy for advanced stages.

Since consistent mutational alteration emerged as critical in tumor development, numerous Phase I–II trials were designed to test targeted molecules in relapsing-metastatic EC population. More recently findings from TCGA gave soundness and new perspective to the clinical and translational exploration, strengthened genetic targets importance, clarifying molecular interactions, and finding novel candidates for target therapies. Studies were initially designed to test molecules in not enriched populations. Latest study designs started to provide this feature as prerequisite.

3.6 Growth Factors

Different molecules from monoclonal antibodies to small molecule inhibitors were demonstrated to be effective n positive expression subset of populations of breast, gastric, and non-small cell lung cancer, establishing one of the most important steps forward regarding personalized medicine in the last years. Given the amount of targetable spots, the concept was translated to EC trials.

These growth factors are also the first actors that activate downstream effectors such as PI3K-AKT-mTOR pathway.

3.6.1 HER2/Neu

Human epidermal growth factor receptor 2 (Her2) alteration is present in several cancers, and through its amplification and overexpression of its encoding gene (ERBB2) it plays an important role in proliferation, metastasis and angiogenesis [64]. However, the clinical significance of HER2 overexpression in endometrial cancer remains unclear. TCGA database (http://www.cbioportal.org/) reported ERBB2 gene alteration rate of 17.2% and also showed that ERBB2-amplified serous-like tumors are often associated with a PIK3CA mutation. These data suggest that agents targeting both ERBB2 and PIK3CA may be a useful combination. Despite these promising biological understandings, the data for HER2-directed agents (e.g., trastuzumab and lapatinib) in EC have been uniformly disappointing [65, 66], with low response rates (0–3.3%). However, more careful selection of patients who overexpress HER2 might be key to identifying the activity of such agents, and research continues on these agents for endometrial cancer.

3.6.2 EGFR

Altered Epidermal Growth Factor Receptor (EGFR) expression has potent downstream effect on tumor growth, and the inhibition of the overexpressed molecule showed efficacy in various solid tumors, such as non-small cell lung cancer and colorectal cancer. As with these tumors, EGFR amplification and overexpression is present in a small subset of EC (7%) in TCGA dataset. However, as with HER2-directed agents, clinical trials of different EGFR inhibitors, such as *Erlotinib* [67] *and Gefitinib* [68], have not been promising, though as small subset of responders appears to be present, ranging from 4 to 12.5% in phase II evaluations. To date, analysis to identify a potentially predictive biomarker, such as EGFR expression level or specific mutation, has not been successful.

3.6.3 FGFR2

The fibroblastic growth factor 2 (FGFR2) appears to play a key role in EC. Studies show that FGF receptor 2 activating mutations are present in 11–16% of patients with EC [69, 70]. Phase II trials evaluating multitargeted tyrosine kinase inhibitors, such as nintedanib [71], brivanib [72], and dovitinib have been performed with some hints of potential benefit. For example, Konecny et al. [73] recruited women with advanced or metastatic endometrial cancer with either FGFR2 mutated (FGF-mut) and FGFR2 wild-type (FGF-wt) patients through a preselection screening. The ORR in the two groups was 5% for FGF-mut and 16% for FGF-wt group with 31.8% and 29.0% patients progression-free at 18 weeks. Adverse events were balanced between groups, where hypertension (17%) and diarrhea (9%) were the most common. Few serious adverse events suspected to be related to study drug were reported to be vomiting (8%), dehydration (6%), and pulmonary embolism (8%) that was also related to the only treatment-related death, occurred due to cardiac arrest.

3.7 PI3K/AKT/mTOR Pathway

TCGA found that PI3KCA mutation and loss of PTEN is one of the most common deregulation in EC. PI3K/AKT/mTOR pathway. This pathway represents one of the most interesting candidate for selective inhibition, as its alteration is an important hallmark in the development of several cancer types [74], and its activation is linked to poor prognosis in EC [75]. Different classes of inhibitors are of interest, though clinical activity has not been entirely promising.

3.7.1 mTOR Inhibitors

The rationale to evaluate agents that inhibit proteins in the PI3K pathway is provided from preclinical models, where it is demonstrated that deregulated PI3K pathway blockade can impair the proliferation of endometrial carcinoma cells [76]. The mammalian target of rapamycin (mTOR), an intracellular serine/threonine protein kinase, represents a key downstream mediator of the PI3K pathway, targeted with numerous rapalogs including everolimus, deforolimus, ridaforolimus, and temsirolimus.

Everolimus was tested in several trials as a single agent [77, 78], with the best response as stable disease in 43% for 8 weeks. A subsequent biomarker analysis of the GOG trial showed no correlation between PTEN mutation and stability of disease, though an activation of the downstream mediator (pS6rp) combined with KRAS mutation was always related to absence of response (Positive Predictive Value: 100%) [79].

Deforolimus and *Ridaforolimus*, were tested in Phase II trials [80–82], and a randomized trial [83], showing an overall response rate of 7.4–11% of patients.

Single study and comprehensive genomic analyses did not provide correlations between PTEN, PI3KCA, AKT mutational status, and response to mTOR inhibitors treatment [84].

Temsirolimus, was tested in a Phase II trial as single agent, in chemotherapy-naïve and -treated EC patients, showing higher effect in chemo-naive vs. -treated patients (14% vs. 4% PR, 69% vs. 48 SD as best response) [85], though independent from PTEN loss status. Asymptomatic pneumonitis was a common event (42%), severe in 8% of these patients, yet not related to efficacy outcome [86]. A separate study evaluated the combination of this drug with *megestrol acetate* and *tamoxifen* [87], but it was stopped due to an elevated risk of thrombosis. Likewise, a combination trial of this agent with bevacizumab was stopped for excessive toxicity [88].

Because of the efficacy of mTOR inhibitors plus aromatase inhibitors in breast cancer [89], the combination was tested in a phase II trial [90] in women with advanced or metastatic endometrial cancer. Objective response rate (RR) was in 32% patients, with a 6-month PFS rate for this cohort of 42% (95% CI, 29.2–62.8%), and a median OS time of 14 months (95% CI, 9.5–24.4 months). Response rates and clinical benefit was correlated to histologies and mutations. Patients carrying CTNNB1 mutations and endometrioid histology had the best response to the treatment, whereas serous histotype was predictor of poor response. Interestingly, the clinical benefit between serous histology and high-grade endometrioid was 11% vs. 50% ($P = 0.018$), maybe suggesting an exquisite recovered hormonal sensitivity for endometrioid tumors.

The ongoing phase II randomized trial (NCT02228681) of everolimus and letrozole vs. hormonal therapy will highlight the additional benefit of the rapalog. Collaterally, in the paper the objective response rate among metformin users was 56% (v 23% for non-users; $P < 0.05$). To study the antitumor activity of metformin, an open-label phase II activity trial evaluating everolimus, letrozole, and metformin in a similar group of patients is ongoing (NCT01797523).

3.7.2 PI3K Inhibitors

PI3K inhibitors selectively target the mutated molecule, previously described as highly mutated in EC.

Preclinical data showed encouraging results regarding a pure inhibitor of PI3K, *BKM-120/Buparlisib*. Patient derived xenografts treated with BKM-120 in combination with standard cytotoxic chemotherapy resulted in significant tumor growth suppression [91]. The molecule has been tested in a Phase II trial (NCT01501604), closed for poor accrual rate. At the last ASCO meeting, poor safety profile and little antitumor activity was showed for the molecule in a French Phase II trial [92].

Pilaralisib, a pan-all class isoforms-PI3K inhibitor, showed antitumor activity in preclinical models. Recently its test in a Phase II trial showed little activity in recurrent metastatic EC [93]. The ORR was lower than other single agent inhibitors (see Table 3.4). Targeted genomic profiling and circular DNA analysis did not show PTEN and PIK3R1 mutational status related to benefit from the treatment. These

Table 3.4 Selected Phase II target agents trials in advanced/recurrent endometrial cancer patients

Cytotoxic agent	Dose	Patients evaluable for response	Response rate (CR + PR) (%)	Stable disease (%)	Reference
mTOR inhibitors					
Temsirolimus	25 mg IV q wk	29	14 (chemo naive), 4 (no chemo naive)	69 (chemo naive), 48 (no chemo naive)	Oza, JCO 2011
Deforolimus	12.5 mg IV q5d, every other week	27	7	27	Colombo, JCO 2007
Ridaforolimus	12.5 mg IV q5d, every other week	45	11	18	Colombo, BJC 2013
Ridaforolimus	40 mg PO q5d	31	8.8	52.9	Tsoref, Gynecol Oncol 2014
Ridaforolimus (vs. progestin or comparator)	40 mg PO q5d	64 (vs. 66)	0 (vs. 4)	35 (vs. 17)	Oza, JCO 2015
Everolimus	10 mg PO qd	28	0	43	Slomovitz, Cancer 2010
Everolimus	10 mg PO qd	44	5, 9	32, 27	ENDORAD, Ray-Coquard, BJC 2013
Temsirolimus, megestrol acetate alternating to tamoxifen (vs. temsirolimus)	25 mg PO, 80 mg PO bid q3w, 20 mg bid q3w (vs. 25 mg PO)	21 (vs. 50)	14.3 (vs. 22)	52 (vs. 52.4)	GOG 248, Fleming, Gynecol Oncol 2014
Everolimus + letrozole	10 mg PO qd + 2.5 mg PO qd	35	32	8.6	Slomovitz, JCO 2015
PI3K inhibitors					
BKM-120/buparlisib	100/60 mg PO qd	24	0	12.5	ENDOPIK, Heudel, JCO suppl 2015
Pilaralisib	400/600 mg PO qd	67	6	37.3	Matulonis, Gynecol Oncol 2015
Anti HER2					
Trastuzumab	2 mg/kg IV q wk	34	0	35	GOG-0181-B, Fleming, Gynecol Oncol 2010
Anti EGFR					
Erlotinib	150 mg po qd	32	12.5	47	Oza, JCO 2008

3 Endometrial Cancer Genetic Classification and Its Clinical Application

Table 3.4 (continued)

Cytotoxic agent	Dose	Patients evaluable for response	Response rate (CR + PR) (%)	Stable disease (%)	Reference
Gefitinib	500 mg po qd	26	3.8	27	GOG 229-C, Leslie, Gynecol Oncol 2013
Lapatinib	1500 mg po qd	30	3.3	23.3	GOG 229-D, Leslie, Gynecol Oncol 2012
Multiple TKI					
Nintedanib	200 × 2 po qd	32	9.4	34	GOG-229-K, Dizon, Gynecol Oncol 2014
Brivanib	800 mg po qd	43	18.6	27.9	GOG 229-, Powell, Gynecol Oncol 2014
Dovitinib	500 mg po qd5—stop d2	22 FGFR2-mut, 31 FGFR2-wt	5 FGFR2-mut, 16 FGFR2-wt	59 FGFR2-mut, 36 FGFR2-wt	Konecny, Lancet Oncol 2015
Antiangiogenics					
Bevacizumab	15 mg/kg IV q3w	52	13.5	50	GOG 229-E, Aghajanian, JCO 2011
Carboplatin and paclitaxel plus bevacizumab; carboplatin and paclitaxel plus temsirolimus; carboplatin and ixabepilone plus bevacizumab; and maintenance	AUC 6 IV, 175 mg/mq, 15 mg/kg IV q3w + maintenance 15 mg/kg IV q3w; AUC 5 IV, 175 mg/mq, 25 mg IV day 1–8 + maintenance 25 mg IV day 1–8—15; AUC 6 IV, 30 mg/mq, 15 mg/kg IV q3w + maintenance 15 mg/kg IV q3w	108; 111; 110	59.5, 55.3, and 52.9	N/A	Aghajanian, JCO suppl 2015
Carboplatin and paclitaxel plus bevacizumab (vs. carboplatin and paclitaxel plus temsirolimus)	AUC 5 IV, 175 mg/mq, 15 mg/kg IV q3w + maintenance 15 mg/kg IV q3w; AUC 5 IV, 175 mg/mq	46 (vs. 46)	71.7 (vs. 54.3)	21.7 (vs. 43.5)	END-2 trial, LoRusso, JCO suppl 2015

findings might suggest the need of a more extensive sequencing to add information on response rate variations.

GDC-980, a dual PI3K/mTOR inhibitor, was tested in another Phase II single-agent study, with poor clinical benefit (9% ORR). A tumor biomarker analysis discovered presence of alteration in PI3K pathway between responders, but overall poorly related to response [94].

Despite of the promising role in inhibiting the tumor activity, single agent activity PI3K-AKT-mTOR pathway inhibitors showed little activity, without clear correlation with mutational status. Speculative reasons may include limited safety and consequent limited drug exposure, insufficient depth and duration of target inhibition, linked to the presence of several PI3K isoforms. Mechanisms of resistance and compensation play a critical role that is has just been found, described and challenged [95].

3.8 PARP Inhibitors

There is interest in the evaluation of poly(ADP-ribose) polymerase (PARP) inhibitors, especially since the drug has just demonstrated effective in ovarian cancer in patients with BRCA1/2 mutation and Olaparib has received approval in the United States. Theoretically, PARPi may act as interesting players, since EC shows similar genetic repair deficiency mutations as ovarian cancer, such as TP53, PIK3CA, K-RAS, and ERBB2. This field is yet to be evaluated, but will warrant interesting therapeutic improvements.

PARP inhibitors showed a greater activity in PTEN-deficient EC cell lines rather than wild-type PTEN endometrioid EC cell lines [96, 97].

Early case reports showed encouraging responses, where a BRCA1/2 negative patient harbored a PTEN mutation in her recurrent EC disease. A dramatic clinical and objective response was noted under olaparib treatment [98]. A Phase II study (PANDA) is currently ongoing to evaluate whether the PARPi *BMN-673*, which has shown to be potentially effective in treating cancers known to behave similar to EC, has therapeutic benefit in the treatment of inoperable advanced EC.

3.9 Antiangiogenic Agents

Antiangiogenic agents has been tested is several trials as single agent and in combination. These molecules may not represent good examples of target based therapies, but due to some promising results these molecules may be incorporated in combinations with targeted molecules.

VEGF expression in EC has clinical and biologic significance. It is associated with higher grade of disease and worse prognosis [99]. Aflibercept and others were also tested, showing little antitumor activity.

The most important trial testing *bevacizumab*, a monoclonal antibody targeting VEGF-A, as single agent in recurrent-metastatic EC [100]. The ORR was 13.4%, and 40% of patients had a 6 months PFS interval. Median PFS was 4 and OS 11 months. No GI perforations, or treatment-related deaths were reported, grade 3–4 hemorrhage episodes happened to two patients, four patients experienced grade 4 hypertension, and others had thrombotic events resulting in an overall acceptable safety profile.

Interestingly, a phase II trial, GOG-86P, presented at the last ASCO meeting [101], compared three arms of chemotherapy and maintenance therapy as a first line treatment for advanced, metastatic or recurrent EC. The three arms were *carboplatin* and *paclitaxel* plus *bevacizumab*, *carboplatin* and *paclitaxel* plus *temsirolimus*, or *carboplatin*, and *ixabepilone* plus *bevacizumab*. For PFS, no difference was showed between groups and compared to historical survival data. However, OS was improved in the first arm compared to historical reference. Hypertension (G 3/4) was more common in the bevacizumab arms (16%) than in the temsirolimus arm (3%), ($P = 0.001$).

A comparison between standard therapy with *carboplatin* and *paclitaxel* with or without *bevacizumab* in not heavily pretreated patients was presented [102]. The MITO END-2 trial showed an ORR 71.7% compared to 54.3% for the controls, and an improvement in median PFS of 13 months versus 8.7 months (HR 0.59, 95% CI 0.35–0.98). No significant adverse events were reported in the trial. These recent positive results may enhance the activity in combination regimens with targeted molecules.

3.10 Other Targets

Multiple other targets have been tested with little antitumor activity. To mention few, *MK-2206*, an AKT inhibitor, was studied in a Phase II single-agent study in recurrent endometrial cancer [103]. Patients carrying PIK3CA mutation or PIK3CA wild-type in their tumors were treated ending in severe side effects (skin) and with limited activity in few of the patients in mutated and wt group. The expansion cohort showed the same small activity, with no correlation to PIK3CA status and response [104].

After not enthusiastic results in not selected populations treated with RAS/MEK/ERK pathway, several trials are still ongoing. Patients with KRAS mutation are tested for a combination treatment in Gynecologic Oncology Group phase II trial (GOG-2290) (NCT01935973), where an inhibitor of the RAS pathway and PI3K/AKT/mTOR pathway are tested in advanced or recurrent EC: *trametinib*, an orally bioavailable MEK 1–2 inhibitor, with or without *GSK2141795*, an AKT inhibitor.

3.11 Conclusion

Despite a better biological understanding of EC, we have yet to translate this information into clinically meaningful progress. The lack of a predictive biomarkers and the low activity of targeted agents likely reflect disease heterogeneity and treatment resistance, due to redundant activated driving pathways in the tumor. This process is deeply discussed in the scientific community [95]. TCGA profiles, exploring chemo-naïve tumors give little help in predicting mutations in pretreated population, where treatment selection give rise to dramatic genomic changes. These data underline the critical need of freshly obtained biopsies to identify alterations of interest. To design trials based on this criteria may allow to enroll enriched population and possibly show the largest drug benefit.

Recently Konecny et al. provided an example of a mutation-based trial design: next generation high-throughput sequencing technologies are helping to introduce in a timely fashion this big amount of information. The failure in showing good response may be related to discussed treatment-resistance, and the promiscuous molecule effect, rather than a multiple anticancer effect, might have carried higher off-target side effects, with shortened drug exposure and impaired responses.

Results from combination therapy trials (e.g.: [90]) show better response rates and give an important proof of treatment-resistance overcoming through a multilevel blockade.

A large field of research is yet to be explored, since the somehow unexpected mechanisms of resistance needs to be elucidated scanning the complexity of curated available genomic datasets, creating ad hoc preclinical models, implementing multilevel blockades to reduce toxicities and optimizing responses, ultimately also implying new molecular methods of drug delivery.

References

1. Siegel RL, Miller KD, Jemal A. Cancer statistics, 2015. CA Cancer J Clin. 2015;65(1):5–29.
2. Silverberg SG, Kurman RJ, Nogales F, et al. Epithelial tumours and related lesions. In: Tavassoli FA, Devilee P, editors. World Health Organization classification of tumours: pathology and genetics—tumours of the breast and female genital organs. Lyon: IARC Press; 2003. p. 217–32.
3. Bokhman JV. Two pathogenetic types of endometrial carcinoma. Gynecol Oncol. 1983;15(1):10–7.
4. Lax SF, Kurman RJ. A dualistic model for endometrial carcinogenesis based on immunohistochemical and molecular genetic analyses. Verh Dtsch Ges Pathol. 1997;81:228–32.
5. Potischman N, et al. Case-control study of endogenous steroid hormones and endometrial cancer. J Natl Cancer Inst. 1996;88:1127–35.
6. Levine RL, Cargile CB, Blazes MS, et al. PTEN mutations and microsatellite instability in complex atypical hyperplasia, a precursor lesion to uterine endometrioid carcinoma. Cancer Res. 1998;58(15):3254–8.
7. Colombo N, Preti E, Landoni F, Carinelli S, et al. Endometrial cancer: ESMO clinical practice guidelines for diagnosis, treatment and follow-up. Ann Oncol. 2013;24(Supplement 6):vi33–8.
8. Hamilton CA, Kapp DS, Chan JK. Clinical aspects of uterine papillary serous carcinoma. Curr Opin Obstet Gynecol. 2008;20(1):26–33.
9. Tashiro H, Isacson C, Levine R, Kurman RJ, Cho KR, Hedrick L. p53 gene mutations are common in uterine serous carcinoma and occur early in their pathogenesis. Am J Pathol. 1997;150:177–85.

10. Jia L, Liu Y, Yi X, et al. Endometrial glandular dysplasia with frequent p53 gene mutation: a genetic evidence supporting its precancer nature for endometrial serous carcinoma. Clin Cancer Res. 2008;14(8):2263–9.
11. Murali R, Soslow RA, Weigelt B. Classification of endometrial carcinoma: more than two types. Lancet Oncol. 2014;15(7):e268–78.
12. Brinton LA, Felix AS, McMeekin DS, et al. Etiologic heterogeneity in endometrial cancer: evidence from a Gynecologic Oncology Group trial. Gynecol Oncol. 2013;129:277–84.
13. Soslow RA, Bissonnette JP, Wilton A, et al. Clinicopathologic analysis of 187 high-grade endometrial carcinomas of different histologic subtypes: similar outcomes belie distinctive biologic differences. Am J Surg Pathol. 2007;31:979–87.
14. Hamilton CA, Cheung MK, Osann K, et al. Uterine papillary serous and clear cell carcinomas predict for poorer survival compared to grade 3 endometrioid corpus cancers. Br J Cancer. 2006;94(5):642–6.
15. Gilks CB, Oliva E, Soslow RA. Poor interobserver reproducibility in the diagnosis of high-grade endometrial carcinoma. Am J Surg Pathol. 2013;37(6):874–81.
16. Lax SF, Kendall B, Tashiro H, Slebos RJ, Hedrick L. The frequency of p53, K-ras mutations, and microsatellite instability differs in uterine endometrioid and serous carcinoma: evidence of distinct molecular genetic pathways. Cancer. 2000;88:814–24.
17. Dedes KJ, Wetterskog D, Ashworth A, Kaye SB, Reis-Filho JS. Emerging therapeutic targets in endometrial cancer. Nat Rev Clin Oncol. 2011;8:261–71.
18. Urick ME, Rudd ML, Godwin AK, Sgroi D, Merino M, Bell DW. PIK3R1 (p85α) is somatically mutated at high frequency in primary endometrial cancer. Cancer Res. 2011;71:4061–7.
19. Cheung LW, Hennessy BT, Li J, et al. High frequency of PIK3R1 and PIK3R2 mutations in endometrial cancer elucidates a novel mechanism for regulation of PTEN protein stability. Cancer Discov. 2011;1:170–85.
20. Santin AD, Bellone S, Van Stedum S, et al. Amplification of c-erbB2 oncogene: a major prognostic indicator in uterine serous papillary carcinoma. Cancer. 2005;104:1391–7.
21. Khalifa MA, Mannel RS, Haraway SD, Walker J, Min KW. Expression of EGFR, HER-2/neu, P53, and PCNA in endometrioid, serous papillary, and clear cell endometrial adenocarcinomas. Gynecol Oncol. 1994;53:84–92.
22. Byron SA, Gartside MG, Wellens CL, et al. Inhibition of activated fibroblast growth factor receptor 2 in endometrial cancer cells induces cell death despite PTEN abrogation. Cancer Res. 2008;68(17):6902–7.
23. Castellano E, Downward J. RAS interaction with PI3K: more than just another effector pathway. Genes Cancer. 2011;2(3):261–74.
24. Schlosshauer PW, Ellenson LH, Soslow RA. β-Catenin and E-cadherin expression patterns in high-grade endometrial carcinoma are associated with histological subtype. Mod Pathol. 2002;15:1032–7.
25. Matias-Guiu X, Prat J. Molecular pathology of endometrial carcinoma. Histopathology. 2013;62:111–23.
26. Kanaya T, Kyo S, Maida Y, Yatabe N, Tanaka M, Nakamura M, Inoue M. Frequent hypermethylation of MLH1 promoter in normal endometrium of patients with endometrial cancers. Oncogene. 2003;22(15):2352–60.
27. Guan B, Wang TL, Shih IM. ARID1A, a factor that promotes formation of SWI/SNF-mediated chromatin remodeling, is a tumor suppressor in gynecologic cancers. Cancer Res. 2011;71(21):6718–27.
28. Perrotti D, Neviani P. Protein phosphatase 2A: a target for anticancer therapy. Lancet Oncol. 2013;14(6):e229–38.
29. Shih Ie M, Panuganti PK, Kuo KT, Mao TL, Kuhn E, Jones S, et al. Somatic mutations of PPP2R1A in ovarian and uterine carcinomas. Am J Pathol. 2011;178(4):1442–7.
30. Pere H, Tapper J, Wahlstrom T, et al. Distinct chromosomal imbalances in uterine serous and endometrioid carcinomas. Cancer Res. 1998;58:892–5.

31. Salvesen HB, MacDonald N, Ryan A, et al. PTEN methylation is associated with advanced stage and microsatellite instability in endometrial carcinoma. Int J Cancer. 2001;91:22–6.
32. Moreno-Bueno G, Hardisson D, Sanchez C, et al. Abnormalities of the APC/beta-catenin pathway in endometrial cancer. Oncogene. 2002;21:7981–90.
33. Liao X, Siu MK, Chan KY, et al. Hypermethylation of RAS effector related genes and DNA methyltransferase 1 expression in endometrial carcinogenesis. Int J Cancer. 2008;123:296–302.
34. Yi TZ, Guo J, Zhou L, et al. Prognostic value of E-cadherin expression and CDH1 promoter methylation in patients with endometrial carcinoma. Cancer Investig. 2011;29:86–92.
35. Lax SF, Kendall B, Tashiro H, Slebos RJ, Hedrick L. The frequency of p53, K-ras mutations, and microsatellite instability differs in uterine endometrioid and serous carcinoma: evidence of distinct molecular genetic pathways. Cancer. 2000;88:814–24.
36. Rudd ML, Price JC, Fogoros S, Godwin AK, Sgroi DC, Merino MJ, Bell DW. A unique spectrum of somatic PIK3CA (p110α) mutations within primary endometrial carcinomas. Clin Cancer Res. 2011;17:1331–40.
37. Cheung LW, Hennessy BT, Li J, Yu S, Myers AP, Djordjevic B, et al. High frequency of PIK3R1 and PIK3R2 mutations in endometrial cancer elucidates a novel mechanism for regulation of PTEN protein stability. Cancer Discov. 2011;1:170–85.
38. Oda K, Stokoe D, Taketani Y, et al. High frequency of coexistent mutations of PIK3CA and PTEN genes in endometrial carcinoma. Cancer Res. 2005;65:10669–73.
39. Forbes SA, Bhamra G, Bamford S, et al. The Catalogue of Somatic Mutations in Cancer (COSMIC). Curr Protoc Hum Genet. 2008;Chapter 10:Unit 10.11.
40. Byron SA, Gartside M, Powell MA, Wellens CL, Gao F, Mutch DG, et al. FGFR2 point mutations in 466 endometrioid endometrial tumors: relationship with MSI, KRAS, PIK3CA, CTNNB1 mutations and clinicopathological features. PLoS One. 2012;7:e30801.
41. Machin P, Catasus L, Pons C, Munoz J, Matias-Guiu X, Prat J. CTNNB1 mutations and β-catenin expression in endometrial carcinomas. Hum Pathol. 2002;33:206–12.
42. Wiegand KC, Lee AF, Al-Agha OM, et al. Loss of BAF250a (ARID1A) is frequent in high-grade endometrial carcinomas. J Pathol. 2011;224:328–33.
43. O'Hara AJ, Bell DW. The genomics and genetics of endometrial cancer. Adv Genomics Genet. 2012;2012:33–47.
44. Kuhn E, Wu RC, Guan B, Wu G, Zhang J, Wang Y, et al. Identification of molecular pathway aberrations in uterine serous carcinoma by genome-wide analyses. J Natl Cancer Inst. 2012;104:1503–13.
45. Zhao S, Choi M, Overton JD, Bellone S, Roque DM, Cocco E, et al. Landscape of somatic singlenucleotide and copy-number mutations in uterine serous carcinoma. Proc Natl Acad Sci U S A. 2013;110:2916–22.
46. Wild PJ, Ikenberg K, Fuchs TJ, Rechsteiner M, Georgiev S, Fankhauser N, et al. p53 suppresses type II endometrial carcinomas in mice and governs endometrial tumour aggressiveness in humans. EMBO Mol Med. 2012;4:808–24.
47. Rudd ML, Price JC, Fogoros S, et al. A unique spectrum of somatic PIK3CA (p110alpha) mutations within primary endometrial carcinomas. Clin Cancer Res. 2011;17(6):1331–40.
48. McConechy MK, Anglesio MS, Kalloger SE, for the Australian Ovarian Cancer Study Group, et al. Subtype-specific mutation of PPP2R1A in endometrial and ovarian carcinomas. J Pathol. 2011;223:567–73.
49. Akhmedkhanov A, Zeleniuch-Jacquotte A, Toniolo P. Role of exogenous and endogenous hormones in endometrial cancer: review of the evidence and research perspectives. Ann N Y Acad Sci. 2001;943:296–315.
50. Henderson BE, Feigelson HS. Hormonal carcinogenesis. Carcinogenesis. 2000;21(3):427–33.
51. Lebeau A, et al. Oestrogen receptor gene (ESR1) amplification is frequent in endometrial carcinoma and its precursor lesions. J Pathol. 2008;216:151–7.
52. Schiff R, Massarweh SA, Shou J, Bharwani L, Mohsin SK, Osborne CK. Cross-talk between estrogen receptor and growth factor pathways as a molecular target for overcoming endocrine resistance. Clin Cancer Res. 2004;10(1 Pt 2):331S–6S.

53. Boulay A, Rudloff J, Ye J, Zumstein-Mecker S, O'Reilly T, Evans DB, Chen S, Lane HA. Dual inhibition of mTOR and estrogen receptor signaling in vitro induces cell death in models of breast cancer. Clin Cancer Res. 2005;11(14):5319–28.
54. Baselga J, Campone M, Piccart M, Burris HA 3rd, Rugo HS, Sahmoud T, Noguchi S, Gnant M, Pritchard KI, Lebrun F, Beck JT, Ito Y, Yardley D, Deleu I, Perez A, Bachelot T, Vittori L, Xu Z, Mukhopadhyay P, Lebwohl D, Hortobagyi GN. Everolimus in postmenopausal hormone-receptor-positive advanced breast cancer. N Engl J Med. 2012;366(6):520–9.
55. Jongen V, Briët J, de Jong R, ten Hoor K, Boezen M, van der Zee A, Nijman H, Hollema H. Expression of estrogen receptor-alpha and -beta and progesterone receptor-A and -B in a large cohort of patients with endometrioid endometrial cancer. Gynecol Oncol. 2009;112(3):537–42.
56. Kohler MF, et al. Mutational analysis of the estrogen-receptor gene in endometrial carcinoma. Obstet Gynecol. 1995;86:33–7.
57. Fiorica JV, Brunetto VL, Hanjani P, Lentz SS, Mannel R, Andersen W, Gynecologic Oncology Group study. Phase II trial of alternating courses of megestrol acetate and tamoxifen in advanced endometrial carcinoma: a Gynecologic Oncology Group study. Gynecol Oncol. 2004;92(1):10–4.
58. The Cancer Genome Atlas Research Network, Kandoth C, Schultz N, Cherniack AD, Akbani R, Liu Y, et al. Integrated genomic characterization of endometrial carcinoma. Nature. 2013;497:67–73.
59. Le Gallo M, Bell DW. The emerging genomic landscape of endometrial cancer. Clin Chem. 2014;60(1):98–110.
60. Liu Y, Patel L, Mills GB, Lu KH, Sood AK, Ding L, Kucherlapati R, Mardis ER, Levine DA, Shmulevich I, Broaddus RR, Zhang W. Clinical significance of CTNNB1 mutation and Wnt pathway activation in endometrioid endometrial carcinoma. J Natl Cancer Inst. 2014;106(9):dju245.
61. The Cancer Genome Atlas Research Network. Integrated genomic analyses of ovarian carcinoma. Nature. 2011;474:609–15.
62. The Cancer Genome Atlas Network. Comprehensive molecular portraits of human breast tumours. Nature. 2012;490:61–70.
63. Lawrence MS, Stojanov P, Polak P, et al. Mutational heterogeneity in cancer and the search for new cancer-associated genes. Nature. 2013;499(7457):214–8.
64. Buza N, Roque DM, Santin AD. HER2/neu in endometrial cancer: a promising therapeutic target with diagnostic challenges. Arch Pathol Lab Med. 2014;138(3):343–50.
65. Fleming GF, Sill MW, Darcy KM, et al. Phase II trial of trastuzumab in women with advanced or recurrent, HER2-positive endometrial carcinoma: a Gynecologic Oncology Group study. Gynecol Oncol. 2010;116(1):15–20. https://doi.org/10.1016/j.ygyno.2009.09.025.
66. Leslie KK, Sill MW, Lankes HA, et al. Lapatinib and potential prognostic value of EGFR mutations in a Gynecologic Oncology Group phase II trial of persistent or recurrent endometrial cancer. Gynecol Oncol. 2012;127:345–50.
67. Oza AM, Eisenhauer EA, Elit L, et al. Phase II study of erlotinib in recurrent or metastatic endometrial cancer: NCIC IND-148. J Clin Oncol. 2008;26(26):4319–25.
68. Leslie KK, Sill MW, Fischer E, et al. A phase II evaluation of gefitinib in the treatment of persistent or recurrent endometrial cancer: a Gynecologic Oncology Group study. Gynecol Oncol. 2013;129:486–94.
69. Dutt A, Salvesen HB, Chen TH, et al. Drug-sensitive FGFR2 mutations in endometrial carcinoma. Proc Natl Acad Sci U S A. 2008;105:8713–7.
70. Pollock PM, Gartside MG, Dejeza LC, et al. Frequent activating FGFR2 mutations in endometrial carcinomas parallel germline mutations associated with craniosynostosis and skeletal dysplasia syndromes. Oncogene. 2007;26:7158–62.
71. Dizon DS, Sill MW, Schilder JM, McGonigle KF, Rahman Z, Miller DS, Mutch DG, Leslie KK. A phase II evaluation of nintedanib (BIBF-1120) in the treatment of recurrent or persistent endometrial cancer: an NRG Oncology/Gynecologic Oncology Group study. Gynecol Oncol. 2014;135(3):441–5.

72. Powell MA, Sill MW, Goodfellow PJ, et al. A phase II trial of brivanib in recurrent or persistent endometrial cancer: an NRG Oncology/Gynecologic Oncology Group study. Gynecol Oncol. 2014;135(1):38–43. https://doi.org/10.1016/j.ygyno.2014.07.083.
73. Konecny GE, Finkler N, Garcia AA, Lorusso D, Lee PS, Rocconi RP, Fong PC, Squires M, Mishra K, Upalawanna A, Wang Y, Kristeleit R. Second-line dovitinib (TKI258) in patients with FGFR2-mutated or FGFR2-non-mutated advanced or metastatic endometrial cancer: a non-randomised, open-label, two-group, two-stage, phase 2 study. Lancet Oncol. 2015;16(6):686–94.
74. Courtney KD, Corcoran RB, Engelman JA. The PI3K pathway as drug target in human cancer. J Clin Oncol. 2010;28(6):1075–83.
75. Salvesen HB, Carter SL, Mannelqvist M, Dutt A, Getz G, Stefansson IM, et al. Integrated genomic profiling of endometrial carcinoma associates aggressive tumors with indicators of PI3 kinase activation. Proc Natl Acad Sci U S A. 2009;106(12):4834–9.
76. Kanamori Y, Kigawa J, Itamochi H, et al. Correlation between loss of PTEN expression and Akt phosphorylation in endometrial carcinoma. Clin Cancer Res. 2001;7:892–5.
77. Slomovitz BM, Lu KH, Johnston T, et al. A phase 2 study of the oral mammalian target of rapamycin inhibitor, everolimus, in patients with recurrent endometrial carcinoma. Cancer. 2010;116:5415–9.
78. Ray-Coquard I, Favier L, Weber B, et al. Everolimus as second- or third-line treatment of advanced endometrial cancer: ENDORAD, a phase II trial of GINECO. Br J Cancer. 2013;108:1771–7.
79. Meyer LA, Slomovitz BM, Djordjevic B, Westin SN, Iglesias DA, Munsell MF, Jiang Y, Schmandt R, Broaddus RR, Coleman RL, Galbincea JM, Lu KH. The search continues: looking for predictive biomarkers for response to mammalian target of rapamycin inhibition in endometrial cancer. Int J Gynecol Cancer. 2014;24(4):713–7.
80. Colombo N, McMeekin S, Schwartz P, Kostka J, Sessa C, Gehrig P, et al. A phase II trial of the mTOR inhibitor AP23573 as a single agent in advanced endometrial cancer. J Clin Oncol. 2007;25:278s. (abstr 5516).
81. Colombo N, McMeekin DS, Schwartz PE, et al. Ridaforolimus as a single agent in advanced endometrial cancer: results of a single-arm, phase 2 trial. Br J Cancer. 2013;108(5):1021–6. https://doi.org/10.1038/bjc.2013.59. Epub 2013 Feb 12.
82. Tsoref D, Welch S, Lau S, Biagi J, Tonkin K, Martin LA, Ellard S, Ghatage P, Elit L, Mackay HJ, Allo G, Tsao MS, Kamel-Reid S, Eisenhauer EA, Oza AM. Phase II study of oral ridaforolimus in women with recurrent or metastatic endometrial cancer. Gynecol Oncol. 2014;135(2):184–9.
83. Oza AM, Pignata S, Poveda A, et al. Randomized phase II trial of ridaforolimus in advanced endometrial carcinoma. J Clin Oncol. 2015;33:3576–82. [Epub ahead of print].
84. Mackay HJ, Eisenhauer EA, Kamel-Reid S, Tsao M, Clarke B, Karakasis K, et al. Molecular determinants of outcome with mammalian target of rapamycin inhibition in endometrial cancer. Cancer. 2014;120(4):603–10.
85. Oza AM, Elit L, Tsao MS, et al. Phase II study of temsirolimus in women with recurrent or metastatic endometrial cancer: a trial of the NCIC clinical trials group. J Clin Oncol. 2011;29:3278–85.
86. Goodwin RA, Jamal R, Tuc D, et al. Clinical and toxicity predictors of response and progression to temsirolimus in women with recurrent or metastatic endometrial cancer. Gynecol Oncol. 2013;13:315–20.
87. Fleming GF, Filiaci VL, Marzullo B, et al. Temsirolimus with or without megestrol acetate and tamoxifen for endometrial cancer: a Gynecologic Oncology Group study. Gynecol Oncol. 2014;132:585–92.
88. Alvarez EA, Brady WE, Walker JL, et al. Phase II trial of combination bevacizumab and temsirolimus in the treatment of recurrent or persistent endometrial carcinoma: a Gynecologic Oncology Group study. Gynecol Oncol. 2013;129:22–7.

89. André F, O'Regan R, Mustafa Ozguroglu M, et al. Everolimus for women with trastuzumab-resistant, HER2-positive, advanced breast cancer (BOLERO-3): a randomised, double-blind, placebo-controlled phase 3 trial. Lancet Oncol. 2014;15:580–91.
90. Slomovitz BM, Jiang Y, Yates MS, et al. Phase II study of everolimus and letrozole in patients with recurrent endometrial carcinoma. J Clin Oncol. 2015;33(8):930–6.
91. Bradford LS, Rauh-Hain A, Clarka RM, et al. Assessing the efficacy of targeting the phosphatidylinositol 3-kinase/AKT/mTOR signaling pathway in endometrial cancer. Gynecol Oncol. 2014;133:346–52.
92. Heudel PE, Fabbro M, Roemer-Becuwe C, et al. Phase II study of the PI3K inhibitor BKM120 monotherapy in patients with advanced or recurrent endometrial carcinoma: ENDOPIK, GINECO study. J Clin Oncol. 2015;33:5588. (suppl; abstr 5588).
93. Matulonis U, Vergote I, Backes F, et al. Phase II study of the PI3K inhibitor pilaralisib (SAR245408; XL147) in patients with advanced or recurrent endometrial carcinoma. Gynecol Oncol. 2015;136(2):246–53.
94. Makker V, Recio FO, Ma L, Matulonis U, O'Hara Lauchle J, Parmar H, et al. Phase II trial of GDC-0980 (dual PI3K/mTOR inhibitor) in patients with advanced endometrial carcinoma: final study results. J Clin Oncol. 2014;32:5513. [Abstr].
95. Rodon J, Dienstmann R, Serra V, Tabernero J. Development of PI3K inhibitors: lessons learned from early clinical trials. Nat Rev Clin Oncol. 2013;10(3):143–53.
96. Mendes-Pereira AM, Martin SA, Brough R, et al. Synthetic lethal targeting of PTEN mutant cells with PARP inhibitors. EMBO Mol Med. 2009;1(6–7):315–22.
97. Dedes KJ, Wetterskog D, Mendes-Pereira AM, et al. PTEN deficiency in endometrioid endometrial adenocarcinomas predict sensitivity to PARP-inhibitors. Sci Transl Med. 2010;2(53):53ra75.
98. Forster MD, Dedes KJ, Sandhu S, Frentzas S, Kristeleit R, Ashworth A, Poole CJ, Weigelt B, Kaye SB, Molife LR. Treatment with olaparib in a patient with PTEN-deficient endometrioid endometrial cancer. Nat Rev Clin Oncol. 2011;8(5):302–6. https://doi.org/10.1038/nrclinonc.2011.42. Epub 2011 Apr 5.
99. Yokoyama Y, Charnock-Jones DS, Licence D, et al. Expression of vascular endothelial growth factor (VEGF)-D and its receptor, VEGF receptor 3, as a prognostic factor in endometrial carcinoma. Clin Cancer Res. 2003;9(4):1361–9.
100. Aghajanian C, Sill MW, Darcy KM, Greer B, McMeekin DS, Rose PG, Rotmensch J, Barnes MN, Hanjani P, Leslie KK. Phase II trial of bevacizumab in recurrent or persistent endometrial cancer: a Gynecologic Oncology Group study. J Clin Oncol. 2011;29(16):2259–65. https://doi.org/10.1200/JCO.2010.32.6397. Epub 2011 May 2.
101. Aghajanian CA, Filaci VL, Dizon DS, et al. A randomized phase II study of paclitaxel/carboplatin/bevacizumab, paclitaxel/carboplatin/temsirolimus and ixabepilone/carboplatin/bevacizumab as initial therapy for measurable stage III or IVA, stage IVB or recurrent endometrial cancer, GOG-86P. J Clin Oncol. 2015;33. (suppl; abstr 5500).
102. Lorusso D, Ferrandina G, Colombo N, et al. Randomized phase II trial of carboplatin-paclitaxel (CP) compared to carboplatin-paclitaxel-bevacizumab (CP-B) in advanced (stage III-IV) or recurrent endometrial cancer: The MITO END-2 trial. J Clin Oncol. 2015;33. (suppl; abstr 5502).
103. Myers AP, Broaddus R, Makker V, Konstantinopoulos PA, Drapkin R, Horowitz NS, et al. Phase II, two-stage, two-arm, PIK3CA mutation stratified trial of MK-2206 in recurrent endometrial cancer (EC). J Clin Oncol. 2013;31:5524. [Suppl.; abstr].
104. Konstantinopoulos P, Makker V, Barry WT, Liu J, Horowitz NS, Birrer MJ, et al. Phase II, single stage, cohort expansion study of MK-2206 in recurrent endometrial serous cancer. J Clin Oncol. 2014;32:5515. [Abstr].

Advances in Endometrial Cancer Diagnosis

Vincent Vandecaveye

Endometrial cancer is staged according to the International Federation of Gynecology and Obstetrics (FIGO) guidelines which are developed independently from imaging [1]. Major prognostic factors for endometrial cancer comprise histologic grade and lymphovascular invasion, local tumor extent including depth of myometrial invasion and cervical stromal involvement, and extrauterine tumor spread including nodal and distant metastatic spread [2]. Although FIGO guidelines do not recommend cross-sectional imaging as routine diagnostic modalities, CT, MRI, and FDG-PET/CT have an increasing role in the management of endometrial cancer patients as they also allow assessment of distant nodal or visceral disease spread [3]. At the time of diagnosis of endometrial cancer, imaging is most important for staging of locoregional and distant tumor extent and for prognostication. The purpose of this chapter is to present a general overview of conventional and newly developed imaging concepts for endometrial cancer.

4.1 Local Staging

Depth of myometrial invasion (Stage IA vs. IB) and cervical stromal invasion are key features in the imaging assessment of local disease extent as both are highly associated with nodal metastases. Deep myometrial invasion >50% is associated with higher frequency of nodal metastases up to 46% [4].

CT has the advantage of widespread availability at a relatively low cost, providing fast and reproducible image acquisition compared to MRI and FDG-PET/CT. CT is usually performed after the injection of iodinated contrast-agent using multidetector technology, which enables data acquisition of large anatomical areas and high-quality thin-slice multiplanar image reformatting. However, the major

V. Vandecaveye (✉)
Radiology, Universitair Ziekenhuis Leuven, Leuven, Belgium
e-mail: vincent.vandecaveye@med.kuleuven.be

disadvantage is the low soft tissue contrast, which hampers the depiction of small endometrial cancers and inhibits accurate assessment of local tumor spread such as myometrial or uterine cervical invasion. For assessment of deep myometrial invasion, a sensitivity of 83% with specificity of 42% and overall staging accuracy between 58 and 76% have been described [5, 6]. A study, using multidetector CT, reported better diagnostic accuracy of 95% for evaluating myometrial invasion and 81% for assessing cervical infiltration. However, the authors acknowledged small patient number and large percentage of cases with deep myometrial invasion [7]. In clinical practice, CT is mostly used to assess extrauterine diseases including regional and para-aortic lymph nodes and shows similar accuracy as MRI for the detection of extrauterine disease spread and identifying nodal metastases [8].

For local staging, MRI benefits from a superior contrast resolution and excellent soft tissue differentiation. Other benefits of MRI include absent radiation exposure, absent need of iodinated contrast-agent and a high flexibility in its performance allowing the adaptation of image protocols to the specific needs of the patient and easy integration of functional imaging sequences such as dynamic contrast-enhanced imaging (DCE-MRI) and diffusion-weighted imaging (DWI). Disadvantages included lower availability compared to CT, lower patient compliance related to longer imaging times, claustrophobia, and contraindications such as pacemakers.

Standardization of the MRI protocol is pivotal to optimize diagnostic accuracy and reproducibility and a protocol has been recommended in the European Society of Urogenital Radiology (ESUR) Endometrial Cancer Staging guidelines [8]. Routine sequences in the imaging protocol consist of T2-weighted images in the sagittal and oblique transverse plane, perpendicular to the endometrial cavity and fat-saturated post-contrast T1-weighted images. Combination with dynamic contrast-enhanced (DCE)-MRI—which is acquired by repetitive imaging with high temporal resolution over a predefined lesion prior to and during the injection of a gadolinium contrast agent—is highly recommended as it allows better delineation of the tumor [9]. Although not routinely recommended, studies have shown that DWI can be of additional value for endometrial characterization, assessment of myometrial invasion, response assessment, and prognostication [9, 10].

DWI distinguishes itself from conventional MRI sequences by detecting water molecule displacements at a cellular scale allowing functional characterization of tissue microstructural properties. The signal intensity of lesions depends on the amount of impediment of water molecule displacements. The more tissue restricts water molecule displacement (e.g. tumoral lesions), the brighter lesions appear at heavily weighted DWI ($b = 800–1000$ s/mm^2), compared to the suppressed background tissue. The typical signal decay with increasing b-value can be quantified using the apparent diffusion coefficient (ADC). In a simplified model, image analysis comprises combined reading of the signal intensity at high b-value images and quantification of ADC to differentiate malignant from benign tissue. Tissue, with a relatively increased cellular density (Tumor) will typically be bright on high b-value images and dark on the ADC-image while tissue with a relatively decreased cellular density (most benign tissues, inflammation and necrosis) will be dark on high b-value images and bright on the ADC-images [11].

Although MRI is considered the most accurate imaging modality for staging and preoperative assessment of endometrial cancer, the value of pretreatment MRI is not unequivocally accepted as the majority of cases are treated by surgery [12]. According to the European Society of Urogenital Radiology (ESUR) Endometrial Cancer Staging guidelines, indications for MRI with proven or suspected endometrial cancer include: high-grade, serous or clear-cell adenocarcinomas; suspicion of advanced disease, including cervical stroma extension and confirmation of stage III and IV disease; screening for lymph node enlargement as a roadmap for lymph node sampling; medical contraindication for surgical staging; and suspected endometrial cancer with inability of curettage (e.g., cervical stenosis) [8].

For assessment of deep myometrial invasion, a meta-analysis in 47 studies aiming to compare the utility of CT, endovaginal ultrasound, and MRI described sensitivity between 78.6% and 100%, respectively, specificity between 71.4% and 100% for contrast-enhanced MRI compared to sensitivity between 40% and 100%, respectively, specificity between 66.7% and 100% for CT and sensitivity between 50% and 100%, respectively, specificity between 65% and 100% for endovaginal ultrasound. For assessment of cervical involvement, sensitivity in the included studies ranged between 55.6 and 100% and specificity between 92.3 and 100% for MRI, compared to 40–71.4% sensitivity with 100% specificity for CT and 66.7–80% sensitivity with 95.2–100% specificity for endovaginal ultrasound [13]. Importantly, the superiority of MRI over endovaginal ultrasound could not be unequivocally shown. However, MRI harbors the important advantage that it is the only modality that allows for simultaneous accurate assessment of myometrial, cervical, and nodal involvement (Fig. 4.1).

Another more recent meta-analysis including 52 eligible studies, showed 80.7% pooled sensitivity and 88.5% pooled specificity for the assessment of deep (>50%) myometrial invasion and 57% pooled sensitivity and 94% pooled specificity for assessment of cervical stromal involvement. Importantly, the addition of the functional MRI sequences, DCE-MRI and DWI, increases sensitivity compared to contrast-enhanced MRI alone [14]. DCE-MRI allows for better differentiation of tumor from blood products and debris as well as tumor from the myometrium due to differential timing of enhancement [9]. Although less established compared to DCE-MRI, DWI improves MR assessment of myometrial invasion with diagnostic accuracies ranging between 62–90% [15, 16]. In a study of Beddy et al., DWI showed superior accuracy over DCE-MRI (90% vs. 71%) for assessment of myometrial invasion [10]. In a study by Rechichi et al., DWI showed not only higher accuracy for tumor staging but also higher interobserver agreement for assessing tumor extension [17]. These findings suggest that DWI adds to the overall diagnostic performance of MRI for local tumor staging, not only by improving diagnostic accuracy but also by improving radiologist confidence. Alternatively, these findings indicate that DWI can obviate the need of contrast-injection, in case of contraindication. An additional important advantage of DWI over conventional MRI for local tumor assessment is the ability for quantification of tissue properties by means of the ADC. This allows DWI to differentiate endometrial cancer from benign endometrial polyps and could be of particular importance in patients difficult to biopsy. A previous study showed that endometrial cancer has significantly lower ADC

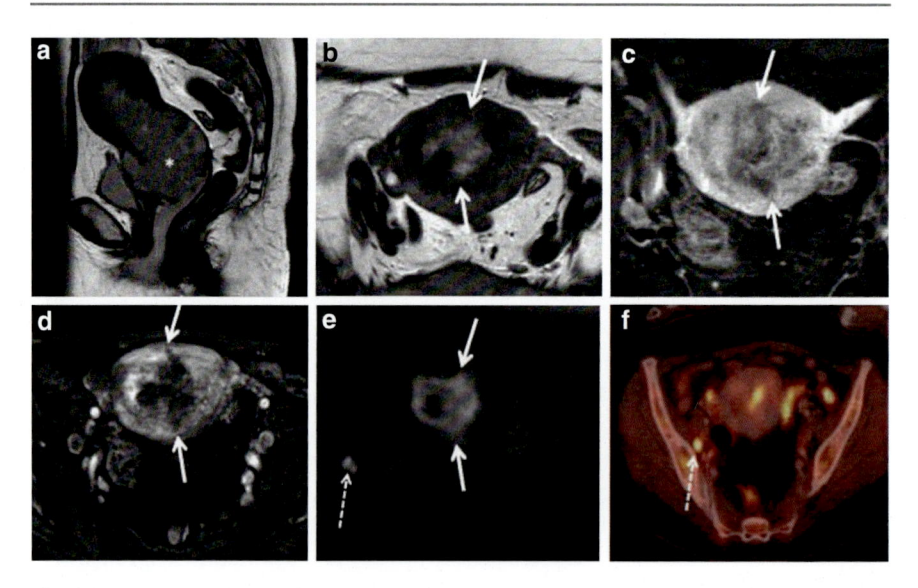

Fig. 4.1 Patient with advanced endometrial cancer: (**a**) Sagittal T2-weighted MRI shows large mass in the endometrial cavity with gross cervical invasion (asterisk). (**b, c**) Transverse T2-weighted and contrast-enhanced T1 image shows multifocal deep myometrial invasion (arrows). (**d, e**) This is better appreciated at DCE-MRI and DWI due to the high tumor-to-background contrast (arrows). DWI also allows the depiction of a bright right iliac lymphadenopathy, confirmed by FDG-PET/CT (**f**, dashed arrow)

compare to benign polyps allowing differentiation with 92% accuracy [18]. Moreover, Studies have shown that the ADC measured over the endometrial mass can predict tumor grade, for which a lower ADC correlates to higher tumor grade [19–21]. However, substantial overlap between ADC of different tumor grades does not allow its clinical application at this time. Recently, a study has shown that tumor volumetry combined with volumetric ADC measurements or ADC histographic analysis may allow accurate preoperative risk stratification of patients with endometrial cancer. ADC histographic analysis depicts the ADC heterogeneity and thus better reflection of the tumoral microstructural heterogeneity. Lower histographic ADC values were shown to correlate significantly with lymphovascular invasion and allow differentiation grade 3 from grade 2 and 1 tumors. Although further development is required, DWI could further help to stratify treatment according to risk of local or distant recurrence [22].

FDG-PET/CT takes advantage of the fact that endometrial cancer demonstrates an increased rate of glycolysis for visualization. In a comparative study, FDG-PET/CT showed 61% accuracy for myometrial invasion and 83% accuracy for cervical invasion similar to MRI [23]. It should however be noted that neither DCE-MRI nor DWI were included in the scan protocol. Overall, FDG-PET/CT has a limited role for local staging whereas it has greater value for staging extrauterine disease. Importantly, similar as for DWI, assessment of the tumoral metabolical properties may hold prognostic information. Previous studies have shown a statistical correlation between the maximum standard uptake value (SUVmax) of the primary tumor and FIGO stage, histological grade, depth of myometrial invasion, lymph nodes metastases and lymphovascular invasion [24, 25]. In a study by Husby et al., Metabolic tumor volume and PET-derived quantitative parameters including the SUVmax were independent predictors of deep myometrial invasion and nodal metastases and may aid in the preoperative identification of high-risk patients and enable the restriction of lymphadenectomy in patient with low risk of aggressive disease [26]. Furthermore, a high SUVmax has been shown to be an independent prognostic factor for overall survival [27].

4.2 Staging of Extrauterine Disease Spread

For detection of nodal metastases, CT and conventional MRI rely on size-related (1 cm threshold) and morphologic criteria like shape or internal architecture. These features are highly variable predictors of nodal involvement and bare the inherent disadvantage that small nodal metastases remain undetected and or that enlarged reactive—and thus benign—lymph nodes are falsely interpreted as malignant. Although the presence of intranodal necrosis at conventional imaging has positive predictive value of 100% for predicting metastatic involvement, its occurrence is too infrequent to significantly influence diagnostic performance [5]. The sensitivity of CT ranges between 52 and 92% for assessing pelvic and para-aortic lymphadenopathy, is not significantly improved by conventional MRI which has described diagnostic accuracy between 55 and 77% [9, 28].

Due to its ability to probe the tissue microstructure—irrespective of lesion size by differences in ADC, DWI has the potential to improve nodal staging compared to conventional MRI.

Differences in ADC between malignant and benign lymph nodes likely result from differences in microstructure with metastatic lymph nodes expected to have increased cellularity, enlarged cell size and nuclei compared to benign lymph nodes. This should result in lower ADC for metastatic lymph nodes due to the restriction of extracellular water molecules.

Reports evaluating DWI quantified by the ADC for nodal staging in patients with endometrial and cervical uterine cancer show variable results. While in the study of Roy et al., ADC values were not statistically different between benign and malignant lymph nodes and thus did not allow for characterization of nodal metastases, Lin et al., showed that adding DWI substantially improved sensitivity compared to conventional MRI while maintaining specificity (83% vs. 25%) [29, 30]. The diverging results likely reflect difficulties encountered in the analysis of DWI. Impeded diffusion with similar low ADC with as for malignancy may be encountered in reactive lymph nodes due to hypercellularity of lymphoid cells. Further refinement of ADC-analysis could overcome this problem and overcome current limitations for differentiation of pelvic lymph nodes. Recently, Rechichi

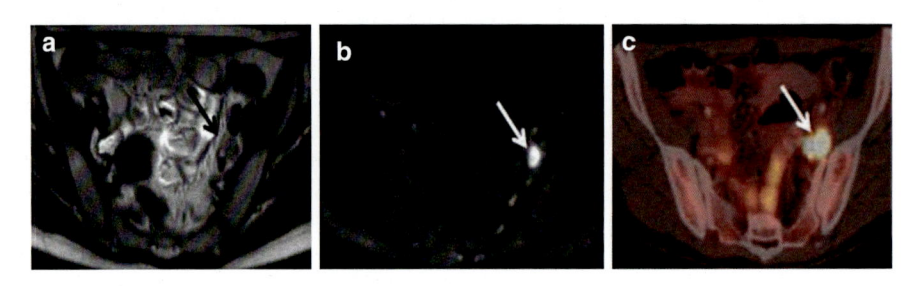

Fig. 4.2 (**a**) T2-weighted MR image shows enlarged lymph node posterior to the right external iliac vein. The lymphadenopathy is markedly hyperintense compared to surrounding lymph nodes on the (**b**) b1000 DWI-image facilitating its detection. The lymphadenopathy was confirmed by (**c**) PET/CT and subsequent lymphadenectomy

et al., found high accuracy for nodal differentiation in endometrial cancer of 98.3% by applying minimum ADC region values compared to 72.9% for the mean ADC—the current standard analysis [31]. Awaiting further development, standardization and larger studies that reproduce initial results, the use of DWI with quantitative ADC for nodal differentiation in endometrial cancer should currently not be considered clinical routine.

Nevertheless, when combined with conventional MRI, qualitative interpretation of high b-value DWI images has been shown to improve the detection of lymphadenopathy in abdominopelvic, compared with conventional imaging [9] (Fig. 4.2).

While the role of FDG-PET/CT seems more limited for local staging, it shows high value for assessing nodal and distant metastases [32]. Several studies have assessed the value of FDG-PET/CT for nodal staging in high-risk endometrial cancer patients. On a per-region based analysis, studies found sensitivities ranging between 36 and 72% with specificities between 88 and 99% [33]. A more recent meta-analysis showed good performance of FDG-PET/CT with an overall accuracy of 89.5% [34]. Currently, the spatial limitation of FDG-PET/CT limits the detection of lesions smaller than 5 mm and sensitivity decreases with lesions size. A study by Kitajima et al., showed 93.3% sensitivity for lesions larger than 1 cm, 66.7% sensitivity for lesions from 0.6 to 0.9 cm, and 16.7% sensitivity for lesions smaller than 0.4 cm [35]. Therefore, FDG-PET/CT is not generally accepted as and an adequate alternative to surgical staging [36]. Therefore, the integration of PET/CT and sentinel lymph node mapping has been proposed in high-risk endometrial cancer patients. The high specificity and positive predictive value of FDG-PET/CT allows to select patients for pelvic and aortic lymphadenectomy. The combination with sentinel lymph node mapping can overcome the spatial resolution limits of FDG-PET/CT and increase the ability to detect small nodal metastases [36]. In addition to nodal staging, FDG-PET also shows value for detecting intra- and extra-abdominal distant metastases with a described accuracy up to 96.9% [37] (Fig. 4.3).

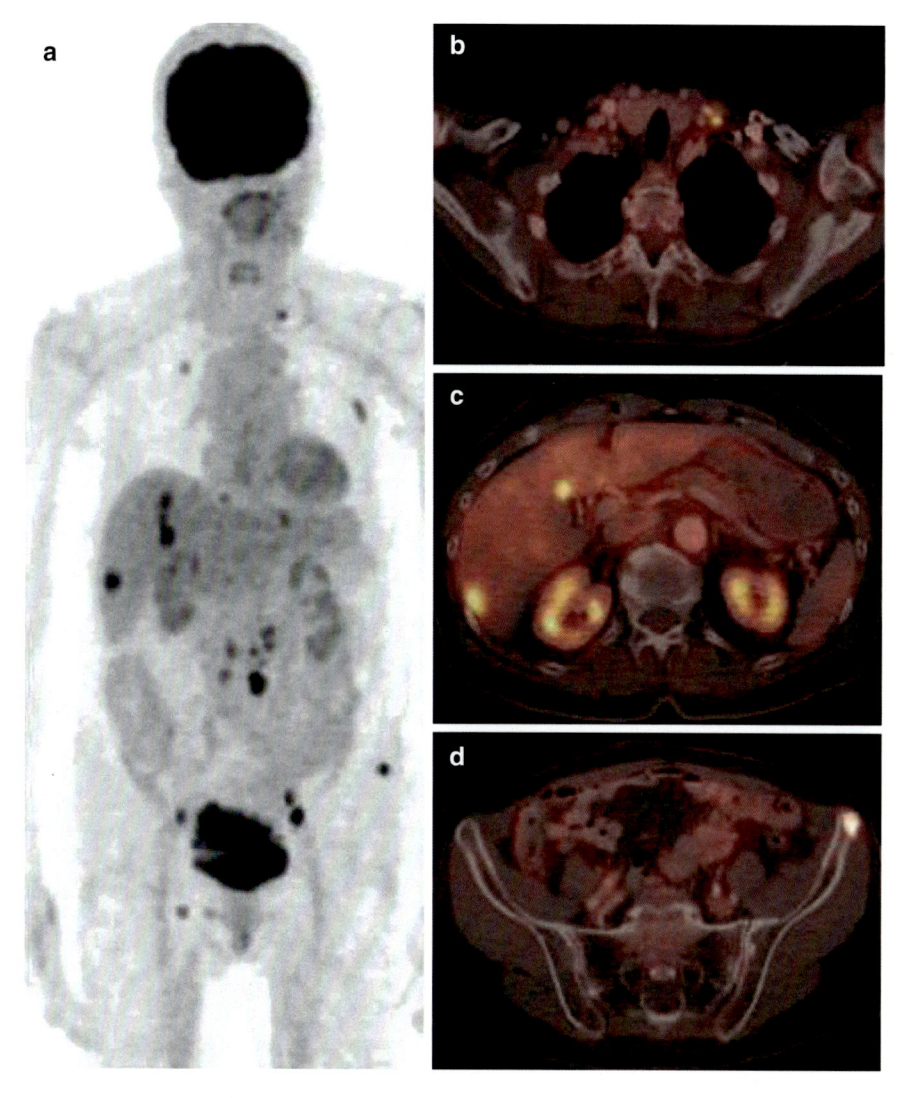

Fig. 4.3 Patient with advanced endometrial cancer: (**a**) MIP reconstruction of PET shows multifocal hypermetabolic lesions in lymph nodes, liver, and bone. Fused PET/CT images show (**b**) left supraclavicular lymphadenopathy, (**c**) liver metastases, and (**d**) bone metastasis in the left iliac crest

4.3 Conclusion

MRI complements clinical examination and ultrasound for local staging of endometrial cancer with the major advantage that it allows for accurate assessment of myometrial invasion. The addition of functional imaging techniques, including DWI and DCE-MRI, improves the accuracy of MRI for characterization of endometrial lesions, local staging including the assessment of myometrial, and cervical involvement. In addition, DWI may also improve the ability of MRI for detection of lymph node metastases but requires further development before it can be reliably implemented as a clinical tool for nodal staging in endometrial cancer. While FDG-PET/CT has relatively low value for local staging it contributes mainly by the assessment of nodal and distant metastases. The high specificity enables adequate selection of patients for pelvic and aortic lymphadenectomy while the lower sensitivity for small nodal metastases can be overcome by additional surgical staging in high-risk endometrial cancer patients with negative nodal staging at FDG-PET/CT.

In addition, quantitative evaluation of DWI by the ADC and FDG-PET by the SUV may help in prognostication and risk stratification but requires validation in larger patient groups to validate its clinical utility. CT can be used as an alternative in endometrial cancer staging but is mostly used for detection of extrauterine disease spread. Due to its widespread availability at a relatively low cost, it is often used as a first d test.

References

1. Creasman W. Revised FIGO staging for carcinoma of the endometrium. Int J Gynaecol Obstet. 2009;105(2):109.
2. Larson DM, Connor GP, Broste SK, Krawisz BR, Johnson KK. Prognostic significance of gross myometrial invasion with endometrial cancer. Obstet Gynecol. 1996;88(3):394–8.
3. Colombo N, Preti E, Landoni F, Carinelli S, Colombo A, Marini C, Sessa C, ESMO Guidelines Working Group. Endometrial cancer: ESMO clinical practice guidelines for diagnosis, treatment and follow-up. Ann Oncol. 2013;24(Suppl 6):vi33–8.
4. Berman ML, Ballon SC, Lagasse LD, Watring WG. Prognosis and treatment of endometrial cancer. Am J Obstet Gynecol. 1980;136(5):679–88.
5. Patel S, Liyanage SH, Sahdev A, Rockall AG, Reznek RH. Imaging of endometrial and cervical cancer. Insights Imaging. 2010;1(5–6):309–28.
6. Connor JP, Andrews JI, Anderson B, Buller RE. Computed tomography in endometrial carcinoma. Obstet Gynecol. 2000;95(5):692–6.
7. Tsili AC, Tsampoulas C, Dalkalitsis N, Stefanou D, Paraskevaidis E, Efremidis SC. Local staging of endometrial carcinoma: role of multidetector CT. Eur Radiol. 2008;18(5):1043–8.
8. Kinkel K, Forstner R, Danza FM, Oleaga L, Cunha TM, Bergman A, Barentsz JO, Balleyguier C, Brkljacic B, Spencer JA. Staging of endometrial cancer with MRI: guidelines of the European Society of Urogenital Imaging. Eur Radiol. 2009;19(7):1565–74.
9. Beddy P, O'Neill AC, Yamamoto AK, Addley HC, Reinhold C, Sala E. FIGO staging system for endometrial cancer: added benefits of MR imaging. Radiographics. 2012;32(1):241–54. https://doi.org/10.1148/rg.321115045.
10. Beddy P, Moyle P, Kataoka M, Yamamoto AK, Joubert I, Lomas D, Crawford R, Sala E. Evaluation of depth of myometrial invasion and overall staging in endometrial cancer: comparison of diffusion-weighted and dynamic contrast-enhanced MR imaging. Radiology. 2012;262(2):530–7.
11. Koh DM, Collins DJ. Diffusion-weighted MRI in the body: applications and challenges in oncology. AJR Am J Roentgenol. 2007;188:1622–35.
12. Spencer JA, Messiou C, Swift SE. MR staging of endometrial cancer: needed or wanted? Cancer Imaging. 2008;8:1–5.
13. Kinkel K, Kaji Y, Yu KK, Segal MR, Lu Y, Powell CB, Hricak H. Radiologic staging in patients with endometrial cancer: a meta-analysis. Radiology. 1999;212(3):711–8.

14. Luomaranta A, Leminen A, Loukovaara M. Magnetic resonance imaging in the assessment of high-risk features of endometrial carcinoma: a meta-analysis. Int J Gynecol Cancer. 2015;25(5):837–42.
15. Lin G, Ng KK, Chang CJ, Wang JJ, Ho KC, Yen TC, Wu TI, Wang CC, Chen YR, Huang YT, Ng SH, Jung SM, Chang TC, Lai CH. Myometrial invasion in endometrial cancer: diagnostic accuracy of diffusion-weighted 3.0-T MR imaging—initial experience. Radiology. 2009;250(3):784–92.
16. Shen SH, Chiou YY, Wang JH, Yen MS, Lee RC, Lai CR, Chang CY. Diffusion-weighted single-shot echo-planar imaging with parallel technique in assessment of endometrial cancer. AJR Am J Roentgenol. 2008;190(2):481–8.
17. Rechichi G, Galimberti S, Signorelli M, Perego P, Valsecchi MG, Sironi S. Myometrial invasion in endometrial cancer: diagnostic performance of diffusion-weighted MR imaging at 1.5-T. Eur Radiol. 2010;20(3):754–62.
18. Fujii S, Matsusue E, Kigawa J, Sato S, Kanasaki Y, Nakanishi J, Sugihara S, Kaminou T, Terakawa N, Ogawa T. Diagnostic accuracy of the apparent diffusion coefficient in differentiating benign from malignant uterine endometrial cavity lesions: initial results. Eur Radiol. 2008;18(2):384–9.
19. Tamai K, Koyama T, Saga T, Umeoka S, Mikami Y, Fujii S, Togashi K. Diffusion-weighted MR imaging of uterine endometrial cancer. J Magn Reson Imaging. 2007;26(3):682–7.
20. Rechichi G, Galimberti S, Signorelli M, Franzesi CT, Perego P, Valsecchi MG, Sironi S. Endometrial cancer: correlation of apparent diffusion coefficient with tumor grade, depth of myometrial invasion, and presence of lymph node metastases. AJR Am J Roentgenol. 2011;197(1):256–62.
21. Bharwani N, Miquel ME, Sahdev A, Narayanan P, Malietzis G, Reznek RH, Rockall AG. Diffusion-weighted imaging in the assessment of tumour grade in endometrial cancer. Br J Radiol. 2011;84(1007):997–1004.
22. Nougaret S, Reinhold C, Alsharif SS, Addley H, Arceneau J, Molinari N, Guiu B, Sala E. Endometrial cancer: combined MR volumetry and diffusion-weighted imaging for assessment of myometrial and lymphovascular invasion and tumor grade. Radiology. 2015;276(3):797–808.
23. Antonsen SL, Jensen LN, Loft A, Berthelsen AK, Costa J, Tabor A, Qvist I, Hansen MR, Fisker R, Andersen ES, Sperling L, Nielsen AL, Asmussen J, Høgdall E, Fagö-Olsen CL, Christensen IJ, Nedergaard L, Jochumsen K, Høgdall C. MRI, PET/CT and ultrasound in the preoperative staging of endometrial cancer—a multicenter prospective comparative study. Gynecol Oncol. 2013;128(2):300–8.
24. Nakamura K, Joja I, Fukushima C, Haruma T, Hayashi C, Kusumoto T, Seki N, Hongo A, Hiramatsu Y. The preoperative SUVmax is superior to ADCmin of the primary tumour as a predictor of disease recurrence and survival in patients with endometrial cancer. Eur J Nucl Med Mol Imaging. 2013;40(1):52–60.
25. Kitajima K, Kita M, Suzuki K, Senda M, Nakamoto Y, Sugimura K. Prognostic significance of SUVmax (maximum standardized uptake value) measured by [18F]FDG PET/CT in endometrial cancer. Eur J Nucl Med Mol Imaging. 2012;39(5):840–5.
26. Husby JA, Reitan BC, Biermann M, Trovik J, Bjørge L, Magnussen IJ, Salvesen ØO, Salvesen HB, Haldorsen IS. Metabolic tumor volume on 18F-FDG PET/CT improves preoperative identification of high-risk endometrial carcinoma patients. J Nucl Med. 2015;56(8):1191–8.
27. Nakamura K, Hongo A, Kodama J, Hiramatsu Y. The measurement of SUVmax of the primary tumor is predictive of prognosis for patients with endometrial cancer. Gynecol Oncol. 2011;123(1):82–7.
28. Lee JH, Dubinsky T, Andreotti RF, Cardenes HR, Dejesus Allison SO, Gaffney DK, Glanc P, Horowitz NS, Jhingran A, Lee SI, Puthawala AA, Royal HD, Scoutt LM, Small W Jr, Varia MA, Zelop CM, Expert Panel on Women's Imaging and Radiation Oncology-Gynecology. ACR appropriateness criteria pretreatment evaluation and follow-up of endometrial cancer of the uterus. Ultrasound Q. 2011;27(2):139–45.

29. Roy C, Bierry G, Matau A, Bazille G, Pasquali R. Value of diffusion-weighted imaging to detect small malignant pelvic lymph nodes at 3 T. Eur Radiol. 2010;20(8):1803–11.
30. Lin G, Ho KC, Wang JJ, Ng KK, Wai YY, Chen YT, Chang CJ, Ng SH, Lai CH, Yen TC. Detection of lymph node metastasis in cervical and uterine cancers by diffusion-weighted magnetic resonance imaging at 3T. J Magn Reson Imaging. 2008;28(1):128–35.
31. Rechichi G, Galimberti S, Oriani M, Perego P, Valsecchi MG, Sironi S. ADC maps in the prediction of pelvic lymph nodal metastatic regions in endometrial cancer. Eur Radiol. 2013;23(1):65–74.
32. Kitajima K, Murakami K, Kaji Y, Sugimura K. Spectrum of FDG PET/CT findings of uterine tumors. AJR Am J Roentgenol. 2010;195(3):737–43.
33. Choi HJ, Ju W, Myung SK, Kim Y. Diagnostic performance of computer tomography, magnetic resonance imaging, and positron emission tomography or positron emission tomography/computer tomography for detection of metastatic lymph nodes in patients with cervical cancer: meta-analysis. Cancer Sci. 2010;101(6):1471–9.
34. Chang MC, Chen JH, Liang JA, Yang KT, Cheng KY, Kao CH. 18F-FDG PET or PET/CT for detection of metastatic lymph nodes in patients with endometrial cancer: a systematic review and meta-analysis. Eur J Radiol. 2012;81(11):3511–7.
35. Kitajima K, Murakami K, Yamasaki E, Fukasawa I, Inaba N, Kaji Y, Sugimura K. Accuracy of 18F-FDG PET/CT in detecting pelvic and paraaortic lymph node metastasis in patients with endometrial cancer. AJR Am J Roentgenol. 2008;190:1652–8.
36. Signorelli M, Crivellaro C, Buda A, Guerra L, Fruscio R, Elisei F, Dolci C, Cuzzocrea M, Milani R, Messa C. Staging of high-risk endometrial cancer with pet/ct and sentinel lymph node mapping. Clin Nucl Med. 2015;40(10):780–5.
37. Picchio M, Mangili G, Samanes Gajate AM, De Marzi P, Spinapolice EG, Mapelli P, Giovacchini G, Sigismondi C, Viganò R, Sironi S, Messa C. High-grade endometrial cancer: value of [(18) F]FDG PET/CT in preoperative staging. Nucl Med Commun. 2010;31(6):506–12.

Part II

Epidemiology and Risk Factors of Endometrial Cancer

Epidemiology, Risk Factors, and Prevention for Endometrial Cancer

5

Johanna Mäenpää

5.1 Epidemiology

Globally, endometrial cancer is the sixth most common cancer in women [1]. The incidence of endometrial cancer is highest in North America and Western Europe. In 2015, the number of new cancers diagnosed in the U.S. was almost 55,000 [2], while in 2012, Europe showed close to 100,000 new cases [3]. Endometrial cancer has, in general, a favorable prognosis. For example, in the U.S, its incidence (25.1/100,000) far exceeds the mortality rate (4.4/100,000) [2]. Endometrial cancer mortality rates throughout 12 European countries are also generally low (shown in Table 5.1). Endometrial cancer is a disease linked to a high standard of living and, thus, the majority of cases are diagnosed in developed countries. Endometrial cancer is predominantly a disease of postmenopausal women, with a median age of 63 years at presentation and less than 10% occurring in women younger than 50 years of age [4].

Asides for geographical differences in the incidence of endometrial cancer, racial differences have also been found. As an example of a country with multiethnic population, the incidence rates of endometrial cancer in England have been documented according to the ethnic background (shown in Table 5.2) [5]. Women with black ethnicity appear to have the highest incidence, while South Asian women tend to have the lowest incidence. Interestingly in the U.S., the incidence of endometrial cancer is lower amongst African Americans compared to the white population [6].

J. Mäenpää (✉)
Faculty of Medicine, Tampere University, Tampere, Finland

Department of Obstetrics and Gynecology, Tampere University Hospital, Tampere, Finland
e-mail: johanna.maenpaa@tuni.fi

© Springer Nature Switzerland AG 2020
M. R. Mirza (ed.), *Management of Endometrial Cancer*,
https://doi.org/10.1007/978-3-319-64513-1_5

Table 5.1 Endometrial cancer mortality rates in 12 European countries in 2000–2004 [1]

Country	Mortality/100,000
Ireland	1.7
United Kingdom	2.0
Italy	2.2
Netherlands	2.2
Spain	2.5
France	2.6
Denmark	2.6
Belgium	2.6
Germany	2.7
Finland	3.0
Austria	3.1
Sweden	3.6

Table 5.2 Age Standardized Incidence Rates of Endometrial Cancer in different ethnic groups in England, 2001–2007, using the incidence in whites as reference [5]

Ethnic group	Incidence/100,00 person-years	Incidence Rate Ratio 99% (FCI/CI)
White	5.3	1.00 (0.98–1.02)
South Asian	4.5	0.90 (0.80–1.01)
Black	6.3	1.16 (1.03–1.31)
Chinese	6.3	1.21 (0.94–1.54)

Eighty percent of women with endometrial cancer have a disease confined to uterine corpus at presentation. For localized disease, the 5-year survival rate exceeds 90%. However, the survival rate is much lower for women having either regional (68%) or especially distant spread (17%), respectively [2].

Most endometrial cancers are sporadic, with Lynch syndrome being the most important familial form. The underlying genetic defect in Lynch syndrome involves mutations in MMR genes. Female members of Lynch syndrome families are at as great risk for endometrial cancer as for colorectal cancer, or 30–70% vs. 25–70%, respectively [7]. Women from Lynch syndrome families get the disease younger (median age 46–62 years) than women in general [8].

Endometrial carcinoma is usually divided into two types: Type I (endometrioid) cancer which is the most prevalent (80–90%), estrogen-dependent, slowly growing, metastasizes late, and has in general, a good prognosis and Type II cancer, estrogen-independent, faster growing, metastasizes early, and has markedly poorer prognosis than Type I [9]. Women with Type II cancer are typically older than women with Type I cancer [4, 10]. Serous and clear-cell carcinomas belong to Type II cancers, as well as approximately 25% of the high grade endometrioid carcinomas [11, 12]. The proportion of Type II cancer is higher in women with Lynch syndrome than in women in general, but also among them, Type I is the prevalent type [13]. The properties of Type I and Type II cancers are summarized in Table 5.3.

5 Epidemiology, Risk Factors, and Prevention for Endometrial Cancer

Table 5.3 Properties of Type I and Type II endometrial cancer

	Type I	Type II
Median age at presentation	63	67 [10]
5-year survival rate	85%	58%
Histology	Endometrioid Grade 1, 2, 3 (75%)	Papillary serous Clear-cell Carcinosarcoma Undifferentiated carcinoma Endometrioid G3 (25%)
Estrogen-dependent	Yes	No
Genetic alterations	PTEN, KRAS, CTNNB1, PIK3CA, MSI and MLH1 [14]	TP53 (mainly serous)
Known risk factors	Metabolic syndrome, obesity, Type II DM, unopposed estrogen	No known risk factors
Sensitivity of vaginal ultrasound in detection	Good [15]	Fair [10]

5.2 Risk Factors

The risk factors of Type I endometrial cancer are listed in Table 5.4. As all risk factors are linked to Type I carcinoma, there are no known risk factors for Type II cancer. Most of the risk factors are either directly or indirectly linked to unopposed estrogen.

Metabolic syndrome is a disorder being increasingly diagnosed in U.S. and EU and characterized by (abdominal) obesity, hyperandrogenism, hyperinsulinemia, and hypertension. Of the components of metabolic syndrome, obesity is the most important as related to endometrial cancer, with a risk ratio (RR) of 2.21 [16]. Also hypertension and hypertriglyceridemia contribute to the risk, although, to a lesser extent. Insulin resistance is prone to the onset of Type II diabetes mellitus (T2DM), which in turn is one of the classical risk factors of endometrial cancer, with an OR of 2.1 [17]. However, a recent epidemiological study implies that the role of T2DM is more indirect, associated rather to the accompanying obesity than to DM per se [20].

Infertility has long been linked to endometrial cancer. Of the causes leading to infertility, polycystic ovary syndrome (PCOS) is the most important one in this respect, with an OR of 2.8 [18]. PCOS is a disorder characterized by unusually thick-walled small follicular cysts situated in a pearl-like pattern (Fig. 5.1) in the periphery of the ovaries. A high luteinizing hormone (LH) to follicle stimulating hormone (FSH) ratio is associated with PCOS, of which patients suffer from chronic anovulation leading to prolonged estrogenic stimulation of endometrium. This stimulation in turn causes hyperplastic changes and, ultimately, endometrial carcinoma. PCOS is

Table 5.4 Risk factors for Type I endometrial carcinoma

Factor	Risk
Metabolic syndrome [16]: – Obesity [16] – Hypertension [16] – Hypertriglyceridemia [16]	RR 1.89 (95% CI 1.34–2.67) – RR 2.21 (95% CI 1.50–3.24) – RR 1.81 (95% CI 1.08–3.03) – RR 1.17 (95% CI 1.10–1.24)
Type II diabetes mellitus: – Unadjusted [17]	– OR 2.1; 95% CI 1.40–3.41
PCOS: – Unadjusted [18] – Adjusted [19]	– OR 2.79–2.89 – OR 2.2 (95% CI 0.9–5.7)
Other: Estrogen-producing ovarian tumors: 20% have simultaneous endometrial cancer Early (<12-year) menarche: RR 2.4 Late (≥55-year) menopause: RR 1.8 Unopposed estrogen (≥5 years) 10–20-fold risk Postmenopausal use of tamoxifen: 4.0 (95% CI 1.70–10.90)	

Fig. 5.1 A typical polycystic ovary (PCO). Courtesy of Dr. Helena Tinkanen

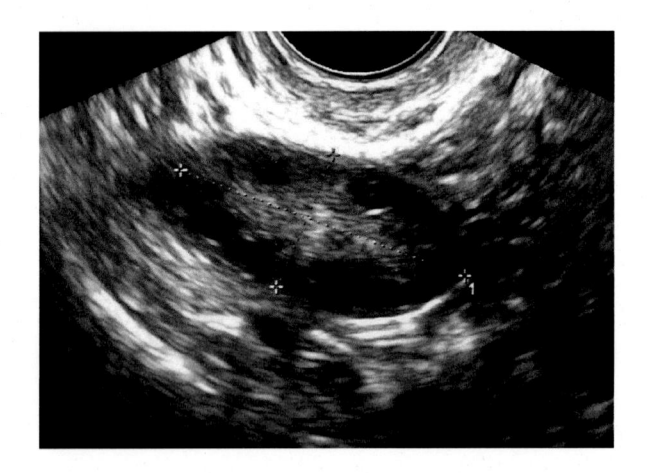

often associated with metabolic syndrome, which is likely to increase the carcinogenic potential; BMI-adjusted OR is lower than unadjusted OR, or 2.2 [19].

Estrogen-producing ovarian tumors, or granulosa and theca cell tumors, are important, yet rare, risk factors of endometrial cancer. In fact, 20% of women carrying these tumors have a simultaneous endometrial cancer [21], undermining the importance of preoperative endometrial sampling. Of constitutional risk factors besides genetic susceptibility (Lynch syndrome), both early menarche and late menopause are associated with approximately double the risk of endometrial cancer [22, 23].

There are also iatrogenic risk factors of endometrial cancer. Unopposed estrogen therapy is associated with up to a 30-fold increased risk, if the duration of the therapy is at least 5 years [24]. Postmenopausal use of tamoxifen in the prevention or treatment of breast cancer is paradoxically associated with a fourfold increased risk of endometrial cancer [25].

5.3 Prevention

Taking into account the risk factors, in general, women should be encouraged to pay attention to weight control if obese, and DM should be kept under careful control. It should, however, be taken into account that these measures merely decrease, and not abolish, the risk of endometrial cancer.

There are also pharmacological measures in the risk reduction. Successful treatment of infertility decreases substantially the risk of endometrial cancer within the anovulating population of women. If conception is not desired, cyclic progestin [26] and preferably, provided no contraindications exist, combined oral contraceptives can be used to counteract the stimulatory effect of estrogen on endometrium [27]. An efficacious alternative is levonorgestrel-releasing intrauterine device (LNG-IUD) [28]. Recent evidence suggests that also nulliparous women can safely use LNG-IUD [29]. Each of these hormonal treatments are also active in preventing endometrial stimulation caused by unopposed estrogen therapy. Moreover, LNG-IUD has been used to oppose the effect of tamoxifen on the endometrium, although its efficacy in this setting is still somewhat controversial [30].

5.4 Cancer Registry

In many countries, Cancer Registries have been founded to facilitate the follow-up of the epidemiology, standardization of the treatment, and collection of survival data of different forms of cancer at national level. In Europe, 60–85% of the funding of the registries comes from governmental sources (http://www.eurocourse.org). Cancer Registries are also a powerful tool for epidemiological research especially in the Nordic Countries, either at national or Nordic level (NORDCAN, or the Association of the Nordic Cancer Registries). From the NORDCAN database, it is easy to find statistical data of cancers at Nordic, national, or even regional level.

References

1. Weiderpass E, Antoine J, Bray FI, Oh J-K, Arbyn M. Trends in corpus uteri cancer mortality in member states of the European Union. Eur J Cancer. 2014;50:1675–84.
2. SEER Database 2005–2011.
3. WHO. GLOBOCAN 2012: Estimated cancer incidence, mortality and prevalence worldwide in 2012. 2012. http://globocan.iarc.fr/Pages/fact_sheets_population.aspx. Accessed 3 Apr 2015.
4. Lee NK, Cheung MK, Shin JY, et al. Prognostic factors for uterine cancer in reproductive-aged women. Obstet Gynecol. 2007;109:655–62.
5. Shirley MH, Barnes I, Sayeed S, Finlayson A, Ali R. Incidence of breast and gynaecological cancers by ethnic group in England, 2001–2007: a descriptive study. BMC Cancer. 2014;14:979.. http://www.biomedcentral.com/1471-2407/14/979
6. Jemal A, Siegel R, Ward E, et al. Cancer statistics, 2008. CA Cancer J Clin. 2008;58(2):71–96.

7. Vasen HFA, Blanco I, Aktan-Collan K, et al. Revised guidelines for the clinical managemen t of Lynch syndrome (HNPCC): recommendations by a group of European experts. Gut. 2013;62(6):812–23.
8. Tzortzatos G, Andersson E, Soller M, et al. The gynecological surveillance of women with Lynch syndrome in Sweden. Gynecol Oncol. 2015;138:717–22.
9. Bokhman JV. Two pathogenetic types of endometrial carcinoma. Gynecol Oncol. 1983;15:10–7.
10. Billingsley CC, Kenne KA, Cansino CD, et al. The use of transvaginal ultrasound in Type II endometrial cancer. Int J Gynecol Cancer. 2015;25(5):858–62.
11. ACOG. ACOG practice bulletin, clinical management guidelines for obstetrician-gynecologists, number 65, August 2005: management of endometrial cancer. Obstet Gynecol. 2005;106:413–25.
12. Kandoth C, Schultz N, Cherniack AD, et al. Integrated genomic characterization of endometrial carcinoma. Nature. 2013;497:67–73.
13. Broaddus RR, Lynch HT, Chen LM, et al. Pathologic features of endometrial carcinoma associated with HNPCC: a comparison with sporadic endometrial carcinoma. Cancer. 2006;106:87–94.
14. O'Hara AJ, Bell DW. The genomics and genetics of endometrial cancer. Adv Genomics Genet. 2012;2012(2):33–47.
15. ACOG. ACOG Committee Opinion No. 426: the role of transvaginal ultrasound in the evaluation of postmenopausal bleeding. Obstet Gynecol. 2009;113:462–4.
16. Esposito K, Chiodini P, Capuano A, et al. Metabolic syndrome and endometrial cancer: a meta-analysis. Endocrine. 2014;45:28–36.
17. Rosato V, Zucchetto A, Bosetti C, et al. Metabolic syndrome and endometrial cancer risk. Ann Oncol. 2011;22:884–9.
18. Barry JA, Azizia MM, Hardiman PJ. Risk of endometrial, ovarian and breast cancer in women with polycystic ovary syndrome: a systematic review and meta-analysis. Hum Reprod Update. 2014;20:748–58.
19. Fader AN, Arriba LN, Frasure HE, von Gruenigen VE. Endometrial cancer and obesity: epidemiology, biomarkers, prevention and survivorship. Gynecol Oncol. 2009;114:121–7.
20. Luo J, Beresford S, Chen C, et al. Association between diabetes, diabetes treatment and risk of developing endometrial cancer. Br J Cancer. 2014;111:1432–9.
21. Peiretti M, Colombo N. Sex cord-stromal tumors of the ovary. In: Textbook of gynaecological oncology. Ankara, Istanbul: Günes; 2012. p. 453–6.
22. Brinton LA, Berman ML, Mortel R, et al. Reproductive, menstrual, and medical risk factors for endometrial cancer: results from a case-control study. Am J Obstet Gynecol. 1992;167:1317–25.
23. Zucchetto A, Serraino D, Polesel J, et al. Hormone-related factors and gynecological conditions in relation to endometrial cancer risk. Eur J Cancer Prev. 2009;18:316–21.
24. Ali AT. Reproductive factors and the risk of endometrial cancer. Int J Gynecol Cancer. 2014;24:384–93.
25. Fisher B, Costantino JP, Wickerham DL, et al. Tamoxifen for prevention of breast cancer: report of the National Surgical Adjuvant Breast and Bowel Project P-1 Study. J Natl Cancer Inst. 1998;90:1371–88.
26. Reed SD, Newton KM, Garcia RL, et al. Complex hyperplasia with and without atypia: Clinical outcomes and implications of progestin therapy. Obstet Gynecol. 2010;116(2 Pt 1):365–73.
27. Collaborative Group on Epidemiological Studies on Endometrial Cancer. Endometrial cancer and oral contraceptives: an individual participant meta-analysis of 27276 women with endometrial cancer from 36 epidemiological studies. Lancet Oncol. 2015;16(9):1061–70. https://doi.org/10.1016/S1470-2045(15)00212-0.

28. Soini T, Hurskainen R, Grénman S, Mäenpää J, Paavonen J, Pukkala E. Cancer risk in women using levonorgestrel-releasing intrauterine system: a nation-wide cohort study. Obstet Gynecol. 2014;124(2 Pt 1):292–9.
29. Kaislasuo J, Heikinheimo O, Lähteenmäki P, Suhonen S. Predicting painful or difficult intrauterine device insertion in nulligravid women. Obstet Gynecol. 2014;124:345–53.
30. Fu Y, Zhuang Z. Long-term effects of levonorgestrel-releasing intrauterine system on tamoxifen-treated breast cancer patients: a meta-analysis. Int J Clin Exp Pathol. 2014;7:6419–29.

Hormone Interactions in Endometrial Cancer

6

Areege Kamal, Nicola Tempest, Alison Maclean, Meera Adishesh, Jaipal Bhullar, Sofia Makrydima, and Dharani K. Hapangama

6.1 Introduction

The human endometrium is the main target organ for the ovarian steroidal hormones. The pivotal role of sex hormones in the development, growth and maintenance of the normal physiological structure of the endometrium is well established. Aberrations in the endometrial hormonal milieu due to endogenous or exogenous factors influence endometrial carcinogenesis and cancer progression. Emerging evidence suggests that other non-steroidal hormones are involved in endometrial carcinogenesis via altering the tumour microenvironment and facilitating tumour progression [1]. Understanding the intricate relationship between these hormones in endometrial carcinogenesis could improve the current therapeutic options and lead to the designing of new strategies for the prevention and treatment of endometrial cancer in the era of evolving hormone therapy. This chapter focuses on the influences of both ovarian steroid hormones and the other non-steroidal hormones in endometrial cancer.

A. Kamal
Department of Women's and Children's Health, Institute of Translational Medicine, University of Liverpool, Liverpool, UK

The National Center for Early Detection of Cancer, Oncology Teaching Hospital, Baghdad Medical City, Baghdad, Iraq

N. Tempest · M. Adishesh · S. Makrydima · D. K. Hapangama (✉)
Department of Women's and Children's Health, Institute of Translational Medicine, University of Liverpool, Liverpool, UK

Liverpool Women's Hospital NHS Foundation Trust, a member of Liverpool Health Partners, Liverpool, UK
e-mail: Nicola.Tempest@liverpool.ac.uk; dharani@liv.ac.uk

A. Maclean · J. Bhullar
Department of Women's and Children's Health, Institute of Translational Medicine, University of Liverpool, Liverpool, UK

© Springer Nature Switzerland AG 2020
M. R. Mirza (ed.), *Management of Endometrial Cancer*,
https://doi.org/10.1007/978-3-319-64513-1_6

6.2 Hormone Regulators of the Endometrium

Our current understanding of the extensively complex female endocrine system through the well-established hypothalamic-pituitary-ovarian axis of the classical hormone pathway, directed at the endometrium, is far from complete (See Fig. 6.1). The following section provides an overview of the steroidal and non-steroidal hormones that influence the endometrium.

6.2.1 Steroid Hormones

Steroid hormones are cholesterol-derived, lipophilic, small molecular weight compounds characterised by a common cyclopentane-perhydro-phenantrene basic structure. The steroid hormone super family includes sex steroids and corticosteroids [2]. Sex steroids are the main regulators of the endometrium, and are classified according to the number of carbon atoms they contain, progestogens (C21), androgens (C19) and oestrogens (C18). The adrenal glands are also responsible for producing corticosteroids, a small amount of androgens and a relatively large amount of androgen precursors, with the ovaries being the primary site of sex steroid synthesis.

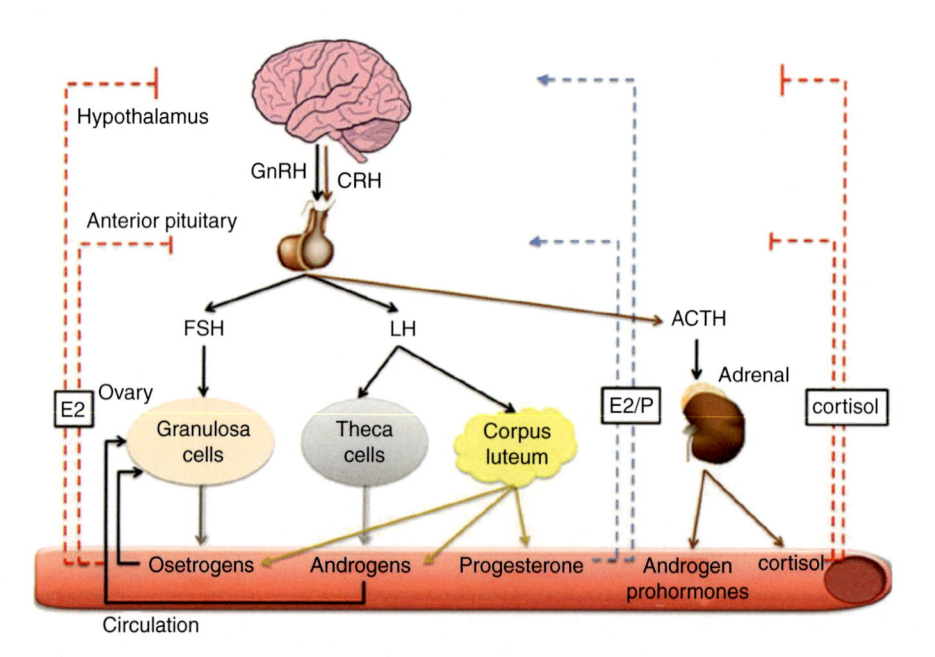

Fig. 6.1 The hypothalamic-pituitary regulation of circulating steroid horemones in premenopausal women. The production of steroid hormones is under the hypothalamo-pituitary regulation; the hypothalamus releases GnRH, which stimulates the release of LH/FSH and corticotrophin releasing hormone (CRH), to signal the ovary and the adrenal glands. Both ovarian estradiol and cortisol in turn have a negative feedback regulatory function at the hypothalamic and pituitary level

Steroid hormones are circulated in blood either as free hormones (less than 3% of the circulating hormones) or bound to proteins. The vast majority of circulatory testosterone and oestradiol are bound to sex-hormone binding globulin (SHBG), whereas cortisol and progesterone are bound to cortisol binding globulin (CBG) with all these hormones also binding to albumin [3]. In women, the sex steroids have a direct, primary effect on the endometrium; the role of corticosteroids and mineralocorticoids on the endometrium is relatively poorly understood.

6.2.1.1 Oestrogens

Oestrogens are the primary "female" sex hormones that regulate endometrial regeneration. In premenopausal non-pregnant women, they are mainly produced by the granulosa cells of the ovary, under the influence of follicle-stimulating hormone (FSH). A smaller amount is produced by extragonadal organs such as the liver, adrenals and fat, which is of a particular importance in postmenopausal women. This chapter focuses on the two major endogenous oestrogens: estradiol (E2), the most potent oestrogen that predominates in the reproductive life, and the weaker estrone (E1) that dominates after the menopause. The least potent oestrogen, the placental-derived estriol (E3), is not discussed further [4].

6.2.1.2 Progesterone

Progesterone produced by the corpus luteum is essential for the endometrial cellular differentiation. It promotes decidualisation, counteracts oestrogen-induced proliferation and, if conception occurs, maintains the pregnancy. Adrenals also produce progesterone, which is largely converted into glucocorticoids and androgens without being released in to the circulation. The half-life of progesterone is as short as 5 min; being either promptly deactivated in the liver or converted in the kidney to a potent mineralocorticoid [5].

6.2.1.3 Androgens

The main circulating forms of androgens in women include the prohormones, dehydroepiandrosterone sulphate (DHEAS), dehydroepiandrosterone (DHEA), androstenedione and testosterone, which are produced primarily by the adrenals and the ovarian theca cells. The subsequent metabolism of these prohormones in peripheral tissue produces the highly potent androgens, testosterone and dihydrotestosterone (DHT), which have a high affinity to androgen receptors (AR) [6]. In addition to being precursors for oestrogen, the available evidence suggests that androgens, via AR are directly involved in stromal decidualisation in the endometrium [7]. The direct function of androgens in the endometrial epithelial cells, however, is less well characterised.

6.2.1.4 Corticosteroids

Two types of corticosteroids are produced by the adrenal cortex, glucocorticoids (e.g. cortisol, produced by the outermost layer, the zona glomerulosa) and mineralocorticoids (e.g. aldosterone produced by the middle layer, the zona fasciculata). Glucocorticoid production is regulated by physical or emotional stress and pain, whilst angiotensin II of renal origin, as part of the renin angiotensin aldosterone system, is the main regulator of mineralocorticoid production. The regulation of carbohydrate and protein metabolism by cortisol and the fluid and electrolyte equilibrium by aldosterone have been well recognised. However, direct regulatory effect of these hormones on human endometrium remains to be fully confirmed. Glucocorticoids may regulate endometrial survival, menstruation and parturition via inflammatory and immunological responses [8]. Mineralocorticoid levels vary during the menstrual cycle being highest during the luteal phase and increasing progressively during pregnancy [9, 10].

6.2.2 Non-steroidal Hormones

Many of the endocrine organs including those of the hypothalamo-pituitary axis produce non-steroidal hormones that may have direct, non-classical effects on the endometrium. These hormones are detailed below.

6.2.2.1 Gonadotrophin Releasing Hormone (GnRH)

GnRH is a decapeptide hormone that is secreted in a pulsatile manner (continuous stimulation downregulates the pituitary), and has at least two isoforms. GnRH I is responsible for both follicle stimulating hormone (FSH) and luteinising hormone (LH) secretion from the anterior pituitary [11], whilst GnRH II may play a role in the behavioural components of reproduction. In endometrial cells, GnRH may have a direct effect on proliferation, apoptosis and tissue remodelling [12].

6.2.2.2 LH and FSH

FSH and LH are glycoprotein hormones with synergistic actions on the ovary. In women, FSH signals the synthesis of the steroid hormones oestradiol, progesterone and testosterone maturation of ovarian follicles, whilst LH triggers ovulation and acts on the theca cells to produce androgens. Gonadotrophins are released in a pulsatile manner according to GnRH pulses, with higher FSH levels observed in the mid-follicular phase of the cycle and LH peaking at the mid-cycle, pre-ovulatory phase. This mid-cycle LH surge is thought to be induced by both oestrogens and progesterone [13]. Although the primary gonadotrophin target is the gonads, they also have extra-ovarian actions in other non-classical target organs such as the endometrium [14, 15].

6.2.2.3 Thyroid Hormones

Thyroid hormones (TH) include the active form, triiodothyronine (T3), and the prohormone, thyroxine (T4), which are tyrosine-based peptides, regulated by thyroid stimulating hormone (TSH) of anterior pituitary origin [16]. Approximately 70% of THs are bound to thyroid-binding globulins (TBGs) in plasma, creating a substantial reserve, whereas the free hormone can diffuse across the plasma membrane of target cells. Although circulatory TH levels do not fluctuate substantially during the menstrual cycle [17], the mean thyroid volume increases by 50% in the luteal phase

[18] implying an altered thyroid function. Importantly, deiodinase 2 (DIO2), which converts T4 to the more potent T3, is present in human endometrium. DIO levels undergo cyclic changes in the human endometrium showing an inverse relationship with progesterone levels [19]. This observation may suggest progesterone suppresses the action of circulating thyroid hormones in the endometrium and merits further investigation. Both thyrotoxicosis and hypothyroidism alter gonadotrophin release, circulatory levels of SHBG and steroid metabolism, resulting in a variety of menstrual disorders [20].

6.2.2.4 Insulin

Insulin is a water-soluble polypeptide anabolic hormone produced by beta cells of the pancreatic islets of langerhans. Insulin promotes the uptake and storage of carbohydrate, amino acids and fat into liver, skeletal muscle and adipose tissue and antagonises the catabolism of these fuel reserves. It also has effects on cell growth, cognition and the vasculature, which are separate from its metabolic actions [21].

The half-life of insulin in the circulation is short (2–3 min), and being water soluble, it can travel freely in the blood to exert its effects via a cell membrane receptor. It has been noted that insulin is higher during the luteal phase of the menstrual cycle but the magnitude of change is rather small and not very relevant in interpreting test results [22].

6.2.2.5 Melatonin

Melatonin, or *N*-acetyle-5-methoxy-tryptamine, is a non-steroidal peptide hormone. It is produced by the pineal gland through metabolism of the hormone serotonin [23] and released under hypothalamic regulation. The suprachiasmatic nucleus communicates with the hypothalamus via sympathetic neurons in the spinal cord resulting in diurnal variation. Melatonin is produced maximally at night and thus plays a role in the sleep–wake cycle [24]. Melatonin also acts as an immune modulator, antioxidant and has anti-angiogenic effects with a role in reproduction [25].

Melatonin interferes with oestrogen signalling pathways and inhibits the activity of aromatase, reducing the conversion of androgens to oestrogen [26]. In female rats, removal of the pineal gland and subsequent decrease in circulating melatonin levels result in an increase in oestrogen, decrease in progesterone and reduced number of successful embryo implantations. This effect is reversed on administration of melatonin [27].

6.3 Steroid Hormones Intracrinology of the Endometrium

Intracrinology refers to the local intracellular biosynthesis and metabolism of hormones in peripheral tissues, followed by local inactivation of these hormones with minimal or no alteration of serum levels [28]. The intracrinology process is mediated by two main classes of proteins: the cytochrome P450 proteins and the hydroxysteroid dehydrogenases [29, 30], most of which have already been characterised in the endometrium (See Fig. 6.2). In physiological settings, this process is

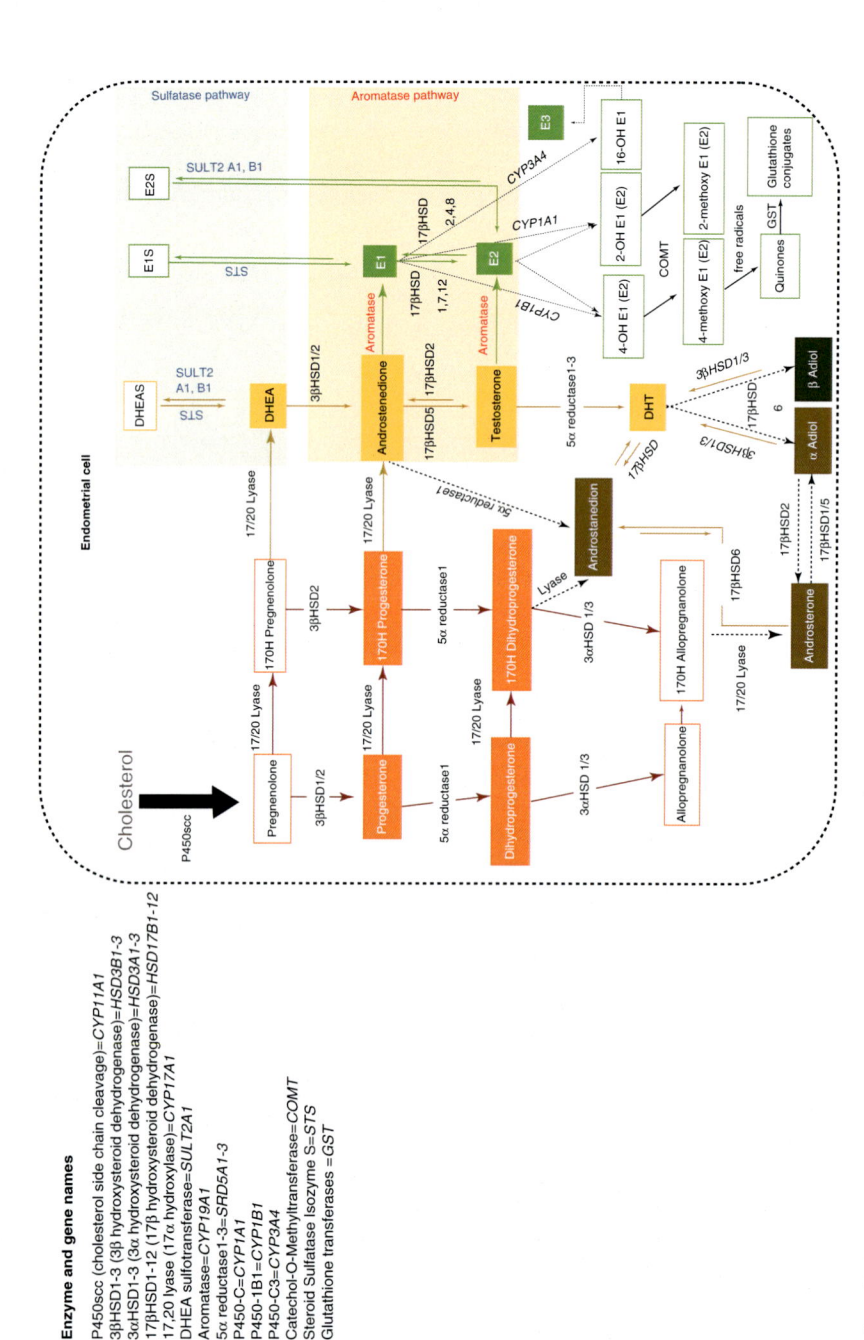

Fig. 6.2 Steroid hormone intracrinology (the local synthesis and metabolism of steroid hormones) in the endometrium. Many enzymes involved in steroid hormone metabolism are expressed in endometrial cells. Active hormones that bind their cognate receptors are in coloured boxes, while those which are inactive or are not a ligand for steroid receptors are in white boxes. Metabolites in black patterned boxes possess steroidal activity and can bind cognate receptors before conjugated to sulphate or glucuronide

essential for fine tuning of the final steroid hormone concentration in the endometrium required for the specific cellular action. An imbalance in the biosynthesis and/or inactivation process of steroid hormones has been described in hormone-dependent tumours such as breast, prostate and endometrial cancers [28] and are expected to play a role in resistance to endocrine therapy. Many different circulating forms of oestrogen, progesterone and androgens occur and they are substrates for the steroid metabolising enzymes expressed in the endometrium.

6.3.1 Progesterone Intracrinology

The general consensus is that the rate-limiting step in progesterone synthesis mediated by steroidogenic acute regulatory protein (STAR) does not take place in intracrine tissues [31]. However, emerging experimental data suggests that endometrium possesses all the enzymes required for *de novo* progesterone synthesis including STAR, P450 side chain cleavage enzyme (CYP11A1) and 3β HSD (See Fig. 6.3) [32]. Endometrial stromal and epithelial cells also express the enzymes that metabolise progesterone into compounds with a low affinity to PR (e.g. 20α-HSDs, 5α-reductases and 3α-HSDs) and progesterone deactivating enzymes [33]. Decreased expression of genes involved in progesterone biosynthesis (STAR and

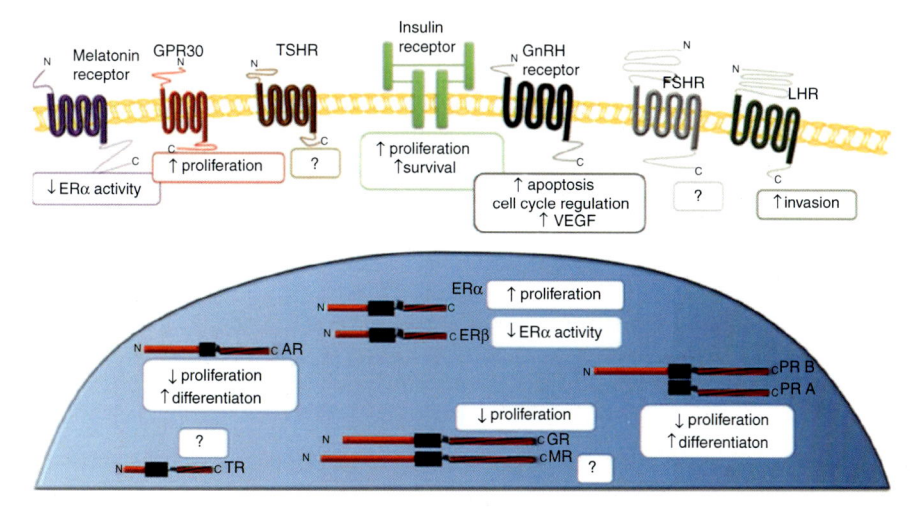

Fig. 6.3 Hormones receptors in endometrial cells. A schematic illustration of the localisation of steroid and non-steroidal hormone receptors and the effects of receptor activation on endometrial cells. Steroid hormone receptors are nuclear and function as ligand-activated transcription factors, whereas non-steroidal receptors are mostly located in the cell membrane. *GPR30* G protein-coupled receptor 30, *TSHR* thyroid stimulating hormone receptor, *GnRH receptor* gonadotropin releasing hormone receptor, *FSHR* follicle stimulating hormone receptor, *LHR* luteinizing hormone receptor, *AR* androgen receptor, *ERα* oestrogen receptor α, *ERβ* oestrogen receptor β, *PR* progesterone receptor, *MR* mineralocorticoid receptor, *TR* thyroid hormone receptor, *GR* glucocorticoid receptor

CYP11A1) has been reported in endometrial cancer tissue compared to the adjacent precancerous tissue [32]. Further studies are required to confirm these findings and to elucidate the role progesterone metabolising enzymes play in altering the intra-tumour bioavailability of exogenous progesterone in endometrial cancer.

6.3.2 Oestrogen Intracrinology

The final intra-tumour oestrogen concentration and activity in endometrial cancer cells are altered due to changes in several hormone metabolic pathways (See Fig. 6.2). These include:

1. The inter-conversion of E2 and E1, regulated by a group of 17βHSD isoforms with different catalytic efficiency [34];

2. Local oestrogen synthesis via two main pathways:

    (a) Aromatase pathway—where androgen prohormones DHEA, androstenedione and testosterone are converted to oestrogens by aromatase and aided by 17βHSDs (See Fig. 6.2) and
    (b) Sulphatase pathway—which activates sulphated precursors estrone sulphate (E1S) and DHEAS to E1 and DHEA, respectively, and then can subsequently be converted to E2 [35];

3. Local inactivation of oestrogens and DNA damage can be initiated by failure of the catechol-oestrogen deactivation in endometrial cancer by catechol-O-methyltransferase (COMT) and glutathione transferase (GT), resulting in the formation of quinone compounds under the effect of peroxidases or via non-enzymatic pathways [36].

6.3.3 Androgen Intracrinology

In addition to the contribution to the local oestrogen synthesis, androgen prohormones serve as important precursors for testosterone and the most potent naturally occurring AR ligand, DHT (See Fig. 6.2). Before terminal inactivation by conjugation with glucuronide and sulphate compounds, metabolites of DHT retain affinity to steroid receptors and can activate ER as a substitute in hormone depravation conditions [37].

6.4 Hormone Receptors

Steroid and non-steroidal hormones exert most of their effect via their respective cognate receptors (See Fig. 6.3). The signalling pathways, structure, isoforms, expression and prognostic value of these receptors in endometrial cancer are discussed in this section.

6.4.1 Steroid Receptors

Steroid hormone receptors (ER, PR, AR and GR) are members of the nuclear hormone receptor superfamily and share the common, evolutionarily conserved structural and functionally distinct domains as the other members of the superfamily (See Fig. 6.3). This includes a central, highly conserved DNA binding domain (DBD) which binds to the same ligand responsive element in the target gene promoters; multifunctional ligand-binding domain (LBD); the ligand-dependent AF-2 at the C-terminal; constitutively active AF-1 at the N-terminal; and flexible-hinge D-domain in between LDB and DBD.

6.4.1.1 Oestrogen Receptors

Cellular signalling of oestrogen is mediated through two receptors: ERα (ESR1) and ERβ (ESR2) [38, 39]. Despite the close homology between the two isoforms, ESR1 gene is located on chromosome 6 whereas ESR2 gene is located on chromosome 14.

The classical pro-proliferative action of oestrogen on the endometrium is exerted via ERα but it also induces ERβ expression. Ligand activated ERβ counteracts ERα action on the same promoter by altering co-activator [40] and key transcription factor recruitments [41]. Hence, the guardian effect of ERβ on the endometrial cellular homeostasis has been of particular interest [42].

The expression of ERα and ERβ is evident in low-grade endometrioid endometrial cancers [43–46], whereas high-grade endometrioid and non-endometrioid cancers have a significantly lower yet persistent expression of both isoforms [45]. The change in the relative expression of these isoforms represented by ERα/ERβ has a prognostic value. ERα/ERβ ratio is reported to be lower in high-grade cancers and associates with a poor patient outcome [47–51].

Alternative splicing of ESR1 and ESR2 pre-mRNA allows these genes to encode diverse proteins which may subsequently regulate the wild-type proteins [52]. The exon skipping variety constitutes the majority of ERα splice variants, out of which ERαΔ5, ERαΔ4, ERα36 and ERαΔ7 are the most studied in the endometrium. Overall, more ERα splice variants are found in malignant tissues compared with normal or premalignant endometrial tissues [53, 54]. ERβ variants (ERβ1, ERβ2, and ERβ5) display similar expression patterns to ERα in endometrioid endometrial cancer (EC) samples. ERβ1 and ERβ2 immunoexpression was higher in low-grade EC, whereas ERβ5 expression was constitutively intense regardless of the grade [55]. Disruption of the subtle equilibrium of these splice variants could be a contributing factor in EC development.

Interestingly, ER expression has been reported as the best predictor of response to sequential endocrine therapy (medroxy progesterone acetate (MPA)/tamoxifen) for patients with advanced or recurrent Endometrial cancer, whereas PR showed limited value [56]. This is likely to be due to the requirement of an active ER to maintain PR expression, which allows MPA action.

6.4.1.2 Progesterone Receptors

PR was first purified and cloned in 1975 [57]. Two protein isoforms have been identified, PR-A and PR-B, produced from a single gene by transcription at two distinct promoters [58–60]. In the endometrium, the ratios of the individual isoforms vary according to the reproductive, hormonal status [61, 62] and during carcinogenesis [63].

PR-B acts as an activator of progesterone-responsive genes, whereas PR-A has a strong repressor effect on PR-B and ER transcriptional activity [64]. The precise mechanism underlying the differential activities of the two PR isoforms is not fully understood. Studies have suggested that the conformational changes of PR-A and PR-B inside the cells alter recruitment of co-activators and co-repressors and therefore transactivation functions [65].

Generally, PR expression is downregulated in less-differentiated endometrial cancers [45]; nonetheless, the debate about the expression of PR isoforms in advanced EC is continuing with studies reporting: (1) the loss of both isoforms in endometrial cancers [56, 66], (2) alteration of the relative expression of the isoforms [67] and (3) a slightly higher PR-B level in advanced endometrial tumours [68].

The prognostic value of PR has long been recognised [69]. Although there is compelling evidence suggesting a significant, independent, prognostic role for PR [70, 71], the predictive value for PR to guide successful endocrine therapy has not yet been fully determined. In this respect, the essential, standard quantification methods and best cut-off points in assessing PR expression in endometrial tumours have not yet been formalised. Such assessment could be of value when progesterone is first-line treatment, for example, in fertility sparing treatment. The recent ESGO-ESMO recommendation, however, limits PR assessment to advanced or recurrent disease [72]. The argument against the assessment of PR in fertility sparing cases is that 2/4 (50%) patients who showed a response to progesterone were PR negative; however, 5/5 (100%) of patients who responded were PR positive and the difference between the two groups was significant ($P = 0.008$) [73]. The small sample size ($n = 9$) included in the referenced trial and the absence of confirmatory studies makes it difficult to form a firm conclusion.

6.4.1.3 Androgen Receptors

AR gained interest in the field of gynaecology with the introduction of danazol as a treatment for endometriosis in the early 1980s [74]. The AR gene is located on the X chromosome at the locus Xq11-Xq12 which encodes a 110-kDa protein consisting of 919 amino acids [75]. The first description of AR expression in the human endometrium was documented by Horie et al. in 1992 [76]. Successive reports characterised AR in the stroma of premenopausal endometrium across the cycle [77–79] and reported its emergence in the postmenopausal glandular epithelium [45]. AR is expressed by low-grade endometrioid endometrial cancers [45, 80, 81] whereas its loss is a feature of high-grade EC, particularly the non-endometrioid subtypes [45]. The association of AR loss with poor EC patient outcomes proposes this protein as a prognostic indicator [45, 82]. Multiple splice variances of AR have been described in prostate cell lines [83], but evidence for their expression in normal and malignant endometrial tissue is lacking.

6.4.1.4 Corticosteroid Receptors (Glucocorticoid and Mineralocorticoid Receptors)

Cortisol activates glucocorticoid receptor (GR) and aldosterone primarily activates mineralocorticoid receptor (MR), although it does have some responsiveness to cortisol [84]. The GR is encoded by the NR3C1 gene located on chromosome 5 (5q31) and both of the GR isoforms, GR-α and GR-β, have been identified in the stromal compartment of the endometrium [85–87]. The active receptor GR-α, controls glucocorticoid-induced cellular apoptosis [88], and may function as a tumour suppressor by ensuring accurate chromosome segregation during mitosis [89]. GR-β isoform, which functions as the main negative inhibitor of GR-α, controls the glucose metabolism through increasing insulin sensitivity, and decreases hepatic gluconeogenesis [90]. The expression of GR is regulated by cortisol catalyzing enzymes, 11β-hydroxy dehydrogenase type 1 (11βHSD1) and type 2 (11βHSD2) [91] via regulating the local cortisol levels. The highest expression of GR and 11βHSD1 are observed in the menstrual phase, allowing cortisol to bind to GR, and thus is postulated to mediate an anti-inflammatory action [87].

6.4.2 Thyroid Hormone Receptor (TR)

Human nuclear TRs, implicated in the genomic pathway, are encoded by TRα and TRβ genes located on human chromosomes 17 and 3, respectively. These receptors function as ligand-dependent transcription factors that form heterodimers with the retinoid X receptor (RXR) or complexes with nuclear co-activator proteins such as p300 and steroid receptor co-activator-1 (SRC-1) and binds to thyroid hormone response elements (TRE) located in the target gene promoters [92].

Non-genomic transcription independent effects are mediated through cell surface αvβ3 receptor, which has a significantly higher affinity for T4. It activates a transporter system within the plasma membrane, resulting in either extracellular actions (involving vascular growth factor receptors and integrins) or intracellular events (cytoplasmic/nuclear trafficking of specific proteins, or activation of signal transducing kinases (MAPK, ERK1/2, Aktd)) [93]. Thyroid receptors therefore can influence a wide range of important regulatory proteins, from basic fibroblast growth factor (βFGF; FGF2), matrix metalloproteinase-9 (MMP-9), to oncogenes or proto-oncogenes. TSH receptor and thyroid hormone receptor are expressed in the human endometrium and their concentration is affected by the menstrual cycle with the highest levels seen during the mid-secretory phase [19].

6.4.3 Insulin Receptors

The insulin receptor is a member of the ligand-activated receptor and tyrosine kinase family of transmembrane signalling proteins. It is located in the plasma membrane and is composed of two pairs of subunits [94, 95]. Insulin receptors are located in primary target cells such as adipocytes, hepatocytes and skeletal muscle cells as well as in non-typical tissues such as the endometrium [94]. The main physiological role of the insulin receptor is metabolic regulation. The ligand activation phosphorylates the insulin receptor resulting in engagement of the effector molecules [95]. High concentrations of insulin downregulate its own receptor in adult cells, and muscular exercise, diet, thyroid hormones, glucocorticoids, androgens, oestrogens and cyclic nucleotides are all able to regulate insulin binding [94]. Interestingly, the insulin-induced downregulation of receptors is reversed in immature foetal cells where a paradoxical upregulation is demonstrated with high insulin. Insulin binding sites are also expressed in the endometrial stroma of women with Endometrial cancer [52]. The association of elevated IR-A levels with cell proliferation and tumourigenicity may be causally linked to its effect on the proportion of cells in S phase and the activation of the Akt pathway [96].

6.4.4 GnRH Receptors

The GnRH receptor (GnRHR) is a member of the G-protein coupled receptor (GPCR) family and functions in the inositol phosphate signalling pathway [97]. GnRHR isoforms, GnRHR I and GnRHR II, are desensitised through GnRH-induced phosphorylation [98]. The GnRHRs are present in the extra-pituitary reproductive tissues like the endometrium [12], placenta, ovary and breast [99–103]. Both GnRHRs have been identified in the endometrium throughout the cycle, and in gynaecological tumours [103–106]. Studies examining physiologic signalling of GnRHR in extrapituitary tissues only used GnRH agonists and/or antagonists with long half-lives, often at pharmacologic levels, and are thus flawed.

6.4.5 FSH/LH Receptors

FSH and LH act through specific 678 and 675 amino acid residues, the long receptors belonging to the leucine-rich-repeat-containing GPCRs (LGR) subfamily [107]. The FSH–FSHR complex forms dimers which may participate in transmembrane signal transduction and thus is more specific, whereas both LH and human chorionic gonadotropin (hCG) act through the single LHR. Activation of both receptors may influence Gs/adenylyl cyclase/cAMP/PKA pathways and their expression in non-gonadal tissues such as the endometrium has been reported [108].

6.4.6 Melatonin Receptors

Melatonin exerts its effects through two high affinity G protein coupled receptors, MT1 and MT2. The MT1 receptor is encoded by MTNR1A gene, located on chromosome 4 (4q35). MT2 receptor is encoded by the MTNR1B gene, located on chromosome 11 (11q21-q22) [109–111].

Rat endometrial stromal cells express MT1 receptors [112], which are responsible for the anti-proliferative effects of melatonin on the growth of these cells in vitro [113]. The ERα positive EC cell line, Ishikawa, expresses the MT1 receptor, but does not express the MT2 receptor. Melatonin upregulates the MT1 receptor, and downregulates ERα receptor, which suggests an anti-proliferative effect of melatonin on the endometrium, possibly via the MT1 receptor [114].

6.4.7 Steroid Receptor Signalling

The molecular action of steroid hormones is mediated through their intracellular receptors [39]. In the absence of the ligand, each receptor monomer is associated with a protein complex that contains a chaperone. This receptor complex is incapable of binding to DNA and is either located in the cytoplasm (AR and GR), loosely bound in the nucleus (ER and PR) or cytoplasmic/membrane bound (ER and PR) [40]. The steroid hormone signalling cascade starts when the hormone diffuses passively across the plasma membrane and binds to the cognate receptor. The hormone–receptor complex induces conformational changes and leads to receptor activation and subsequent molecular changes. Several signalling pathways have been postulated which can be broadly classified into [39];

1. *Genomic pathway*: is the standard and the best characterised pathway via which steroid receptors act as ligand-inducible transcription factors. Inside the nucleus, activated steroid receptors bind as homodimers to the respective hormone responsive element located in the relevant gene promoters and initiate recruitment of co-activators, co-repressors and chromatin-remodelling factors and directly regulate gene transcription (classical pathway). Steroid receptors can also initiate gene transcription indirectly by interacting with other transcriptional factors such as specificity protein 1 (SP-1) and this is termed as the non-classical pathway
2. *Non-genomic pathway*: is a less well characterised pathway that mediates a more rapid and reversible response without the need for nuclear translocation. Activated steroid receptor in the cytoplasm or plasma membrane can stimulate second messenger cascades which subsequently interact with several signalling pathways such as phosphatidyl-inositol 3-kinase (PI3K)/Akt.

In addition to these main ligand-induced signalling pathways, sex steroid hormone receptors can initiate signal transduction in the absence of their ligands (hormone-independent pathway). The activation of this pathway is influenced by several factors such as the type of the cell, promoter and activator [115].

6.4.8 The Normal Endometrial Response to Steroid Hormones

6.4.8.1 Premenopausal
Premenopausal endometrium is characterised by the presence of two functionally diverse layers, the superficial functionalis and the deeper basalis [116]. The

functionalis is proposed to be exceptionally sensitive to hormones, exemplified by the regular monthly cyclical changes of proliferation, differentiation, followed by menstrual shedding and regeneration when pregnancy is not established, all of which are meticulously regulated by the ovarian hormones [117]. The basalis on the other hand, is thought to be less responsive to these hormones. It exists throughout a woman's life and is postulated to be the germinal layer of the endometrium from which a new functionalis is generated from [117, 118]. Further studies are required to explain the different responsiveness to the hormones by these two endometrial layers in which hormone intracrinology is expected to play a role.

6.4.8.2 Postmenopausal (PM)

The PM hormonal milieu supporting the thin PM endometrium (the remaining basalis) is characterised by the presence of low oestrogen, adrenal androgens and the absence of progesterone [1, 42]. Compared with many other reproductive tissues, the endometrium does not undergo senescence and a fully operational functionalis can be restored with the administration of the appropriate exogenous hormones even decades after the menopause [119]. This apparent preservation of both the hormone responsiveness and the regenerative potential, however, is likely to be the basis for the high incidence of carcinogenesis observed in the PM endometrium.

The hypothesis of hormone-induced carcinogenesis was first documented by Bittner [120] in 1948 and refined by Henderson et al. [121] in 1982. The hypothesis states that "neoplasia is the consequence of excessive hormonal stimulation of a particular target organ, the normal growth and function of which are under hormonal control. The response of this end organ (e.g., endometrium, breast) to the proliferative effects of the hormone is a progression from normal growth to hyperplasia to neoplasia" [122]. Over the past three decades, researchers have been trying to understand the mechanisms, circumstances and consequences of hormone-induced neoplasia, and several hormonal factors were found to contribute to the malignant transformation of endometrial cells.

6.4.9 Oncogenic Roles of Oestrogen

The basic impact of oestrogens on proliferation and growth of reproductive tissues was recognised in the 1950s [123], predating the identification of oestrogen receptors [124].

The most plausible theory of oestrogen-induced carcinogenesis remains to be the mitotic action of oestrogen via the classical [125] or non-classical [126–130] nuclear ERα pathways, unopposed by progesterone. Progesterone counteracts this trophic drive of E2, therefore a relative increase in E2 over progesterone levels (due to endogenous or exogenous factors) is associated with an excessive and prolonged proliferation of endometrial cells.

Non-genomic oestrogen signalling is another oestrogen pro-oncogenic pathway. The non-transcriptional response to oestrogen via membrane located ER activates the extracellular signal-related kinase (Erk) 1/2 signalling pathway which plays a critical role in cell proliferation by regulating cell growth and cell cycle progression [131]. G protein-coupled receptor 30 (GPR30), an orphan membrane receptor, has also been implicated in this pathway [132]. GPR30–oestrogen complex was shown to stimulate EC cell proliferation and promote invasion by increasing the production and activity of matrix metalloproteinase-2 (MMP-2) and matrix metalloproteinase-9 (MMP-9) via the MEK/ERK MAPK pathway [133].

Emerging evidence has advocated the involvement of DNA methylation status in oestrogen signalling as a possible pathway in endometrial carcinogenesis. Defective chromatin architecture at the ER target locus may have a key role in endometrial proliferative disease [134]. Age independent hypermethylation of ESR1 promoter has been reported in 90% of Endometrial cancer in contrast to observations in breast cancer [135–137] (See Fig. 6.4). This further highlights the differences in hormone regulatory mechanisms between various hormonally active tissues, which to some extent preclude the possibility of generalising the findings in one tissue to others. Oestrogen-associated genotoxicity is another emerging theory in oestrogen-induced carcinogenesis. Endometrial tumour initiation has been proposed to be a consequence of metabolic activation of catechol-oestrogens, semiquinolones and quinolones [138]. Several studies have shown that 4-hydroxylated oestrogen, catalysed by cytochrome P450 1B1, is able to induce DNA damage [139–142]. Importantly, this is not a product of the main hepatic and extrahepatic metabolic pathway of E2, but occurs in organs prone to oestrogen-associated cancer such as the endometrium [143, 144]. An increase in carcinogenic catechol oestrogens is associated with DNA damage at a specific DNA region (codon 130/131) on the tumour suppressor gene PTEN, which is frequently found to be mutated in EC [145–147].

6.4.10 The Tumour Suppressive Role of Progesterone

The clinical implementation of progesterone as an inhibitor of endometrial carcinogenesis has emerged from the strong association between conditions associated with higher progesterone exposure, such as ovulation and high parity and lower EC risk [148]. The lack of endogenous progesterone synthesis, consequent to anovulation with unperturbed oestrogen production, can lead to excessive and prolonged proliferation of the endometrial cells which may progress to hyperplasia [149].

Direct antiproliferative action of progesterone on the endometrial epithelial cells is exerted via the classical genomic action of PR (See Fig. 6.4). PR isoforms sensitise EC cells to apoptosis; induce cell cycle arrest [150]; regulate p53 via non-classical genomic action [151]; regulate several transcriptional factors and adhesion molecules involved in tumour progression and metastasis (AP-1, NFκB, integrins and cadherins); and PR-B promotes cell differentiation by inducing Wnt inhibitory proteins such as FOXO1 [152].

The crosstalk between epithelial and stromal cells is essential for the normal endometrial function of progesterone. Evidence from tissue recombination studies

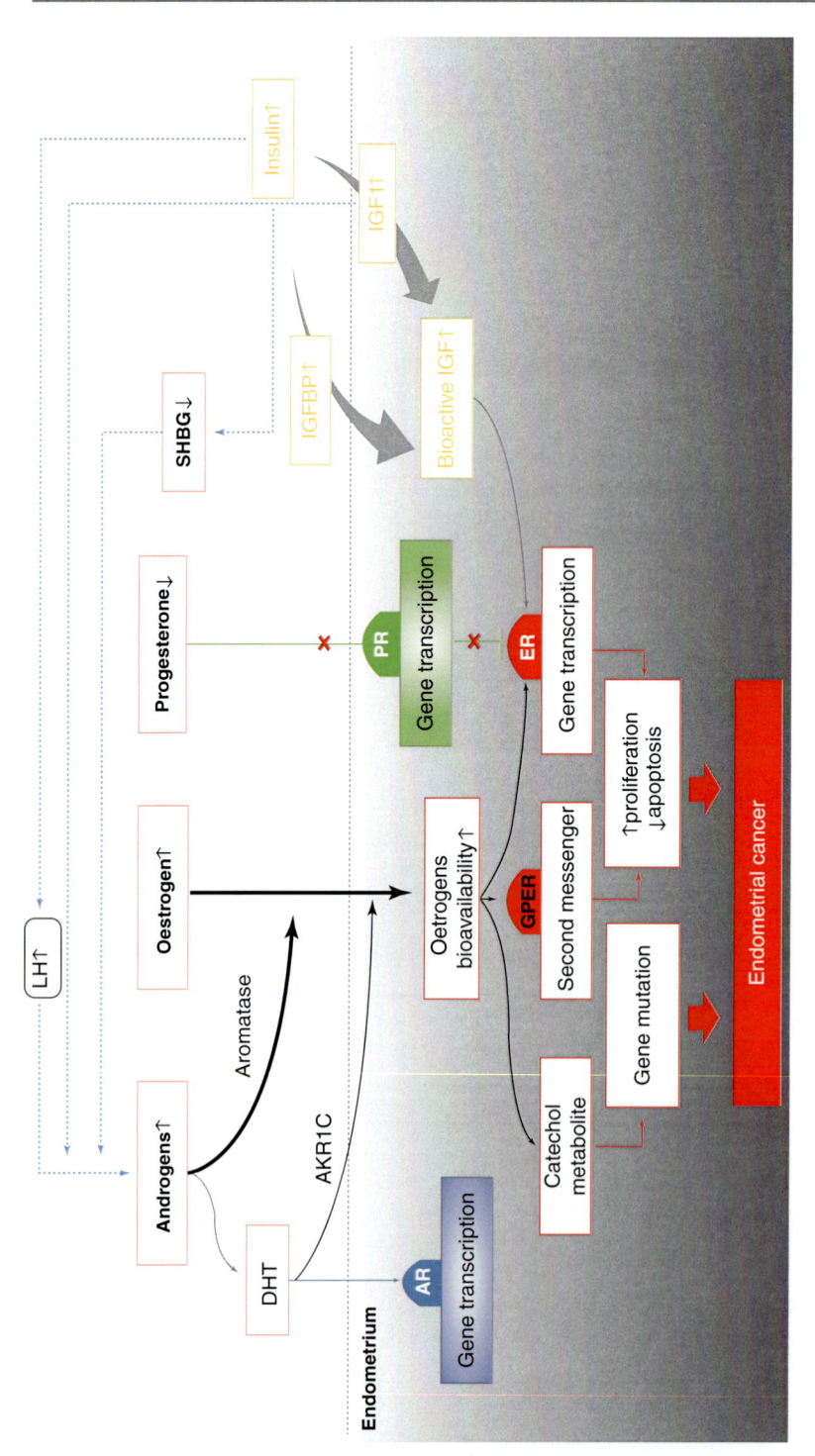

Fig. 6.4 Different hormonal and metabolic pathways associated with disturbed steroid hormones homeostasis in favour of oestrogen pro-oncogenic pathway [1]. *AKR1C* aldoketoreductase 1C, *DHT* dihydrotestosterone, *GPER* G protein coupled oestrogen receptor, *IGF-1* insulin-like growth factor 1, *IGFBP* insulin-like growth factor binding protein, *LH* luteinizing hormone, *SHBP* steroid hormone binding protein

utilising PR knockout (PRKO) mice with selective inactivation of endometrial epithelial and stromal PR suggests that stromal PR is a prerequisite for the antioestrogenic effect of progesterone and regulates epithelial cell apoptosis [153–155]. Progesterone suppresses the production of stromal growth factors that act as paracrine mediators of the mitogenic effects of oestrogen on the epithelium by inducing the basic helix-loop-helix transcription factor, Hand2, expression in the endometrial stromal cells [156].

Epigenetic modification of PR is one of the suggested mechanisms of impaired progesterone protective function in EC either by methylation of PR-B promoter or post transcriptional deactivation of PR isoforms via miRNA or small ubiquitin-like modifier proteins [137, 157]. In conclusion, progesterone's insufficiency as well as aberrant cognate receptor expression and activity have a pivotal role in EC development.

6.4.11 Hyperinsulinism

Hyperinsulinism, associated with either diabetes mellitus or polycystic ovarian syndrome (PCOS), plays an important role in endometrial carcinogenesis as it potentiates mitotic activity in the glands and stroma by increasing the activity of insulin-like growth factor 1 (IGF-1) [158–160] (See Fig. 6.4). Excess insulin stimulates the androgenic activity of the theca cells; elevates serum-free testosterone levels through decreased hepatic sex hormone-binding globulin (SHBG) production; amplifies LH and IGF-I-stimulated androgen production; and enhances serum IGF-I bioactivity through suppressed IGF binding protein production [159, 161, 162]. The two isoforms of IR-A and IR-B are co-expressed in EC, but the overexpression of IR-A promote the proliferation of Endometrial cancer cells by insulin [96, 163, 164]. Therefore, an excess in insulin signalling can result in endometrial changes with a pro-proliferative, pro-survival phenotype and inflammatory changes akin to unopposed oestrogen.

6.4.12 Hyperandrogenism

The association between high circulating androgen levels and EC is well established [165–169], however the *in vivo* and *in vitro* evidence to support the carcinogenesis effect of androgens in the endometrium is weak [170]. Administration of exogenous testosterone and androstenedione either to PM [171] or transgender women [172] has not increased the EC risk. By contrast, emerging evidence suggests AR to be a favourable prognostic indicator [45, 82]. Along these lines, the expression of 5α reductase enzyme, which is responsible for the conversion of testosterone to the most potent endogenous androgen DHT, is associated with better patient outcomes in EC [82]. *In vitro* studies show different androgens to have antiproliferative effects on primary premenopausal endometrial cells [173] and EC cell lines [174].

Therefore the most plausible explanation for the positive association between serum androgens and EC is the increased bioavailability of unopposed oestrogens via peripheral conversion of androstenedione and testosterone, to E1 and E2 (See Fig. 6.2). Studies have shown higher levels of aromatase [175, 176] and aldoketoreductase (AKR1C) [177] enzymes expression in neoplastic endometrial cells compared with normal endometrium. This may increase the local production of oestrogenic compounds with relatively higher affinity to ER instead of AR and therefore augment an oestrogenic pathway [178]. This pathway is not limited to type I EC, since high expression of aromatase is also observed in type II, which may allow this subtype of EC to increase local oestrogen biosynthesis and hence proliferation [179].

6.4.13 The Role of Other Hormones in Endometrial Carcinogenesis

6.4.13.1 GnRH

GnRH may regulate the endometrium via autocrine or paracrine routes. Endogenous GnRH may have a negative role in the autocrine system interfering with the growth factors. GnRH-2 has a direct effect on EC cells by inducing apoptosis, arresting the cell cycle and inhibiting the cellular proliferation [101, 180]. Activation of ERK1/2 and p38 MAPK via integrin beta 3 and focal adhesion kinase (FAK) is one of the suggested pathways [181]. Therefore, GnRH ligands may be useful for treating EC. Controversially, a recent study has shown that GnRH-2 increases EC cells proliferation by stimulating epidermal growth factor release [182] and others concluded that GnRH-2 promotes cell migration and invasion by inducing different metastasis related proteinase and vascular endothelial growth factor (VEGF) resulting in neo-angiogenesis [183]. Endometrial epithelial GnRH mRNA levels appear to be upregulated by progesterone, and about 80% of endometrial cancers express both GnRH and GnRHR as a part of the autocrine system [184]. Therefore, further studies clarifying the controversies associated with the role of this hormone and its therapeutic potential in EC are needed.

6.4.13.2 Luteinizing Hormone/Human Chorionic Gonadotrophin

The literature on gonadotrophin levels associated with EC is contradictory, some report lower FSH levels suggesting an altered hypothalamic function [185] whilst others report high gonadotropin levels in endometrial hyperplasia and carcinoma [186].

LH/hCG receptors (LH-R) are expressed in 80% of endometrial cancers [187, 188] in a grade specific manner and may regulate the invasiveness of EC cells [189]. The *in vitro* work examining the direct effect of LH-R and LH has shown that the over-expression of the LH-R increases the ability of EC cells to undergo local invasion and metastatic spread in animal models. Likewise, LH withdrawal strongly inhibits local and distant metastatic spread of tumours [190]. LH upregulates its own receptor, therefore it is an important target in relation to the PM period where the levels of LH remain elevated (See Fig. 6.4).

6.4.13.3 Thyroid Stimulating Hormone (TSH) and Thyroid Hormones (TH)

Elevated TSH levels in patients with EC have been independently associated with poor disease-specific survival [191]. TSH may influence endometrial carcinogenesis and invasiveness via its action on adipose tissue and the subsequent release of leptin [192]. However, TSH and TH receptors have been identified in endometrial tissues, supporting a more direct effect on cell proliferation. T4 can bind to integrin $\alpha v\beta 3$ and cause MAP kinase-dependent phosphorylation of the nuclear oestrogen receptor [193]. Simultaneously, the complex T3/TR initiates the genomic pathway and regulates lipocalin 2, a tumour-associated protein, that enhances tumour cell migration and invasion [194]. These remarks warrant further studies examining a direct role for TSH and thyroid hormone on endometrial carcinogenesis [195–197].

6.4.13.4 Melatonin

The anti-tumour effect of melatonin has been demonstrated in many cancers, through interacting with membrane and nuclear receptors [198]. In breast cancer, this is related to the oestrogen receptor status and therefore may be relevant to most endometrial cancers, which are also oestrogen-dependent. In the ERα positive EC cell line Ishikawa, treatment with melatonin significantly inhibits cell growth and the effect is reversed by administration of 17-b estradiol [199], inferring that melatonin acts via the oestrogen receptor to decrease EC proliferation.

Melatonin levels have been shown to decrease in the postmenopausal period [200] when EC commonly occurs. Women with EC have lower melatonin levels. Night shift workers who have a lower level of melatonin also appear to have an increased risk of developing EC [201]. Melatonin administration in addition to harmone replacement therapy (HRT) was associated with reduced body mass, intraperitoneal fat, reduced endometrial proliferation and prevented the appearance of histological atypia of the endometrium in an ovariectomised rat model. This indicates that melatonin may have a prophylactic role in preventing EC in postmenopausal women [202].

6.4.13.5 Corticosteroids

Glucocorticoids have anti-inflammatory, immunosuppressive effects, and cause cellular apoptosis [203]. Glucocorticoid receptors have inhibitory effects on the growth of lymphoid cancer cells, and other solid tumours [204]. These anti-proliferative effects may also be applicable to EC. In the GR-positive EC cell line, Ishikawa, treatment with dexamethasone causes downregulation of the cellular adhesion molecule N-cadherin, and upregulation of the anti-proliferative factor, upstream c-fos relating transcription factor (USF-2), suggesting glucocorticoids to have a similar growth inhibitory action as progesterone in EC [205]. Further examination of GR and glucocorticoid treatment in EC will help to examine their therapeutic implication further.

6.5 Hormonal Aberrations Relevant to EC Risk Factors

6.5.1 Endogenous Hormones

Many of the well-known high-risk endogenous conditions (See Table 6.1) for developing EC are associated with one or more of the specific hormonal aberrations mentioned above [209]. Early age at menarche, late age of menopause, nulliparity, anovulation, history of infertility and presence of oestrogen-producing tumours increase the risk of EC, presumably due to the prolonged or unopposed exposure to oestrogen [209, 210]. Conversely, pregnancy, including termination of pregnancy, decreases the risk by prolonged exposure to progesterone [211].

Polycystic ovarian syndrome (PCOS) has been defined as the strongest independent endogenous risk factor for the development of EC [208]. Anovulation, hyperandrogenism and hyperinsulinemia that commonly associate with PCOS, create a vicious cycle of hormonal abnormalities that can induce endometrial carcinogenesis [212]. Diabetes and obesity, both independent risk factors for EC, are associated with hyperinsulineamia [207] and alter hormonal homeostasis at several levels. Peripheral aromatisation of oestrogen remains the main carcinogenic pathway in obesity; however, the involvement of cytokines and adipokines is increasingly being reported [206]. The premalignant precursor of endometrioid EC, endometrial

Table 6.1 The known high-risk conditions for developing EC and their associated hormonal aberrations

Factor	Risk	Hormone-associated mechanism
Obesity	RR: 1.59 for every 5 kg/m² increase [206]	↑ Peripheral oestrogens production ↑ Insulin and growth factors ↑ Inflammatory cytokines ↑ Leptin/adiponectin ratio
Diabetes	RR: 1.89 [207]	Obesity → oestrogen/progesterone imbalance Hyperinsulinism and IGF-1
PCOS	OR: 2.79 OR: 4.05 for young women <54 years old [208]	Unopposed oestrogens Obesity → ↑ oestrogen Hyperinsulinism, Hyperandrogenism
Hyperplasia	Without cytological atypia RR: 1.01–1.03 With cytological atypia RR: 14–45 [187]	Unopposed oestrogens Obesity → ↑oestrogen ↑ Insulin ↑ LH/FSH ratio ↑ Endometrial aromatase activity ↓ Melatonin

hyperplasia, with cytological atypia is almost invariably associated with unopposed oestrogen and co-exists with EC in up to 50% of cases [213, 214].

6.5.2 Exogenous Hormones

The main pharmacological agent that has been associated with an increased risk of endometrial carcinogenesis is unopposed exogenous oestrogens or agents that mimic oestrogens. Potent oestrogens are never indicated in isolation without sequential or concomitant progesterone in hormone replacement for women having an intact uterus. Yet there are several non-steroidal non-hormonal compounds, termed selective oestrogen receptor modulators (SERMs), licenced for osteoporosis or as adjuvant treatment/chemoprevention of breast cancer. They bind to ER causing either an agonistic or antagonistic effect depending on the availability of oestrogen [215]. Although the earlier SERMs, such as tamoxifen, cause endometrial proliferation with pathological changes ranging from hyperplasia and polyps to invasive carcinomas and sarcomas in the endometrium due to its ER agonist activity in the uterus [216], the newer SERMS (Raloxifene, Bazedoxifene and Ospemifene) are reported to have neutral effects on the endometrium [217, 218]. Furthermore, the trophic effect of tamoxifen is only seen in postmenopausal women and no robust evidence for increasing EC in premenopausal women exists. Therefore tamoxifen treatment in these women requires no additional monitoring beyond routine gynaecological care [219].

Tibolone, a synthetic steroid with oestrogenic, some progestogenic and androgenic properties, is commonly used to prevent climacteric symptoms and osteoporosis, but has also been reported to increase the risk of EC [220]. However, a previous Cochrane Systematic Review failed to depict any clear evidence of association given the low number of events [221].

Selective progesterone receptor modulators (SPRM), such as mifepristone, have partial agonist/antagonist activity and the observed endometrial effect depends on the availability of progesterone [77]. Long-term use of high-dose mifepristone thickens the endometrium, although the associated histology shows cystic glandular atrophy with a reduction in glandular mitosis. Nevertheless, concerns have been raised regarding a potential trophic effect of SPRMs on the endometrium [222]. Second generation SPRM, ulipristal acetate, licenced for preoperative or intermittent treatment of moderate-to-severe symptoms of uterine fibroids in adult women of reproductive age does not increase the occurrence of endometrial features of concerns [223]. There are reports of hyperplasia without atypia and polyps with prolonged treatment, yet the endometrium reverted back to normal 6 months after treatment (PEARL III). Therefore, until further conclusive data is available, clinicians using high-dose prolonged therapy with SPRMs in women need to be aware of possible endometrial changes similar to the ones following tamoxifen treatment [224, 225].

6.6 Conclusion

EC is a common hormonally responsive gynaecological malignancy. Being a target organ for ovarian steroid hormones and a plethora of other hormones, the normal and pathological human endometrial function is likely to be relevant to the levels and action of these hormones. The development of novel preventative and diagnostic strategies as well as stratifying women for post-surgical treatment requires our full and detailed understanding of intertwined action of these hormones on the endometrial cell subtypes. Thus accelerated efforts by EC researchers to answer many unclear areas highlighted in this chapter are needed to improve the outcome of millions of women suffering from this devastating condition.

Acknowledgement The authors would like to acknowledge the support from Wellbeing of Women project grant RG1487 (DKH), Higher Committee for Education Development in Iraq (AK), Wellbeing of Women Clinical Training Fellowship RTF510 (NT), Liverpool Women's Hospital (SM, MA), and Institute of Translational medicine, University of Liverpool (AK, MA, DKH). All authors declare that there is no conflict of interest.

References

1. Kamal A, et al. Hormones and endometrial carcinogenesis. Horm Mol Biol Clin Invest. 2016;25(2):129–48.
2. Miller WL, Auchus RJ. The molecular biology, biochemistry, and physiology of human steroidogenesis and its disorders. Endocr Rev. 2011;32(1):81–151.
3. Hammond GL. Plasma steroid-binding proteins: primary gatekeepers of steroid hormone action. J Endocrinol. 2016;230(1):R13–25.
4. Cui J, Shen Y, Li R. Estrogen synthesis and signaling pathways during aging: from periphery to brain. Trends Mol Med. 2013;19(3):197–209.
5. Taraborrelli S. Physiology, production and action of progesterone. Acta Obstet Gynecol Scand. 2015;94(Suppl 161):8–16.
6. Longcope C, Baker R, Johnston CC Jr. Androgen and estrogen metabolism: relationship to obesity. Metabolism. 1986;35(3):235–7.
7. Cloke B, Christian M. The role of androgens and the androgen receptor in cycling endometrium. Mol Cell Endocrinol. 2012;358(2):166–75.
8. Terada N, et al. Effect of dexamethasone on uterine cell death. J Steroid Biochem Mol Biol. 1991;38(1):111–5.
9. Ahmed AH, et al. Are women more at risk of false-positive primary aldosteronism screening and unnecessary suppression testing than men? J Clin Endocrinol Metab. 2011;96(2):E340–6.
10. Szmuilowicz ED, et al. Relationship between aldosterone and progesterone in the human menstrual cycle. J Clin Endocrinol Metab. 2006;91(10):3981–7.
11. Guillemin R. The adenohypophysis and its hypothalamic control. Annu Rev Physiol. 1967;29:313–48.
12. Wu HM, et al. GnRH signaling in intrauterine tissues. Reproduction. 2009;137(5):769–77.
13. Hapangama DK. Mifepristone: the multi-faceted anti-hormone. J Drug Eval. 2003;1:149–75.
14. Chang CC, et al. Effects of gonadotropins (Gonal-F and Puregon) on human endometrial cell proliferation in vitro. Taiwan J Obstet Gynecol. 2011;50(1):42–7.
15. Ku SY, et al. Effect of gonadotropins on human endometrial stromal cell proliferation in vitro. Arch Gynecol Obstet. 2002;266(4):223–8.

16. Miot F, et al. Thyroid hormone synthesis and secretion. In: De Groot LJ, et al., editors. Endotext. South Dartmouth: MDText.com; 2000.
17. Girdler SS, Pedersen CA, Light KC. Thyroid axis function during the menstrual cycle in women with premenstrual syndrome. Psychoneuroendocrinology. 1995;20(4):395–403.
18. Hegedüs L, Karstrup S, Rasmussen N. Evidence of cyclic alterations of thyroid size during the menstrual cycle in healthy women. Am J Obstet Gynecol. 1986;155(1):142–5.
19. Aghajanova L, et al. Thyroid-stimulating hormone receptor and thyroid hormone receptors are involved in human endometrial physiology. Fertil Steril. 2011;95(1):230–7, 237.e1–2.
20. Doufas AG, Mastorakos G. The hypothalamic-pituitary-thyroid axis and the female reproductive system. Ann N Y Acad Sci. 2000;900:65–76.
21. Strachan M, Frier B. Insulin therapy. London: Springer; 2013.
22. Masuda S, et al. Evaluation of menstrual cycle-related changes in 85 clinical laboratory analytes. Ann Clin Biochem. 2016;53(Pt 3):365–76.
23. Axelrod J, Weissbach H. Enzymatic O-methylation of N-acetylserotonin to melatonin. Science. 1960;131(3409):1312.
24. Brown GM. Light, melatonin and the sleep-wake cycle. J Psychiatry Neurosci. 1994;19(5):345–53.
25. Macchi MM, Bruce JN. Human pineal physiology and functional significance of melatonin. Front Neuroendocrinol. 2004;25(3–4):177–95.
26. Martínez-Campa C, et al. Melatonin inhibits aromatase promoter expression by regulating cyclooxygenases expression and activity in breast cancer cells. Br J Cancer. 2009;101(9):1613–9.
27. Dair EL, et al. Effects of melatonin on the endometrial morphology and embryo implantation in rats. Fertil Steril. 2008;89(5 Suppl):1299–305.
28. Labrie F. Intracrinology in action: importance of extragonadal sex steroid biosynthesis and inactivation in peripheral tissues in both women and men. J Steroid Biochem Mol Biol. 2015;145:131–2.
29. Payne AH, Hales DB. Overview of steroidogenic enzymes in the pathway from cholesterol to active steroid hormones. Endocr Rev. 2004;25(6):947–70.
30. Payne AH, Hales DB. Overview of steroidogenic enzymes in the pathway from cholesterol to active steroid hormones. Endocr Rev. 2011;25:947–70. https://doi.org/10.1210/er.2003-0030.
31. Luu-The V. Assessment of steroidogenesis and steroidogenic enzyme functions. J Steroid Biochem Mol Biol. 2013;137:176–82.
32. Sinreih M, Hevir N, Rizner TL. Altered expression of genes involved in progesterone biosynthesis, metabolism and action in endometrial cancer. Chem Biol Interact. 2013;202(1–3):210–7.
33. Arici A, et al. Progesterone metabolism in human endometrial stromal and gland cells in culture. Steroids. 1999;64(8):530–4.
34. Rižner TL. Estrogen biosynthesis, phase I and phase II metabolism, and action in endometrial cancer. Mol Cell Endocrinol. 2013;381(1–2):124–39.
35. Ito K, et al. Biological roles of estrogen and progesterone in human endometrial carcinoma—new developments in potential endocrine therapy for endometrial cancer. Endocr J. 2007;54(5):667–79.
36. Bochkareva NV, et al. Enzymes of estrogen metabolism in endometrial cancer. Bull Exp Biol Med. 2006;141(2):240–2.
37. Aspinall SR, et al. The proliferative effects of 5-androstene-3 beta,17 beta-diol and 5 alpha-dihydrotestosterone on cell cycle analysis and cell proliferation in MCF7, T47D and MDAMB231 breast cancer cell lines. J Steroid Biochem Mol Biol. 2004;88(1):37–51.
38. Walter P, et al. Cloning of the human estrogen receptor cDNA. Proc Natl Acad Sci U S A. 1985;82(23):7889–93.
39. Mosselman S, Polman J, Dijkema R. ER beta: identification and characterization of a novel human estrogen receptor. FEBS Lett. 1996;392(1):49–53.
40. Routledge EJ, et al. Differential effects of xenoestrogens on coactivator recruitment by estrogen receptor (ER) alpha and ERbeta. J Biol Chem. 2000;275(46):35986–93.

41. Saville B, et al. Ligand-, cell-, and estrogen receptor subtype (alpha/beta)-dependent activation at GC-rich (Sp1) promoter elements. J Biol Chem. 2000;275(8):5379–87.
42. Hapangama DK, Kamal AM, Bulmer JN. Estrogen receptor β: the guardian of the endometrium. Hum Reprod Update. 2015;21(2):174–93.
43. Fujimoto J, et al. Clinical implications of the expression of estrogen receptor-alpha and -beta in primary and metastatic lesions of uterine endometrial cancers. Oncology. 2002;62(3):269–77.
44. Zannoni GF, et al. The expression ratios of estrogen receptor α (ERα) to estrogen receptor β1 (ERβ1) and ERα to ERβ2 identify poor clinical outcome in endometrioid endometrial cancer. Hum Pathol. 2013;44(6):1047–54.
45. Kamal AM, et al. Androgen receptors are acquired by healthy postmenopausal endometrial epithelium and their subsequent loss in endometrial cancer is associated with poor survival. Br J Cancer. 2016;114(6):688–96.
46. Critchley HO, et al. Wild-type estrogen receptor (ERbeta1) and the splice variant (ERbetacx/beta2) are both expressed within the human endometrium throughout the normal menstrual cycle. J Clin Endocrinol Metab. 2002;87(11):5265–73.
47. Jazaeri AA, et al. Well-differentiated endometrial adenocarcinomas and poorly differentiated mixed mullerian tumors have altered ER and PR isoform expression. Oncogene. 2001;20(47):6965–9.
48. Takama F, et al. Oestrogen receptor beta expression and depth of myometrial invasion in human endometrial cancer. Br J Cancer. 2001;84(4):545–9.
49. Jongen V, et al. Expression of estrogen receptor-alpha and -beta and progesterone receptor-A and -B in a large cohort of patients with endometrioid endometrial cancer. Gynecol Oncol. 2009;112(3):537–42.
50. Smuc T, Rizner TL. Aberrant pre-receptor regulation of estrogen and progesterone action in endometrial cancer. Mol Cell Endocrinol. 2009;301(1–2):74–82.
51. Fujimoto J, et al. Review: steroid receptors and metastatic potential in endometrial cancers. J Steroid Biochem Mol Biol. 2000;75:209–12.
52. Taylor SE, Martin-Hirsch PL, Martin FL. Oestrogen receptor splice variants in the pathogenesis of disease. Cancer Lett. 2010;288(2):133–48.
53. Witek A, et al. Quantitative analysis of estrogen receptor-alpha and -beta and exon 5 splicing variant mRNA in endometrial hyperplasia in perimenopausal women. Folia Histochem Cytobiol. 2001;39(Suppl 2):119–21.
54. Taylor SE, et al. Elevated oestrogen receptor splice variant ERαΔ5 expression in tumour-adjacent hormone-responsive tissue. Int J Environ Res Public Health. 2010;7(11):3871–89.
55. Collins F, et al. Expression of oestrogen receptors, ERalpha, ERbeta, and ERbeta variants, in endometrial cancers and evidence that prostaglandin F may play a role in regulating expression of ERalpha. BMC Cancer. 2009;9:330.
56. Singh M, et al. Relationship of estrogen and progesterone receptors to clinical outcome in metastatic endometrial carcinoma: a Gynecologic Oncology Group Study. Gynecol Oncol. 2007;106(2):325–33.
57. Smith RG, et al. Purification of human uterine progesterone receptor. Nature. 1975;253(5489):271–2.
58. Conneely OM, et al. Reproductive functions of the progesterone receptor isoforms: lessons from knock-out mice. Mol Cell Endocrinol. 2001;179(1–2):97–103.
59. Conneely OM, et al. The chicken progesterone receptor A and B isoforms are products of an alternate translation initiation event. J Biol Chem. 1989;264(24):14062–4.
60. Kastner P, et al. Two distinct estrogen-regulated promoters generate transcripts encoding the two functionally different human progesterone receptor forms A and B. EMBO J. 1990;9(5):1603–14.
61. Duffy DM, et al. The ratio of progesterone receptor isoforms changes in the monkey corpus luteum during the luteal phase of the menstrual cycle. Biol Reprod. 1997;57(4):693–9.
62. Mangal RK, et al. Differential expression of uterine progesterone receptor forms A and B during the menstrual cycle. J Steroid Biochem Mol Biol. 1997;63(4–6):195–202.

63. Graham JD, et al. Progesterone receptor A and B protein expression in human breast cancer. J Steroid Biochem Mol Biol. 1996;56(1–6 Spec No):93–98.
64. Vegeto E, et al. Human progesterone receptor A form is a cell- and promoter-specific repressor of human progesterone receptor B function. Mol Endocrinol. 1993;7(10):1244–55.
65. Giangrande PH, et al. The opposing transcriptional activities of the two isoforms of the human progesterone receptor are due to differential cofactor binding. Mol Cell Biol. 2000;20(9):3102–15.
66. Tangen IL, et al. Loss of progesterone receptor links to high proliferation and increases from primary to metastatic endometrial cancer lesions. Eur J Cancer. 2014;50(17):3003–10.
67. Arnett-Mansfield RL, et al. Relative expression of progesterone receptors A and B in endometrioid cancers of the endometrium. Cancer Res. 2001;61(11):4576–82.
68. Fujimoto J, et al. Expression of progesterone receptor form A and B mRNAs in gynecologic malignant tumors. Tumour Biol. 1995;16(4):254–60.
69. Martin JD, et al. The effect of estrogen receptor status on survival in patients with endometrial cancer. Am J Obstet Gynecol. 1983;147(3):322–4.
70. Zhang Y, et al. Prognostic role of hormone receptors in endometrial cancer: a systematic review and meta-analysis. World J Surg Oncol. 2015;13:208.
71. Yanli Z, et al. Prognostic role of hormone receptors in endometrial cancer: a systematic review and meta-analysis. World J Surg Oncol. 2015;13(1):1–12.
72. Colombo N, et al. ESMO-ESGO-ESTRO consensus conference on endometrial cancer: diagnosis, treatment and follow-up. Radiother Oncol. 2015;117(3):559–81.
73. Yamazawa K, et al. Fertility-preserving treatment with progestin, and pathological criteria to predict responses, in young women with endometrial cancer. Hum Reprod. 2007;22(7):1953–8.
74. Traish AM, Feeley RJ, Guay AT. Testosterone therapy in women with gynecological and sexual disorders: a triumph of clinical endocrinology from 1938 to 2008. J Sex Med. 2009;6(2):334–51.
75. Lubahn DB, et al. Cloning of human androgen receptor complementary DNA and localization to the X chromosome. Science. 1988;240(4850):327–30.
76. Horie K, et al. Immunohistochemical localization of androgen receptor in the human endometrium, decidua, placenta and pathological conditions of the endometrium. Hum Reprod. 1992;7(10):1461–6.
77. Slayden OD, et al. Progesterone antagonists increase androgen receptor expression in the rhesus macaque and human endometrium. J Clin Endocrinol Metab. 2001;86(6):2668–79.
78. Mertens HJ, et al. Androgen, estrogen and progesterone receptor expression in the human uterus during the menstrual cycle. Eur J Obstet Gynecol Reprod Biol. 2001;98(1):58–65.
79. Critchley HO, Saunders PT. Hormone receptor dynamics in a receptive human endometrium. Reprod Sci. 2009;16(2):191–9.
80. Ito K, et al. Expression of androgen receptor and 5alpha-reductases in the human normal endometrium and its disorders. Int J Cancer. 2002;99(5):652–7.
81. Sasaki M, et al. Inactivation of the human androgen receptor gene is associated with CpG hypermethylation in uterine endometrial cancer. Mol Carcinog. 2000;29(2):59–66.
82. Tanaka S, et al. The role of 5α-reductase type 1 associated with intratumoral dihydrotestosterone concentrations in human endometrial carcinoma. Mol Cell Endocrinol. 2015;401:56–64.
83. Sprenger CC, Plymate SR. The link between androgen receptor splice variants and castration-resistant prostate cancer. Horm Cancer. 2014;5(4):207–17.
84. Nicolaides NC, et al. The human glucocorticoid receptor: molecular basis of biologic function. Steroids. 2010;75(1):1–12.
85. Bamberger AM, et al. The glucocorticoid receptor is specifically expressed in the stromal compartment of the human endometrium. J Clin Endocrinol Metab. 2001;86(10):5071–4.
86. Henderson TA, et al. Steroid receptor expression in uterine natural killer cells. J Clin Endocrinol Metab. 2003;88(1):440–9.
87. McDonald SE, et al. 11Beta-hydroxysteroid dehydrogenases in human endometrium. Mol Cell Endocrinol. 2006;248(1–2):72–8.

88. Wu I, et al. Selective glucocorticoid receptor translational isoforms reveal glucocorticoid-induced apoptotic transcriptomes. Cell Death Dis. 2013;4:e453.
89. Matthews LC, et al. Glucocorticoid receptor regulates accurate chromosome segregation and is associated with malignancy. Proc Natl Acad Sci U S A. 2015;112(17):5479–84.
90. He B, et al. Human glucocorticoid receptor β regulates gluconeogenesis and inflammation in mouse liver. Mol Cell Biol. 2016;36(5):714–30.
91. Smith RE, et al. 11 beta-Hydroxysteroid dehydrogenase type II in the human endometrium: localization and activity during the menstrual cycle. J Clin Endocrinol Metab. 1997;82(12):4252–7.
92. Mondal S, et al. Chemistry and biology in the biosynthesis and action of thyroid hormones. Angew Chem Int Ed Engl. 2016;55(27):7606–30.
93. Davis PJ, Goglia F, Leonard JL. Nongenomic actions of thyroid hormone. Nat Rev Endocrinol. 2016;12(2):111–21.
94. Kaplan SA. The insulin receptor. J Pediatr. 1984;104(3):327–36.
95. Lee J, Pilch PF. The insulin receptor: structure, function, and signaling. Am J Physiol. 1994;266(2 Pt 1):C319–34.
96. Wang CF, et al. Overexpression of the insulin receptor isoform A promotes endometrial carcinoma cell growth. PLoS One. 2013;8(8):e69001.
97. Maggi R, et al. GnRH and GnRH receptors in the pathophysiology of the human female reproductive system. Hum Reprod Update. 2016;22(3):358–81.
98. Perrett RM, McArdle CA. Molecular mechanisms of gonadotropin-releasing hormone signaling: integrating cyclic nucleotides into the network. Front Endocrinol. 2013;4:180.
99. Islami D, et al. Comparison of the effects of GnRH-I and GnRH-II on HCG synthesis and secretion by first trimester trophoblast. Mol Hum Reprod. 2001;7(1):3–9.
100. Chou CS, MacCalman CD, Leung PC. Differential effects of gonadotropin-releasing hormone I and II on the urokinase-type plasminogen activator/plasminogen activator inhibitor system in human decidual stromal cells in vitro. J Clin Endocrinol Metab. 2003;88(8):3806–15.
101. Gründker C, et al. Gonadotropin-releasing hormone (GnRH) agonist triptorelin inhibits estradiol-induced serum response element (SRE) activation and c-fos expression in human endometrial, ovarian and breast cancer cells. Eur J Endocrinol. 2004;151(5):619–28.
102. Limonta P, et al. The biology of gonadotropin hormone-releasing hormone: role in the control of tumor growth and progression in humans. Front Neuroendocrinol. 2003;24(4):279–95.
103. Clayton RN, Catt KJ. Gonadotropin-releasing hormone receptors: characterization, physiological regulation, and relationship to reproductive function. Endocr Rev. 1981;2(2):186–209.
104. Raga F, et al. Quantitative gonadotropin-releasing hormone gene expression and immunohistochemical localization in human endometrium throughout the menstrual cycle. Biol Reprod. 1998;59(3):661–9.
105. Raga F, et al. Independent regulation of matrix metalloproteinase-9, tissue inhibitor of metalloproteinase-1 (TIMP-1), and TIMP-3 in human endometrial stromal cells by gonadotropin-releasing hormone: implications in early human implantation. J Clin Endocrinol Metab. 1999;84(2):636–42.
106. Kang SK, et al. Differential expression of human gonadotropin-releasing hormone receptor gene in pituitary and ovarian cells. Mol Cell Endocrinol. 2000;162(1–2):157–66.
107. Fan QR, Hendrickson WA. Structure of human follicle-stimulating hormone in complex with its receptor. Nature. 2005;433(7023):269–77.
108. Telikicherla D, et al. A comprehensive curated resource for follicle stimulating hormone signaling. BMC Res Notes. 2011;4:408.
109. Singh M, Jadhav HR. Melatonin: functions and ligands. Drug Discov Today. 2014;19(9):1410–8.
110. Slaugenhaupt SA, et al. Mapping of the gene for the Mel1a-melatonin receptor to human chromosome 4 (MTNR1A) and mouse chromosome 8 (Mtnr1a). Genomics. 1995;27(2):355–7.
111. Reppert SM, et al. Molecular characterization of a second melatonin receptor expressed in human retina and brain: the Mel1b melatonin receptor. Proc Natl Acad Sci U S A. 1995;92(19):8734–8.

112. Zhao H, Poon AM, Pang SF. Pharmacological characterization, molecular subtyping, and autoradiographic localization of putative melatonin receptors in uterine endometrium of estrous rats. Life Sci. 2000;66(17):1581–91.
113. Zhao H, Pang SF, Poon AM. mt(1) Receptor-mediated antiproliferative effects of melatonin on the rat uterine antimesometrial stromal cells. Mol Reprod Dev. 2002;61(2):192–9.
114. Watanabe M, et al. Expression of melatonin receptor (MT1) and interaction between melatonin and estrogen in endometrial cancer cell line. J Obstet Gynaecol Res. 2008;34(4):567–73.
115. Weigel NL, Zhang Y. Ligand-independent activation of steroid hormone receptors. J Mol Med. 1998;76(7):469–79.
116. Hapangama DK, Drury J, Da Silva L, Al-Lamee H, Earp A, Valentijn AJ, Edirisinghe DP, Murray PA, Fazleabas AT, Gargett CE. Abnormally located SSEA1+/SOX9+ endometrial epithelial cells with a basalis-like phenotype in the eutopic functionalis layer may play a role in the pathogenesis of endometriosis. Hum Reprod. 2019;34(1):56–68.
117. Tempest N, Maclean A, Hapangama DK. Endometrial stem cell markers: current concepts and unresolved questions. Int J Mol Sci. 2018;19(10):3240. https://doi.org/10.3390/ijms19103240.
118. Valentijn AJ, et al. SSEA-1 isolates human endometrial basal glandular epithelial cells: phenotypic and functional characterization and implications in the pathogenesis of endometriosis. Hum Reprod. 2013;28(10):2695–708.
119. Paulson RJ, et al. Pregnancy in the sixth decade of life: obstetric outcomes in women of advanced reproductive age. JAMA. 2002;288(18):2320–3.
120. Bittner JJ. Some enigmas associated with the genesis of mammary cancer in mice. Cancer Res. 1948;8(12):625–39.
121. Henderson BE, et al. Endogenous hormones as a major factor in human cancer. Cancer Res. 1982;42(8):3232–9.
122. Henderson BE, Ross R, Bernstein L. Estrogens as a cause of human cancer: the Richard and Hinda Rosenthal Foundation award lecture. Cancer Res. 1988;48(2):246–53.
123. Jensen EV. The contribution of "alternative approaches" to understanding steroid hormone action. Mol Endocrinol. 2005;19(6):1439–42.
124. Toft D, Gorsk J. A receptor molecule for estrogens: isolation from the rat uterus and preliminary characterization. Proc Natl Acad Sci U S A. 1966;55(6):1574–81.
125. O'Malley BW. A life-long search for the molecular pathways of steroid hormone action. Mol Endocrinol. 2005;19(6):1402–11.
126. O'Lone R, et al. Genomic targets of nuclear estrogen receptors. Mol Endocrinol. 2004;18(8):1859–75.
127. Umayahara Y, et al. Estrogen regulation of the insulin-like growth factor I gene transcription involves an AP-1 enhancer. J Biol Chem. 1994;269(23):16433–42.
128. Pietras R, Mrquez-Garbn D. Membrane-associated estrogen receptor signaling pathways in human cancers. Clin Cancer Res. 2007;13(16):4672–6.
129. Kushner PJ, et al. Estrogen receptor pathways to AP-1. J Steroid Biochem Mol Biol. 2000;74(5):311–7.
130. Ray A, Prefontaine KE, Ray P. Down-modulation of interleukin-6 gene expression by 17 beta-estradiol in the absence of high affinity DNA binding by the estrogen receptor. J Biol Chem. 1994;269(17):12940–6.
131. Zhang L, et al. Nongenomic effect of estrogen on the MAPK signaling pathway and calcium influx in endometrial carcinoma cells. J Cell Biochem. 2009;106(4):553–62.
132. Thomas P, et al. Identity of an estrogen membrane receptor coupled to a G protein in human breast cancer cells. Endocrinology. 2005;146(2):624–32.
133. Yin-Yan H. Estrogenic G protein-coupled receptor 30 signaling is involved in regulation of endometrial carcinoma by promoting proliferation, invasion potential, and interleukin-6 secretion via the MEK/ERK mitogen-activated protein kinase pathway. Cancer Sci. 2009;100(6):1051–61.
134. Koike N, et al. Epigenetic dysregulation of endometriosis susceptibility genes (review). Mol Med Rep. 2015;12(2):1611–6.

135. Sasaki M, et al. Cytosine-phosphoguanine methylation of estrogen receptors in endometrial cancer. Cancer Res. 2001;61(8):3262–6.
136. Campan M, Weisenberger DJ, Laird PW. DNA methylation profiles of female steroid hormone-driven human malignancies. Curr Top Microbiol Immunol. 2006;310:141–78.
137. Sasaki M, et al. Progesterone receptor B gene inactivation and CpG hypermethylation in human uterine endometrial cancer. Cancer Res. 2001;61(1):97–102.
138. Liehr JG. Role of DNA adducts in hormonal carcinogenesis. Regul Toxicol Pharmacol. 2000;32(3):276–82.
139. Martin FL, et al. Constitutive expression of bioactivating enzymes in normal human prostate suggests a capability to activate pro-carcinogens to DNA-damaging metabolites. Prostate. 2010;70(14):1586–99.
140. Zhang Y, et al. Cytochrome P450 isoforms catalyze formation of catechol estrogen quinones that react with DNA. Metabolism. 2007;56(7):887–94.
141. Belous AR, et al. Cytochrome P450 1B1-mediated estrogen metabolism results in estrogen-deoxyribonucleoside adduct formation. Cancer Res. 2007;67(2):812–7.
142. Hayes CL, et al. 17 beta-estradiol hydroxylation catalyzed by human cytochrome P450 1B1. Proc Natl Acad Sci U S A. 1996;93(18):9776–81.
143. Aoyama T, et al. Estradiol metabolism by complementary deoxyribonucleic acid-expressed human cytochrome P450s. Endocrinology. 1990;126(6):3101–6.
144. Kerlan V, et al. Nature of cytochromes P450 involved in the 2-/4-hydroxylations of estradiol in human liver microsomes. Biochem Pharmacol. 1992;44(9):1745–56.
145. Benecke A, Chambon P, Gronemeyer H. Synergy between estrogen receptor alpha activation functions AF1 and AF2 mediated by transcription intermediary factor TIF2. EMBO Rep. 2000;1(2):151–7.
146. Teng Y, et al. Catechol-O-methyltransferase and cytochrome P-450 1B1 polymorphisms and endometrial cancer risk: a meta-analysis. Int J Gynecol Cancer. 2013;23(3):422–30.
147. Ke H, et al. 4-hydroxy estrogen induces DNA damage on codon 130/131 of PTEN in endometrial carcinoma cells. Mol Cell Endocrinol. 2015;400:71–7.
148. Yang S, Thiel KW, Leslie KK. Progesterone: the ultimate endometrial tumor suppressor. Trends Endocrinol Metab. 2011;22(4):145–52.
149. Hapangama DK, Bulmer JN. Pathophysiology of heavy menstrual bleeding. Womens Health (Lond). 2016;12(1):3–13. https://doi.org/10.2217/whe.15.81.
150. Dai D, et al. Progesterone inhibits human endometrial cancer cell growth and invasiveness: down-regulation of cellular adhesion molecules through progesterone B receptors. Cancer Res. 2002;62(3):881–6.
151. Dai D, et al. Progesterone regulation of activating protein-1 transcriptional activity: a possible mechanism of progesterone inhibition of endometrial cancer cell growth. J Steroid Biochem Mol Biol. 2003;87(2–3):123–31.
152. Wang Y, et al. Progesterone inhibition of Wnt/β-catenin signaling in normal endometrium and endometrial cancer. Clin Cancer Res. 2009;15(18):5784–93.
153. Kurita T, et al. Stromal progesterone receptors mediate the inhibitory effects of progesterone on estrogen-induced uterine epithelial cell deoxyribonucleic acid synthesis. Endocrinology. 1998;139(11):4708–13.
154. Franco HL, et al. Epithelial progesterone receptor exhibits pleiotropic roles in uterine development and function. FASEB J. 2012;26(3):1218–27.
155. Kurtita T, Wang YZ, Donjacour AA, Zhao C, Lydon JP, O'Malley BW, Isaacs JT, Dahiya R, Cunha GR. Paracrine regulation of apoptosis by steroid hormones in the male and female reproductive system. Cell Death Differ. 2001;8(2):192–200.
156. Li Q, Kannan A, DeMayo FJ, Lydon JP, Cooke PS, Yamagishi H, Srivastava D, Bagchi MK, Bagchi IC. The antiproliferative action of progesterone in uterine epithelium is mediated by Hand2. Science. 2011;331(6019):912–6.
157. Campan M, Weisenberger D, Laird P. Microbiology compans; 2001. p. 111.
158. Fanta M. Is polycystic ovary syndrome, a state of relative estrogen excess, a real risk factor for estrogen-dependent malignancies? Gynecol Endocrinol. 2013;29(2):145–7.

159. Holm NS, et al. The prevalence of endometrial hyperplasia and endometrial cancer in women with polycystic ovary syndrome or hyperandrogenism. Acta Obstet Gynecol Scand. 2012;91(10):1173–6.
160. Park JC, et al. Endometrial histology and predictable clinical factors for endometrial disease in women with polycystic ovary syndrome. Clin Exp Reprod Med. 2011;38(1):42–6.
161. Dumesic DA, Lobo RA. Cancer risk and PCOS. Steroids. 2013;78(8):782–5.
162. Goodarzi MO, et al. Polycystic ovary syndrome: etiology, pathogenesis and diagnosis. Nat Rev Endocrinol. 2011;7(4):219–31.
163. Zhang G, et al. Preliminary investigation of the expression and functions of insulin receptor isoforms in endometrial carcinoma. Zhonghua Fu Chan Ke Za Zhi. 2012;47(11):839–45.
164. Wang CF, et al. Effects of insulin, insulin-like growth factor-I and -II on proliferation and intracellular signaling in endometrial carcinoma cells with different expression levels of insulin receptor isoform A. Chin Med J (Engl). 2013;126(8):1560–6.
165. Potischman N, et al. Case-control study of endogenous steroid hormones and endometrial cancer. J Natl Cancer Inst. 1996;88(16):1127–35.
166. Kaaks R, Lukanova A, Kurzer MS. Obesity, endogenous hormones, and endometrial cancer risk: a synthetic review. Cancer Epidemiol Biomarkers Prev. 2002;11(12):1531–43.
167. Lukanova A, et al. Circulating levels of sex steroid hormones and risk of endometrial cancer in postmenopausal women. Int J Cancer. 2004;108(3):425–32.
168. Allen NE, et al. Endogenous sex hormones and endometrial cancer risk in women in the European Prospective Investigation into Cancer and Nutrition (EPIC). Endocr Relat Cancer. 2008;15(2):485–97.
169. Audet-Walsh E, et al. Profiling of endogenous estrogens, their precursors, and metabolites in endometrial cancer patients: association with risk and relationship to clinical characteristics. J Clin Endocrinol Metab. 2011;96(2):E330–9.
170. Gibson DA, et al. Evidence of androgen action in endometrial and ovarian cancers. Endocr Relat Cancer. 2014;21(4):T203–18.
171. Kalantaridou SN, Calis KA. Testosterone therapy in premenopausal women. Semin Reprod Med. 2006;24(2):106–14.
172. Mueller A, Gooren L. Hormone-related tumors in transsexuals receiving treatment with cross-sex hormones. Eur J Endocrinol. 2008;159(3):197–202.
173. Tuckerman EM, et al. Do androgens have a direct effect on endometrial function? An in vitro study. Fertil Steril. 2000;74(4):771–9.
174. Hackenberg R, Schulz KD. Androgen receptor mediated growth control of breast cancer and endometrial cancer modulated by antiandrogen- and androgen-like steroids. J Steroid Biochem Mol Biol. 1996;56(1–6 Spec No):113–117.
175. Bulun SE, et al. Regulation of aromatase expression in estrogen-responsive breast and uterine disease: from bench to treatment. Pharmacol Rev. 2005;57(3):359–83.
176. Gao C, et al. The therapeutic significance of aromatase inhibitors in endometrial carcinoma. Gynecol Oncol. 2014;134(1):190–5.
177. Zakharov V, et al. Suppressed expression of type 2 3alpha/type 5 17beta-hydroxysteroid dehydrogenase (AKR1C3) in endometrial hyperplasia and carcinoma. Int J Clin Exp Pathol. 2010;3(6):608–17.
178. Pereira de Jésus-Tran K, et al. Comparison of crystal structures of human androgen receptor ligand-binding domain complexed with various agonists reveals molecular determinants responsible for binding affinity. Protein Sci. 2006;15(5):987–99.
179. Berstein L, et al. Aromatase and comparative response to its inhibitors in two types of endometrial cancer. J Steroid Biochem Mol Biol. 2005;95(1–5):71–4.
180. Morgan K, et al. Gonadotropin-releasing hormone receptor levels and cell context affect tumor cell responses to agonist in vitro and in vivo. Cancer Res. 2008;68(15):6331–40.
181. Park DW, et al. Gonadotropin-releasing hormone (GnRH)-I and GnRH-II induce cell growth inhibition in human endometrial cancer cells: involvement of integrin beta3 and focal adhesion kinase. Reprod Biol Endocrinol. 2009;7:81.

182. Cho-Clark M, et al. GnRH-(1-5) transactivates EGFR in Ishikawa human endometrial cells via an orphan G protein-coupled receptor. Mol Endocrinol. 2014;28(1):80–98.
183. Wu HM, et al. Gonadotropin-releasing hormone type II (GnRH-II) agonist regulates the invasiveness of endometrial cancer cells through the GnRH-I receptor and mitogen-activated protein kinase (MAPK)-dependent activation of matrix metalloproteinase (MMP)-2. BMC Cancer. 2013;13:300.
184. Emons G, et al. GnRH antagonists in the treatment of gynecological and breast cancers. Endocr Relat Cancer. 2003;10(2):291–9.
185. Benjamin F, Deutsch S. Plasma levels of fractionated estrogens and pituitary hormones in endometrial carcinoma. Am J Obstet Gynecol. 1976;126(6):638–47.
186. Jänne O, et al. Female sex steroid receptors in normal, hyperplastic and carcinomatous endometrium. The relationship to serum steroid hormones and gonadotropins and changes during medroxyprogesterone acetate administration. Int J Cancer. 1979;24(5):545–54.
187. Emons G, et al. Efficacy and safety of AEZS-108 (LHRH agonist linked to doxorubicin) in women with advanced or recurrent endometrial cancer expressing LHRH receptors: a multicenter phase 2 trial (AGO-GYN5). Int J Gynecol Cancer. 2014;24(2):260–5.
188. Engel JB, et al. Targeted chemotherapy of endometrial, ovarian and breast cancers with cytotoxic analogs of luteinizing hormone-releasing hormone (LHRH). Arch Gynecol Obstet. 2012;286(2):437–42.
189. Noci I, et al. hLH/hCG-receptor expression correlates with in vitro invasiveness in human primary endometrial cancer. Gynecol Oncol. 2008;111(3):496–501.
190. Pillozzi S, Fortunato A. Over-expression of the LH receptor increases distant metastases in an endometrial cancer mouse model. Front Oncol. 2013;3:285.
191. Seebacher V, et al. Does thyroid-stimulating hormone influence the prognosis of patients with endometrial cancer? A multicentre trial. Br J Cancer. 2013;109(1):215–8.
192. Liu Y, et al. Leptin activates STAT3 and ERK1/2 pathways and induces endometrial cancer cell proliferation. J Huazhong Univ Sci Technolog Med Sci. 2011;31(3):365–70.
193. Tang HY, et al. Thyroid hormone causes mitogen-activated protein kinase-dependent phosphorylation of the nuclear estrogen receptor. Endocrinology. 2004;145(7):3265–72.
194. Chung IH, et al. Thyroid hormone-mediated regulation of lipocalin 2 through the Met/FAK pathway in liver cancer. Oncotarget. 2015;6(17):15050–64.
195. Yurkovetsky Z, et al. Development of multimarker panel for early detection of endometrial cancer. High diagnostic power of prolactin. Gynecol Oncol. 2007;107(1):58–65.
196. Fader AN, et al. Endometrial cancer and obesity: epidemiology, biomarkers, prevention and survivorship. Gynecol Oncol. 2009;114(1):121–7.
197. Yamazawa K, et al. A case-control study of endometrial cancer after antipsychotics exposure in premenopausal women. Oncology. 2003;64(2):116–23.
198. Ekmekcioglu C. Expression and putative functions of melatonin receptors in malignant cells and tissues. Wien Med Wochenschr. 2014;164(21–22):472–8.
199. Kanishi Y, et al. Differential growth inhibitory effect of melatonin on two endometrial cancer cell lines. J Pineal Res. 2000;28(4):227–33.
200. Sack RL, et al. Human melatonin production decreases with age. J Pineal Res. 1986;3(4):379–88.
201. Viswanathan AN, Hankinson SE, Schernhammer ES. Night shift work and the risk of endometrial cancer. Cancer Res. 2007;67(21):10618–22.
202. Ciortea R, et al. Effect of melatonin on intra-abdominal fat in correlation with endometrial proliferation in ovariectomized rats. Anticancer Res. 2011;31(8):2637–43.
203. Yudt MR, Cidlowski JA. The glucocorticoid receptor: coding a diversity of proteins and responses through a single gene. Mol Endocrinol. 2002;16(8):1719–26.
204. King KL, Cidlowski JA. Cell cycle regulation and apoptosis. Annu Rev Physiol. 1998;60:601–17.
205. Davies S, et al. Gene regulation profiles by progesterone and dexamethasone in human endometrial cancer Ishikawa H cells. Gynecol Oncol. 2006;101(1):62–70.

206. De Pergola G, Silvestris F. Obesity as a major risk factor for cancer. J Obes. 2013;2013:291546.
207. Hernandez AV, et al. Insulin resistance and endometrial cancer risk: a systematic review and meta-analysis. Eur J Cancer. 2015;51(18):2747–58.
208. Barry JA, Azizia MM, Hardiman PJ. Risk of endometrial, ovarian and breast cancer in women with polycystic ovary syndrome: a systematic review and meta-analysis. Hum Reprod Update. 2014;20(5):748–58.
209. Gong TT, Wang YL, Ma XX. Age at menarche and endometrial cancer risk: a dose-response meta-analysis of prospective studies. Sci Rep. 2015;5:14051.
210. Colombo N, et al. ESMO-ESGO-ESTRO consensus conference on endometrial cancer: diagnosis, treatment and follow-up. Int J Gynecol Cancer. 2016;26(1):2–30.
211. Xu WH, et al. Menstrual and reproductive factors and endometrial cancer risk: results from a population-based case-control study in urban Shanghai. Int J Cancer. 2004;108(4):613–9.
212. Navaratnarajah R, Pillay OC, Hardiman P. Polycystic ovary syndrome and endometrial cancer. Semin Reprod Med. 2008;26(1):62–71.
213. Boruban MC, et al. From endometrial hyperplasia to endometrial cancer: insight into the biology and possible medical preventive measures. Eur J Cancer Prev. 2008;17(2):133–8.
214. Emons G, et al. New WHO classification of endometrial hyperplasias. Geburtshilfe Frauenheilkd. 2015;75(2):135–6.
215. Ellis AJ, et al. Selective estrogen receptor modulators in clinical practice: a safety overview. Expert Opin Drug Saf. 2015;14(6):921–34.
216. Cohen I. Endometrial pathologies associated with postmenopausal tamoxifen treatment. Gynecol Oncol. 2004;94(2):256–66.
217. Mirkin S, Pickar JH. Selective estrogen receptor modulators (SERMs): a review of clinical data. Maturitas. 2015;80(1):52–7.
218. Nakamura K, et al. Efficacy of raloxifene hydrochloride for the prevention of health care problems in patients who undergo surgery for endometrial cancer: a multicenter randomized clinical trial. Int J Gynecol Cancer. 2015;25(2):288–95.
219. Committee Opinion No. 601: tamoxifen and uterine cancer. Obstet Gynecol. 2014;123(6):1394–7.
220. Mørch LS, et al. The influence of hormone therapies on type I and II endometrial cancer: a nationwide cohort study. Int J Cancer. 2016;138(6):1506–15.
221. Formoso G, et al. Short and long term effects of tibolone in postmenopausal women. Cochrane Database Syst Rev. 2012;(2):CD008536.
222. Spitz IM, et al. Management of patients receiving long-term treatment with mifepristone. Fertil Steril. 2005;84(6):1719–26.
223. Donnez J, et al. Long-term medical management of uterine fibroids with ulipristal acetate. Fertil Steril. 2016;105(1):165–173.e4.
224. Grunberg SM, et al. Long-term administration of mifepristone (RU486): clinical tolerance during extended treatment of meningioma. Cancer Invest. 2006;24(8):727–33.
225. Ramondetta LM, et al. Phase 2 trial of mifepristone (RU-486) in advanced or recurrent endometrioid adenocarcinoma or low-grade endometrial stromal sarcoma. Cancer. 2009;115(9):1867–74.

Hereditary Cancers

7

Lorenzo Ceppi, Don S. Dizon, and Michael J. Birrer

7.1 Introduction

Every year, epithelial endometrial cancer (EC) incidence accounts for 7% of all cancers in women worldwide, representing the fourth most common malignancy arising in women. In the United States alone, over 61,800 new cases are expected and over 12,160 women will die of this disease in 2019 [1].

According to the Division of Cancer Prevention and Control, the incidence of endometrial cancer in the United States is likely to increase more than for many other types of cancers [2]: the number of cases per year will rise from 48,301 in 2010 to 63,119 in 2020 (+30.7%). Much of this increase is likely as a result of an aging population and more sedentary behaviors and the associated impact from obesity. However, there is a subset of patients (up to 5% [3]) in whom endometrial cancer is a manifestation of a familial syndrome, due to a genetic predisposition.

Familial risk for endometrial cancer is classically seen in patients impacted by Lynch Syndrome (formerly known as the Hereditary Non-polyposis Colorectal Cancer [HNPCC] syndrome), which has an estimated prevalence of 2–5% of newly diagnosed EC [4] and Cowden Syndrome, which is associated with a PTEN

L. Ceppi
Center for Cancer Research, The Gillette Center for Gynecologic Oncology, Massachusetts General Hospital, Harvard Medical School, Boston, MA, USA

Department of Medicine and Surgery, Milano-Bicocca University, ASST-Monza, Desio Hospital, Monza, Italy

D. S. Dizon
Center for Cancer Research, The Gillette Center for Gynecologic Oncology, Massachusetts General Hospital, Harvard Medical School, Boston, MA, USA

M. J. Birrer (✉)
Center for Cancer Research, The Gillette Center for Gynecologic Oncology, Massachusetts General Hospital, Harvard Medical School, Boston, MA, USA

O'Neal Cancer Center, Birmingham, AL, USA
e-mail: mbirrer@uab.edu

Table 7.1 Familial syndromes classically associated with endometrial cancer

Syndrome	Gene	Chromosome
Lynch		
Mismatch repair genes	MSH2	2p21
	MLH1	3p21.3
	MSH6	2p16
	PMS2	7p22.2
Other genes	EPCAM	2p21
Cowden	PTEN	10q23.3

mutation. Although some reports suggest that mutations in BRCA1 or BRCA2, which are associated with Hereditary Breast Ovarian Cancer Syndrome (HBOCS), increase the risk of endometrial cancer, the data are controversial at best and no conclusive evidence is available to inform this question (Table 7.1).

The mutations in these syndromes are grounded in the germline inheritance of a single mutated allele of a tumor-suppressor gene. As one allele is inherited as mutated, the patient is more likely to develop a mutation or a loss of the function in the remaining allele. The loss of function of a cellular control is the basis of cancer development through lifetime [5].

In this chapter, we review the familial syndromes associated with an increased endometrial cancer risk.

7.2 Lynch Syndrome (LS)

Lynch syndrome, named after Dr. Henry Lynch, is a familial cancer syndrome manifest by cancers affecting patients at an early age. In the general population, LS is present in about 1–600 to 1–3000 individuals [6]. Classically, it is associated with colorectal cancer although it is recognized now that EC is also a common manifestation among women affected. LS is the most common cause of hereditary endometrial cancer [7] and accounts for 2–5% of all EC diagnoses. While HNPCC was used interchangeably with LS, it is no longer used [8] because of the heterogeneity on which it was applied to families who may or may not have had evidence of microsatellite instability on genomic testing.

The major phenotype of LS is colorectal cancer (CRC), and patients with LS have an estimated cumulative risk by age of 70 years of up to 55% of being affected. Beyond this, women with LS face a 30–45% lifetime risk of developing EC and a 4–20% risk of ovarian cancer (OC), highlighting the importance of gynecologic screening in these patients [9–11]. Indeed, several datasets indicate that for women, the risk of EC may exceed the risk of colorectal cancer [12]. Beyond these tumors, patients with LS are also at increased risk of other tumors compared to the general population, including tumors of the stomach, urinary tract, pancreatic or hepatobiliary tract, small bowel, brain, and skin (Table 7.2). Even though LS screening diagnostics and therapeutics are also related to other cancers (colorectal and ovarian cancer mainly), the discussion of these other associations are beyond the scope of the present review and will not be discussed.

Table 7.2 Cumulative risks of cancer by age 70 years in Lynch syndrome

Cancer	Risk in general population, %	Risk in LS, %	Mean age at diagnosis, years
Colon	5.5	35–55%	69
MLH1/MSH2		Female: 22–53	27–46
MSH6		Female: 10	54–63
PMS2		Female: 15	47–66
Endometrium	2.7	30–45%	65
MLH1/MSH2		14–54	48–62
MSH6		17–71	54–57
PMS2		15	49
Stomach	<1	0.2–13	49–55
Ovary	1.6	4–20	43–45
Hepato-biliary tract	<1	0.02–4	54–57
Urinary tract	<1	0.2–25	52–60
Small bowel	<1	0.4–12	46–49
Brain/central nervous system	<1	1–4	50
Sebaceous neoplasm	<1	1–9	NA
Pancreas	1.5	0.4–4.0	63–65

7.3 Genetics

LS is characterized by germline mutations in mismatch repair (MMR) genes: every individual that inherits the mutation is at an increased risk of developing cancer during their lifetime. The function of MMR system is to maintain genomic integrity by correcting base substitution mismatches and small insertion–deletion mismatches that are generated by errors in base pairing during DNA replication. The reported distribution of specific mutations in LS is 32, 39, 15, and 14% for MLH1 (MutL homolog 1), MSH2 (MutS homolog 2), MSH6 (MutS homolog 6), and PMS2 (postmeiotic segregation 2) [13]. Recently, mutation in EPCAM (formerly known as TACSTD1) was associated with Lynch syndrome. EPCAM 3′ end deletions act through a mechanism of tissue-specific epigenetic silencing causing MSH2 gene primer hypermethylation and loss of expression [14].

Mismatch repair deficiency leads to an accumulation of genetic mutations and genomic instability. The most common event is base-pair mismatch in the microsatellite regions, represented of repetitive nucleotide sequences (microsatellites) throughout the whole genome in coding and noncoding regions. This occurrence is known as microsatellite instability (MSI), a characteristic feature of LS-associated cancers. Mismatch repair can affect cell growth genes (TGFβR2 [15]) and of the DNA MMR genes themselves (hMSH3, hMSH6) that possibly drive the tumorigenesis in Lynch-related tumors.

Table 7.2 shows cumulative lifetime risk to age 70 of EC described in published reports.

The largest published dataset to date shows higher EC risk for mMLH1 carriers (54%) rather than for mMSH2 [16] (21%), with lower risk for mMSH6 carriers (16%). Even a much lower EC risk is related to PMS2 mutations [17]. EPCAM mutation carriers yield a very low EC risk compared to mMSH2 patients [18].

7.4 Clinical Features

LS-associated EC has a mean age of incidence in the late fourth decade, approximately 10 years earlier than the age of onset of sporadic EC [19]. For this reason, women with young onset EC (i.e., before 50) should be evaluated for LS, which impacts up to 10% of cases [20]. When such a tumor is diagnosed before 50 years it should be considered as a sentinel event [21], which often predates other cancer diagnoses by a decade.

Despite this younger age at diagnosis, there are few features to distinguish LS-associated and sporadic EC. Broaddus [22] compared 50 women with LS-associated EC to 42 women with sporadic EC diagnosed at a young age (<50 years) and 26 women who had EC with MSI associated with MLH1 promoter methylation (not Lynch-related genetic alteration). Among women with LS-associated EC, only three carried a mutation in MLH1, 94% of these cancers were associated with an MSH2 mutation. LS-associated EC appeared to have less endometrioid histology tumors, compared to women with sporadic EC and those with disease associated with MLH1 promoter methylation (86% versus 98 and 96%, respectively), were less likely to have tumor associated with lymph-vascular invasion (24% versus 40 and 52%, P, 0.005), were more likely to be stage I at diagnosis (78% versus 67 and 60%) and less likely to be stage III/IV at diagnosis (12% versus 26 and 36%). In addition, there appeared to be a trend among LS patients to have non-endometrioid histology. However, undifferentiated histology was only observed in EC associated with an MLH1 methylation. These reported differences had no statistical significance, if not otherwise reported, but they represent the only available comparison to date.

Some data suggest that the disease may arise from the lower uterine segment. In a study by Westin, et al. 29% of patients with LS-associated disease arose in the lower uterine segment, compared to only 1.8% in those with sporadic disease [23]. Finally, there does not appear to be any prognostic impact of EC based on whether or not it is associated with LS. This was illustrated by Boks et al. [24] who reported not only a similar distribution of histologic subtypes but also similar 5 years overall survival between the groups.

7.5 Genetic Risk Assessment

The purpose of a genetic risk assessment is to identify unaffected women at an elevated risk of cancer related to LS and to identify patients with EC who may be at increased risk of second malignancies. Multiple organizations have developed criteria to identify patients at an increased risk based on history and clinical factors (Table 7.3).

The International Collaborative Group on Hereditary Non-polyposis Colorectal Cancer established criteria to identify HNPCC families in 1991 first (known as the Amsterdam I criteria) [25]. These criteria were developed for research purpose and included history of three cancer cases involving relatives with at least one first relative of the other two, cancer diagnoses in at least two generations, and one cancer diagnosed before 50 years. The specificity of these criteria was high, but the sensitivity was low as colonic malignancies only were considered.

The original criteria were broadened to include also extra colonic cancer diagnoses in an attempt to make identification of patients more sensitive in 1999 (Amsterdam II) [26], although these criteria were criticized as because in several studies, only 13–36% of mutation carrier families met these criteria [27, 28]. In addition, sensitivity remained low (0.22, range 0.13–0.67), though it was associated with high specificity (0.98, range 0.97–1.0).

In 1997, the Bethesda guidelines [29] were developed as an alternative to Amsterdam criteria and were revised to incorporate all cancer types seen with LS in

Table 7.3 Comparison between Revised Amsterdam and Bethesda criteria for Lynch Syndrome screening

Revised Amsterdam criteria for diagnosis of hereditary non-polyposis colorectal cancer	Revised Bethesda guidelines
1. Three or more relatives with histologically verified HNPCC-associated cancer (colorectal cancer, cancer of the endometrium, small bowel, ureter, or renal pelvis), one of which is a first-degree relative of the other two. Familial adenomatous polyposis should be excluded	1. CRC diagnosed at younger than 50 years
2. Cancer involving at least two generations	2. Presence of synchronous or metachronous CRC or other LS-associated tumors
3. One or more cancer cases diagnosed before the age of 50 years	3. CRC with MSI-high pathologic-associated features (Crohn-like lymphocytic reaction, mucinous/signet cell differentiation, or medullary growth pattern) diagnosed in an individual younger than 60 years old
	4. Patient with CRC and CRC or LS-associated tumor a diagnosed in at least one first-degree relative younger than 50 years old
	5. Patient with CRC and CRC or LS-associated tumor at any age in two first-degree or second-degree relatives
	a: LS-associated tumors include tumor of the colorectum, endometrium, stomach, ovary, pancreas, ureter, renal pelvis, biliary tract, brain, small bowel, sebaceous glands, and kerotoacanthomas

2004 [30]. Features were added to the original Amsterdam criteria, including age of diagnosis, tumor features, and personal and family cancer history. These guidelines have less strict criteria used to identify potential patients who might carry LS, but result in a higher sensitivity of 0.82 (0.78–0.91) although specificity is lower at 0.77 (0.75–0.79) [31]. Despite the different criteria, neither appears able to identify all patients with mismatch repair gene mutations. Revised Amsterdam criteria and Bethesda guidelines are listed in Table 7.3.

In 2007, the Society of Gynecologic Oncologists (SGO) aimed to provide further guidance on the role of genetic risk assessment based on clinical criteria (Table 7.4) [32]. In contrast to the Amsterdam I and Bethesda criteria, the SGO sought to stratify at-risk individuals into those in whom there is a 20–25% versus 5–10% chance of having LS, for whom testing would be recommended or helpful, respectively. The society listed cancer affected patients, but also not affected high risk patients. The proposed approach is to offer genetic testing to women with a first- or second-degree relative with a known mismatch repair gene mutation, secondly to women with a first- or second-degree relative with a LS-related tumor, regardless of age.

Table 7.4 SGO Education Committee statement on risk assessment for inherited gynecologic cancer predispositions

Patients with greater than approximately 20–25% chance of having an inherited predisposition to endometrial, colorectal, and related cancers and for whom genetic risk assessment is recommended	Patients with greater than approximately 5–10% chance of having an inherited predisposition to endometrial, colorectal, and related cancers and for whom genetic risk assessment may be helpful
1. Patients with endometrial or colorectal cancer who meet the Amsterdam II criteria	1. Patients with endometrial or colorectal cancer diagnosed prior to age 50
2. Patients with synchronous or metachronous endometrial and colorectal cancer with the first cancer diagnosed prior to age 50	2. Patient with endometrial or ovarian cancer with a synchronous or metachronous colon or other Lynch/HNPCC-associated tumor[a] at any age
3. Patients with synchronous or metachronous ovarian and colorectal cancer with the first cancer diagnosed prior to age 50	3. Patients with endometrial or colorectal cancer and a first-degree relative with a Lynch/HNPCC-associated tumor[a] diagnosed prior to age 50
4. Patients with colorectal or endometrial cancer with evidence of a mismatch repair defect (i.e. microsatellite instability (MSI) or immunohistochemical loss of expression of MLH1, MSH2, MSH6, or PMS2)	4. Patients with colorectal or endometrial cancer diagnosed at any age with two or more first- or second-degree relatives[b] with Lynch/HNPCC-associated tumors[a], regardless of age
5. Patients with a first- or second-degree relative with a known mismatch repair gene mutation	5. Patients with a first- or second-degree relative[b] that meets the above criteria[a]

[a]Lynch/HNPCC-related tumors include colorectal, endometrial, stomach, ovarian, pancreas, ureter and renal pelvis, biliary tract, and brain (usually glioblastoma as seen in Turcot syndrome) tumors, sebaceous gland adenomas and keratoacanthomas in Muir–Torre syndrome, and carcinoma of the small bowel
[b]First- and second-degree relatives are parents, siblings, aunts, uncles, nieces, nephews, grandparents, and grandchildren

7.6 Computational Models

In addition to clinical criteria, computational models are also available. These use algorithms that take into account clinical features to calculate individual risk for having an LS gene mutation. They are most often employed if clinical criteria suggest the presence of LS. Commonly used models are described below.

MMR predict model [33] uses sex and age at diagnosis of CRC, location of tumor (proximal vs. distal), multiple CRCs (synchronous or metachronous), diagnosis of EC in any first-degree relative, and age at diagnosis of CRC in first-degree relatives. http://hnpccpredict.hgu.mrc.ac.uk/.

MMRpro model [34] uses personal and family history of colorectal and endometrial cancer age at diagnosis and molecular testing results for MMR genes, if available. This calculator determines the risk divided for germline mutation and also indicated the risk for future cancer in presymptomatic gene carriers and other unaffected individuals. http://bcb.dfci.harvard.edu/bayesmendel/software.php.

PREMM$_{1,2,6}$ model [35] uses sex, personal, and family history of colorectal, endometrial, or other LS cancers. This calculator estimates for germline mutation risk. This model can be found at: http://premm.dfci.harvard.edu/.

It has been published that this model would be cost-effective improving health outcomes as primary screening of individuals between the ages of 25 and 35, followed by genetic testing of those whose risk exceeds 5% [36].

These models, developed with different methods for different purposes and with the primary aim to distinguish patients at risk for LS-related CRC, included also LS-related EC risk assessment. Mercado [37] assessed the area under the curve, sensitivity and specificity of the abovementioned prediction models among 563 population-based and 129 clinic-based endometrial cancer cases. Although the models were able to detect affected population (AUCs of 0.77, 0.76, and 0.77, respectively), in the clinic-based cohort the accuracy was lower (AUCs of 0.67, 0.64, and 0.54, respectively). The conclusion was that computational models have limited clinical utility in determining which patients with endometrial cancer should undergo genetic testing for Lynch syndrome. Immunohistochemical analysis and microsatellite instability testing may be the best currently available tools to screen for Lynch syndrome in endometrial cancer patients.

7.7 Tumor Testing

For affected patients in whom LS risk is strongly suspected, genomic testing of the tumor should be performed [38] to identify MMR system mutations, and to guide the next germline mutation genetic test.

Immunohistochemistry (IHC) can recognize mismatch repair deficiency through the test of MMR panel (MLH1, MSH2, MSH6, PMS2) on endometrial or colorectal tumor tissue, showing protein loss of expression. As a complementary tool, microsatellite instability can be tested through a polymerase chain reaction (PCR) assay [39]. Depending on the distribution of DNA fragments between tumor and normal tissue, samples can be identified as MSI-high, -low, or stable, if no difference is shown. MSI-H is defined as instability in ≥30% of the examined microsatellites. Both MMR IHC and MSI testing have a high accuracy performance. IHC is preferred as a diagnostic tool, MSI testing can be considered in rare cases were no protein expression loss is shown in an individual with LS likely familiar history. Cases like that are when missense mutations occurs were a not functional MMR protein is produced. Indeed it is reported for MMR IHC and MSI testing [40] a sensitivity of 0.83 (0.75–0.89) and 0.85 (0.75–0.93), and a specificity of 0.89 (0.68–0.95) and 0.90 (0.87–0.93) respectively.

It is important to note that MLH1 loss with or without PMS2 protein loss can be the result of MLH1 promoter methylation, which occurs in 20–30% of endometrial cancers and up to 20% of colorectal cancers. This is not an hereditary mutation and the differential diagnosis must be ruled out. Several available tools for testing methylation based on fluorescence-based real-time PCR [41, 42], or on gene sequencing methods (pyrosequencing) [43] are available to perform such an analysis.

For patients with colorectal or endometrial cancer, a practice bulletin endorsed by the SGO suggests that testing of all affected women irrespective of age of diagnosis is perhaps the most sensitive approach to the identification of women with LS [44]. However, it is also acknowledged this would increase the patients' number tested by a factor of 3–4. Therefore, acknowledging that most women with either of these LS-related cancers present at a younger age, they ultimately recommend molecular screening of every CRC and EC diagnosed before age 60 years for LS when resources are available [45], and at least one subsequent report found that it was cost-effective [46]. SGO in a clinical practice statement [47] recommends universal screening to overcome lack of familiar history diagnoses, considering for screening also women older than 60 years.

To confirm the diagnosis, germline DNA mutation represent the definitive test. Also for unaffected patients where clinical suspect has to be confirmed, MMR and/or MSI testing can be performed on peripheral blood, which can be used to screen for large rearrangements.

In all cases where genetic testing is concerned, careful pre- and posttest counseling is critical and full informed consent should be given. This includes resources to provide psychosocial support, information regarding financial repercussions, and frank discussions regarding ethical implications of testing (e.g., testing of minors), and options for cancer prevention (including the role of risk-reducing surgeries). In the US, the Genetic Information Non-discrimination Act (GINA) (http://frwebgate.access.gpo.gov/cgibin/getdoc.cgi?dbname=110_cong_public_laws&docid=f:publ233.110.pdf) bars discrimination from employment or medical insurance coverage on the basis of genetic risk. However, this protection does not yet extend to other insurance types, including life and long-term care insurance.

7.8 Screening and Prevention

For patients with LS, screening is focused on gastrointestinal and gynecologic cancer. In one study, gastrointestinal screening with colonoscopy or sigmoidoscopy and barium enema every 3 years resulted in a lower incidence of colorectal cancer incidence and death due to disease compared to a population that did not undergo screening [48]. These results were corroborated by a subsequent systematic review [49].

Although methods for screening for endometrial cancer are available, none have shown benefits in either earlier detection or survival. Dove-Edwin et al. [50] evaluated the role of transvaginal ultrasound in women from one of 292 LS families over a period of 13 years. Only two cases of endometrial carcinoma were reported and neither was detected by surveillance screening. Renkonen-Sinisalo et al. [51] reported their experience involving 175 women with MMR mutations using pelvic exam with endometrial biopsy. EC occurred in 14 cases, 11 of which were diagnosed by surveillance, 8 by intrauterine biopsies. Transvaginal ultrasound detected only 4 EC patients but missed 6 other cases. Intrauterine sampling detected 14 cases of potentially premalignant hyperplasia. Because of the potential for endometrial biopsy to detect disease, current guidelines suggest that this be performed every 1–2 years, starting at age 30–35 years [44].

7.9 Prophylactic Surgery

For women, hysterectomy is reasonable option for cancer prevention. If performed, a bilateral salpingo-oophorectomy should also be done as women with LS are also at risk for ovarian cancer.

The benefit of prophylactic pelvic surgery was shown in one study where women with documented MMR mutations underwent prophylactic hysterectomy and bilateral salpingo-oophorectomy were matched with controls without any surgery performed. The reduction of risk was substantial: no tumor occurred in the surgery group (61 patients) versus 69 cases of EC among 210 patients. A comparable risk reduction was demonstrated for ovarian cancer occurrence, where no ovarian or primary peritoneal tumor occurred versus 12 cases among 223 patients [52]. The incidence of endometrial in those who did not undergo prophylactic surgery was 33%. Of note, as discussed before, there are reports of intraoperative diagnoses of EC during prophylactic surgery in this population [51, 53].

A modeling study evaluated different screening strategies with risk reducing surgery and concluded that annual screening starting at age 30 years followed by prophylactic surgery at age 40 years was the most effective gynecologic cancer prevention strategy, but incremental benefit over prophylactic surgery at age 40 years alone was attained at substantial cost [54]. Patients should be counseled telling that the substantial increase of cancer risk occurs after 40s, and that the prophylactic approach before then is the most effective.

7.10 Chemoprevention

Chemoprevention against endometrial cancer may be provided by progestin-based oral contraceptives. These agents have a known impact on the overall incidence of EC [55] and are effective in preventing endometrial hyperplasia and early endometrial cancer treatment [56]. Studies demonstrated an increased breast cancer risk related to combined hormonal replacement therapy (estrogens and progestins), but this evidence is not related to combined OCP.

Lu et al. reported evidence of effect of progestin-containing OCPs or depo-medroxyprogesterone acetate (depoMPA) on endometrial proliferation in LS women [57], but the impact on subsequent cancer risk has not been adequately evaluated.

Although the data are limited, SGO/ACOG guidelines suggest the use of progestin-based contraception for chemoprevention in LS patients based on expert opinion.

NSAIDs and Cox-2 inhibitors have been tested as potential chemo preventative options in LS patients although most data come from studies to prevent colorectal cancer. For example, the CAPP2 [58] trial enrolled patients with LS and randomly assigned them to treatment with aspirin 600 mg per day or Novelose (resistant starch) for 4 years. The long-term analysis [59] showed a survival advantage for patients completing at least 2 years of aspirin treatment with a hazard ratio of 0.41 (95% CI, 0.19–0.86, $P = 0.02$). In addition, there was a trend towards a lower incidence of cancers, including those of the endometrium and ovary. Finally, there were no differences in adverse events reported and no protection for patients who underwent chemoprevention for less than 2 years was evident.

Currently, no sufficiently indication should be made to extend this treatment to LS population [60] to decrease cancer risk. There is a recommendation to discuss an individual patient treatment choice, taking into account risks and benefits [61].

7.11 Other Cancer Syndromes Associated with an Increased Risk of Endometrial Cancer

7.11.1 Muir-Torre Syndrome

Muir-Torre Syndrome is an autosomal-dominant inherited skin condition characterized by sebaceous skin adenoma, epithelioma or and carcinoma, multiple keratoacantomas, and visceral diseases such as colorectal, endometrial, urological, and upper gastrointestinal cancers. It is considered a Lynch variant due to the same underlying mutations that drive these tumors as LS: MSH2 and MLH1 [62, 63]. As such, the cancer risk in this population is the same as LS. However, given the risk of skin carcinomas, screening for Muir-Torre syndrome-associated skin lesions among LS patients is recommended.

7.11.2 Cowden Syndrome

Cowden Syndrome is associated with an autosomic germline mutation in PTEN gene, and it is part of the PTEN hamartoma tumor syndrome. As its description, individuals with Cowden Syndrome are at increased risk for benign and malignant neoplasias including skin and mucosal hamartomas, as well as intestine polyps. The greatest risk for women with CS is breast cancer with a lifetime risk of 85%, followed by thyroid 35%, kidney 33%, endometrial 28%, and colorectal 9% cancers, and melanoma 6% [64, 65]. It is estimated that CS affects 1 in 20,000 individuals. The median occurrence of these diseases is 20–30 years. While general cancer screening is recommended [66], there are none specific to endometrial cancer. Instead, patients who develop abnormal uterine bleeding (menorrhagia or any bleeding other than normal period) should be referred for further evaluation.

7.11.3 Hereditary Breast Ovarian Cancer Syndrome

At this time, whether patients with hereditary breast and ovarian cancer syndrome (HBOCS), most commonly associated with mutations in BRCA genes, have an increased risk of endometrial cancer is controversial. Levine et al. studied a consecutive series of 199 Ashkenazi Jewish population with EC. He found that among this population, only three EC cases had BRCA1 or 2 mutations [67]. Notably, not even the 17 cases of papillary serous endometrial carcinoma were associated with a BRCA mutation. A separate prospective study showed that only 6 of 857 BRCA1 and BRCA2 mutation carriers developed EC after an average follow-up time of 3.3 years and in 4 of these cases, EC was also associated with tamoxifen use [68]. The low incidence of EC in BRCA carriers was underscored in a separate study which reported 17 cases of EC among 4456 women with a BRCA mutation after a mean follow-up of 5.7 years [69]. In this study, the Standardized Incidence Ratio (SIR) for BRCA1 carriers was 1.91 (95% CI: 1.06–3.19, $p = 0.03$) and for BRCA2 carriers was 1.75 (95% CI: 0.55–4.23, $p = 0.2$). The SIR for women who received tamoxifen was 4.14 (95% CI: 1.92–7.87) and was 1.67 (95% CI: 0.81–3.07) for women who did not. The authors concluded that the higher endometrial cancer risk in BRCA1 mutation carriers was attributable to a history of tamoxifen use. For this reason hysterectomy at the time of prophylactic BSO may be a reasonable option, but only if subsequent treatment with tamoxifen is being considered. At present, there is no guidance on the role of hysterectomy or the risk management for EC in women with a BRCA mutation.

7.11.3.1 Recommendations for Lynch Syndrome, from SGO/ACOG Guidelines [43]

Limited or Inconsistent Scientific Evidence (Level B)
1. Genetic risk assessment should be considered for unaffected women who have a first-degree relative affected with endometrial or colorectal cancer who was either diagnosed before age 60 years or who is identified to be at risk of Lynch syndrome by one of the systematic clinical screens that incorporates a focused personal and family medical history.
2. Whenever possible, molecular evaluation for Lynch syndrome should begin with tumor testing.

3. Obstetric and gynecologic physicians and practices should adopt one of the following three approaches for assessing the possibility of Lynch syndrome in a woman personally affected with colorectal or endometrial cancer:
   (a) Perform tumor testing on any endometrial or colorectal tumor from a woman identified to be at risk of Lynch syndrome through a systematic clinical screen that includes a focused personal and family medical history.
   (b) Perform tumor testing on all endometrial or colorectal tumors irrespective of age of diagnosis.
   (c) Perform tumor testing on all endometrial or colorectal tumors diagnosed before age 60 years.

Consensus and Expert Opinion (Level C)
– Progestin-based contraception, including oral contraceptives, may be considered for chemoprevention of endometrial cancer in women with Lynch syndrome.

References

1. Siegel RL, et al. Cancer statistics, 2015. CA Cancer J Clin. 2015;65:5–29.
2. Weir HK. The past, present, and future of cancer incidence in the United States: 1975 through 2020. Cancer. 2015;121:1827.
3. Gruber SB, Thompson WD. A population-based study of endometrial cancer and familial risk in younger women. cancer and steroid hormone study group. Cancer Epidemiol Biomark Prev. 1996;5(6):411–7.
4. Watson P, Lynch H. Extracolonic cancer in hereditary non poliposis colon rectal cancer. Cancer. 1993;71:677.
5. Knudson AG Jr. Hereditary cancer, oncogenes, and antioncogenes. Cancer Res. 1985;45:1437–43.
6. Dunlop MG, Farrington SM, Nicholl I, et al. Population carrier frequency of hMSH2 and hMLH1 mutations. Br J Cancer. 2000;83(12):1643–5.
7. Hendriks YM, De Jong AE, Morreau H, et al. Diagnostic approach and management of Lynch syndrome (hereditary nonpolyposis colorectal carcinoma): a guide for clinicians. CA Cancer J Clin. 2006;56:213–25.
8. Jass JR. Hereditary non-polyposis colorectal cancer: the rise and fall of a confusing term. World J Gastroenterol. 2006;12:4943–50.
9. Dunlop MG, Farrington SM, Carothers AD, et al. Cancer risk associated with germline DNA mismatch repair gene mutations. Hum Mol Genet. 1997;6(1):105–10.
10. Barrow E, Alduaij W, Robinson L, Shenton A, Clancy T, Lalloo F, Hill J, Evans DG. Colorectal cancer in HNPCC: cumulative lifetime incidence, survival and tumour distribution. A report of 121 families with proven mutations. Clin Genet. 2008;74(3):233–42.
11. Stoffel E, Mukherjee B, Raymond VM, et al. Calculation of risk of colorectal and endometrial cancer among patients with Lynch syndrome. Gastroenterology. 2009;137(5):1621–7.
12. Barrow E, Hill J, Evans DG. Cancer risk in Lynch syndrome. Familial Cancer. 2013;12(2):229–40.
13. Palomaki GE, et al. EGAPP supplementary evidence review: DNA testing strategies aimed at reducing morbidity and mortality from Lynch syndrome. Genet Med. 2009;11(1):42–65.

14. Ligtenberg MJ, Kuiper RP, Chan TL, et al. Heritable somatic methylation and inactivation of MSH2 in families with Lynch syndrome due to deletion of the 3′ exons of TACSTD1. Nat Genet. 2009;41:112–7.
15. Kim TM, Laird PW, Park PJ. The landscape of microsatellite instability in colorectal and endometrial cancer genomes. Cell. 2013;155(4):858–68.
16. Bonadona V, Bonaiti B, Olschwang S, et al. Cancer risks associated with germline mutations in MLH1, MSH2 and MSH6 genes in Lynch syndrome. JAMA. 2011;305:2304.
17. Senter L, Clendenning M, Sotamaa K, et al. Th e clinical phenotype of Lynch syndrome due to germ-line PMS2 mutations. Gastroenterology. 2008;135:419–28.
18. Ligtenberg MJ, Kuiper RP, Geurts van Kessel A, Hoogerbrugge N. EPCAM deletion carriers constitute a unique subgroup of Lynch syndrome patients. Familial Cancer. 2013;12(2):169.
19. Aarnio M, et al. Clinicopathological features and management of cancers in lynch syndrome. Pathol Res Int. 2012:350309.
20. Lu KE, Schorge JO, et al. Prospective determination of prevalence of Lynch syndrome in young women with endometrial cancer. J Clin Oncol. 2007;25(33):5158–64.
21. Lu KH, Dinh M, Kohlmann W, et al. Gynecologic malignancy as a "sentinel cancer" for women with HNPCC. Obstet Gynecol. 2005;105:569–74.
22. Broaddus RR, Lynch HT, Chen LM, et al. Pathologic features of endometrial carcinoma associated with HNPCC: a comparison with sporadic endometrial carcinoma. Cancer. 2006;106:87.
23. Westin SN, Lacour RA, Urbauer DL, Luthra R, Bodurka DC, Lu KH, Broaddus RR. Carcinoma of the lower uterine segment: a newly described association with Lynch syndrome. J Clin Oncol. 2008;26:5965.
24. Boks DE, Trujillo AP, Voogd AC, et al. Survival analysis of endometrial carcinoma associated with hereditary nonpolyposis colorectal cancer. Int J Cancer. 2002;102(2):198–200.
25. Vasen HFA, Mecklin JP, Meera Khan P, et al. The international collaborative group on hereditary non-polyposis colorectal cancer. Dis Colon Rectum. 1991;34:424–5.
26. Vasen HFA, Watson P, Mecklin JP, et al. New criteria for hereditary non-polyposis colorectal cancer (HNPCC, Lynch syndrome) proposed by the International Collaborative Group on HNPCC (ICG-HNPCC). Gastroenterology. 1999;116:1453–6.
27. Hampel H, Frankel WL, Martin E, Arnold M, Khanduja K, Kuebler P, et al. Screening for the Lynch syndrome (hereditary nonpolyposis colorectal cancer). N Engl J Med. 2005;352:1851–60.
28. Lindor NM, Rabe K, Petersen GM, et al. Lower cancer incidence in Amsterdam-I criteria families without mismatch repair deficiency: familial colorectal cancer type X. JAMA. 2005;293:1979–85.
29. American Gastroenterological Association. American Gastroenterological Association medical position statement: hereditary colorectal cancer and genetic testing. Gastroenterology. 2001;121(1):195.
30. Umar A, et al. Revised Bethesda guidelines for hereditary nonpolyposis colorectal cancer (Lynch syndrome) and microsatellite instability. J Natl Cancer Inst. 2004;96:261–8.
31. Giardiello FM, Allen JI, Axilbund JE, et al. Guidelines on genetic evaluation and management of Lynch syndrome: a consensus statement by the US Multi-society Task Force on colorectal cancer. Am J Gastroenterol. 2014;109(8):1159–79.
32. Lancaster JM, et al. SGO Committee statement Society of Gynecologic Oncologists Education Committee statement on risk assessment for inherited gynecologic cancer predispositions. Gynecol Oncol. 2007;107:159–62.
33. Green RC, Parfrey PS, Woods MO, et al. Prediction of Lynch syndrome in consecutive patients with colorectal cancer. J Natl Cancer Inst. 2009;101:331–40.
34. Barnetson RA, Tenesa A, Farrington SM, et al. Identification and survival of carriers of mutations in DNA mismatch-repairs genes in colon cancer. N Engl J Med. 2006;354:2751–63.
35. Kastrinos F, Steyerberg EW, Mercado R, et al. The PREMM(1,2,6) model predicts risk of MLH1, MSH2, and MSH6 germline mutations based on cancer history. Gastroenterology. 2011;40:73–81.

36. Dinh TA, Rosner BI, Atwood JC, et al. Health benefits and cost-effectiveness of primary genetic screening for Lynch syndrome in the general population. Cancer Prev Res. 2010;4:9–22.
37. Mercado RC, Hampel H, Kastrinos F, et al. Performance of PREMM1,2, 6, MMRpredict, and MMRpro in detecting Lynch syndrome among endometrial cancer cases. Genet Med. 2012;14(7):670–80.
38. Backes FJ, Leon ME, Ivanov I, et al. Prospective evaluation of DNA mismatch repair protein expression in primary endometrial cancer. Gynecol Oncol. 2009;114:486–90.
39. Umar A, Boland CR, Terdiman JP, et al. Revised Bethesda guidelines for hereditary nonpolyposis colorectal cancer (Lynch syndrome) and microsatellite instability. J Natl Cancer Inst. 2004;96(4):261–8.
40. Palomaki GE, McClain MR, Melillo S, et al. EGAPP supplementary evidence review: DNA testing strategies aimed at reducing morbidity and mortality from Lynch syndrome. Genet Med. 2009;11:42–65.
41. Eads CA, Danenberg KD, Kawakami K, Saltz LB, Blake C, Shibata D, Danenberg PV, Laird PW. MethyLight: a high-throughput assay to measure DNA methylation. Nucleic Acids Res. 2000;28:E32.
42. Nygren AO, Ameziane N, Duarte HM, Vijzelaar RN, Waisfisz Q, Hess CJ, Schouten JP, Errami A. Methylation-specific MLPA (MS-MLPA): simultaneous detection of CpG methylation and copy number changes of up to 40 sequences. Nucleic Acids Res. 2005;33:e128.
43. Newton K, Jorgensen NM, Wallace AJ, et al. Tumour MLH1 promoter region methylation testing is an effective prescreen for Lynch syndrome (HNPCC) et al. J Med Genet. 2014;51:789–96.
44. American College of Obstetricians and Gynecologists. Lynch syndrome. Practice Bulletin No. 147. Obstet Gynecol. 2014;124:1042–54.
45. Society of Gynecologic Oncology. SGO clinical practice statement: screening for Lynch syndrome in endometrial cancer. Chicago: SGO; 2014. https://www.sgo.org/clinical-practice/guidelines/screeningfor-lynch-syndrome-in-endometrial-cancer/. Retrieved 22 July 2014.
46. Resnick KE, Hampel H, Fishel R, et al. Lynch syndrome screening strategies among newly diagnosed endometrial cancer patients. Gynecol Oncol. 2009;114(1):128–34.
47. Society of Gynecologic Oncology. SGO clinical practice statement: screening for Lynch syndrome in endometrial cancer. Chicago: SGO; 2014. https://www.sgo.org/clinical-practice/guidelines/screeningfor-lynch-syndrome-in-endometrial-cancer/. Retrieved May 2015.
48. Jarvinen HJ, Aarnio M, Mustonen M, et al. Controlled 15-year trial on screening for colorectal cancer in families with hereditary nonpolyposis colorectal cancer. Gastroenterology. 2000;118(5):829.
49. Lindor NM, et al. Lower cancer incidence in Amsterdam-I criteria families without mismatch repair deficiency: familial colorectal cancer type X. JAMA. 2005;293:1979–85.
50. Dove-Edwin I, Boks D, Goff S, et al. The outcome of endometrial carcinoma surveillance by ultrasound scan in women at risk of hereditary nonpolyposis colorectal carcinoma and familial colorectal carcinoma. Cancer. 2002;94:1708.
51. Renkonen-Sinisalo L, Bützow R, Leminen A, et al. Surveillance for endometrial cancer in hereditary nonpolyposis colorectal cancer syndrome. Int J Cancer. 2007;120(4):821.
52. Schmeler KM, Lynch HT, Chen LM, et al. Prophylactic surgery to reduce the risk of gynecologic cancers in the Lynch syndrome. N Engl J Med. 2006;354(3):261–9.
53. Chung L, Broaddus R, Crozier M, Luthraa R, Levenback C, Lu K. Unexpected endometrial cancer at prophylactic hysterectomy in a woman with hereditary nonpolyposis colon cancer. Obstet Gynecol. 2003;102(5 Pt 2):1152–5.
54. Kwon JS, Sun CC, Peterson SK, et al. Cost-effectiveness analysis of prevention strategies for gynecologic cancers in Lynch syndrome. Cancer. 2008;113:326–35.
55. Weiss NS, Sayvetz TA. Incidence of endometrial cancer in relation to the use of oral contraceptives. N Engl J Med. 1980;302:551–4.
56. Baker J, Obermair A, Gebski V, Janda M. Efficacy of oral or intrauterine device-delivered progestin in patients with complex endometrial hyperplasia with atypia or early endometrial adenocarcinoma: a meta-analysis and systematic review of the literature. Gynecol Oncol. 2012;125:263–70.

57. Lu KH, Loose DS, Yates MS, Nogueras-Gonzalez GM, Munsell MF, Chen LM, et al. Prospective, multi-center randomized intermediate biomarker study of oral contraceptive vs. Depo-Provera for prevention of endometrial cancer in women with Lynch syndrome. Cancer Prev Res. 2013;6:774–81.
58. Burn J, Bishop DT, Mecklin JP, et al. Effect of aspirin or resistant starch on colorectal neoplasia in the Lynch syndrome. N Engl J Med. 2008;359:2567–78.
59. Burn J, Gerdes AM, Macrae F, et al. Long-term effect of aspirin on cancer risk in carriers of hereditary colorectal cancer: an analysis from the CAPP2 randomized controlled trial. Lancet. 2011;378:2081–7.
60. Rothwell PM, Fowkes FG, Belch JF, et al. Effect of daily aspirin on long-term risk of death due to cancer: analysis of individual patient data from randomized trials. Lancet. 2011;377:31–41.
61. National Comprehensive Cancer Network. Clinical practice guidelines in oncology genetic/familial high risk assessment: colorectal (Version 3.2019). https://www.nccn.org/professionals/physician_gls/pdf/genetics_colon.pdf. Accessed June 2019.
62. Ponti G, Ponz de Leon M. Muir-Torre syndrome. Lancet Oncol. 2005;6:980.
63. South CD, et al. The frequency of Muir-Torre syndrome among Lynch syndrome families. J Natl Cancer Inst. 2008;100(4):277.
64. Gustafson S, Zbuk KM, Scacheri C, et al. Cowden syndrome. Semin Oncol. 2007;34(5):428–34.
65. Tan M-H, Mester JL, Ngeow J, Rybicki LA, Orloff MS, Eng C. Lifetime Cancer risks in individuals with germline PTEN mutations. Clin Cancer Res. 2012;18(2):400–7. https://doi.org/10.1158/1078-0432.CCR-11-2283.
66. National Comprehensive Cancer Network. Clinical practice guidelines in oncology genetic/familial high risk assessment: breast and ovarian (Version 2.2014). https://www.nccn.org/professionals/physician_gls/pdf/genetics_screening.pdf. Accessed 22 June 2019.
67. Levine D, Lin O, Barakat R, et al. Risk of endometrial cancer associated with BRCA mutation. Gynecol Oncol. 2001;80(3):395–8.
68. Biener M, Fich A, Rosen B, et al. The risk of endometrial cancer in women with BRCA1 and BRCA2 mutations. A prospective study. Gynecol Oncol. 2007;104:7.
69. Segev Y1, Iqbal J, Lubinski J, et al. The incidence of endometrial cancer in women with BRCA1 and BRCA2 mutations: an international prospective cohort study. Gynecol Oncol. 2013;130(1):127–31.

Part III
International Clinical Guidelines

The Need for Level 1 Clinical Evidence in Daily Practice

8

Athina Koutouleas and Mansoor Raza Mirza

8.1 What Is Evidence-Based Medicine?

It is difficult to begin to describe evidence-based medicine (EBM) without first mentioning Dr. David Sackett. A Chicago-born and bred internal medical physician who quickly switched his career path to clinical epidemiology, Dr. Sackett went on to make enormous contributions to clinical community. By placing importance on the understanding and measurement of patient adherence to prescribed treatments, the methodology of randomized control trials (RCTs), Dr. Sackett's influence has led to the improvements in patient care across indications beyond his own specialty field [1]. Fundamentally, his work led to a mind-set shift in the way clinicians and academic authorities thought about the role of evidence in clinical care. In doing so, he laid the foundation for EBM, which is defined as the process of systematically reviewing, appraising, and using clinical research findings to aid the delivery of optimum clinical care to patients [1]. Dr. Sackett himself describes this practice as the conscientious, explicit, and judicious use of current best evidence in making decisions about the care of individual patients [2]. Since its early definitions in clinical epidemiology, the concept of EBM has been recognized by hundreds of thousands of clinicians across the globe and across various medical disciplines [3]. In light of the importance of grading clinical evidence in everyday practice and care, this chapter highlights EBM in the context of endometrial cancer. This chapter describes how good gyne-oncologists use both clinical expertise and the best available external evidence to guide treatment choices for their patients with endometrial cancer.

A. Koutouleas
OvaCure, Hellerup, Denmark

M. R. Mirza (✉)
Department of Oncology, Rigshospitalet, Nordic Society of Gynaecological Oncology (NSGO), Copenhagen, Denmark
e-mail: Mansoor.Raza.Mirza@regionh.dk

8.2 Defining Level 1 Evidence

Evidence-based care requires critical review of published resources for evidence to help direct and guide care for the specific clinical question. These resources are commonly obtained from searches in databases such as PubMed, EBSCO, Cochrane Consumer Network (CCN), field-specific association resources, government sites, and other electric resources. The clinician or practitioner must be able to systematically evaluate the evidence obtained for its relevance and validity as related to the specific clinical question.

There are a number of different hierarchies of evidence available which can be used to rank the strength and validity of the evidence from expert opinion to systematic reviews and meta-analyses (see Tables 8.1 and 8.2, Fig. 8.1). Efficacy is defined as the capacity or power to produce a clinical effect. This can be assessed based on meta-analyses and systematic reviews (Level 1 according to CCN). Evidence guidelines, randomized clinical trials, observational studies, cohort, case control, case series, and case reports address effectiveness—the quality or amount of the effect in practice, outside the laboratory or other controlled environment (Level 2 evidence). Evidence from expert committees, opinions, or clinical experience is considered the lowest grade of evidence due to the higher probability for bias (Level 3).

The clinician or practitioner can incorporate the published evidence, the individual patient's case and their own clinical expertise to develop an appropriate plan of care. Additionally, clinical guidelines or algorithms may be available to assist in care planning. These guidelines are generally developed by a multidisciplinary team with support from professional organizations, institutions, or governmental agencies that publish the guidelines (i.e. ESMO, ASCO, NIH/NCI, EMA etc.).

Table 8.1 Example of grading of evidence

Level	Type of Evidence
I	Evidence is obtained from meta-analysis of multiple, well-designed, controlled studies. Randomized trials with low false-positive and low false-negative errors (high power).
II	Evidence is obtained from at least one well-designed experimental study, Randomized trials with high false-positive and/or negative errors (low power).
III	Evidence is obtained from well-designed, quasi-experimental studies such as non-randomized, controlled single-group, pre-post, cohort, time, or matched case-control series.
IV	Evidence is obtained from well-designed, non-experimental studies such as comparative and correlational descriptive and case studies.
V	Evidence from case reports and clinical examples.

8 The Need for Level 1 Clinical Evidence in Daily Practice

Table 8.2 Grades of evidence as per the Oxford Centre for Evidence-Based Medicine (OCEBM)

Level	Type of evidence
1a	Systematic review with homogeneity of randomized control trials
1b	Individual randomized control trial with a narrow confidence interval
1c	All or none related outcome
2a	Systematic review with homogeneity of cohort studies
2b	Individual cohort study (including low-quality randomized control trials, e.g., <80% follow-up)
2c	"Outcomes" Research; Ecological studies
3a	Systematic review with homogeneity of case-control studies
3b	Individual case–control study
4	Case-series (and poor-quality cohort and case–control studies)
5	Expert opinion without explicit critical appraisal, or based on physiology, bench research or "first principles"
Grades of recommendation	
A	Consistent level 1 studies
B	Consistent level 2 or 3 studies or extrapolations from level 1 studies
C	Level 4 studies or extrapolations from level 2 or 3 studies
D	Level 5 evidence or troublingly inconsistent or inconclusive studies of any level

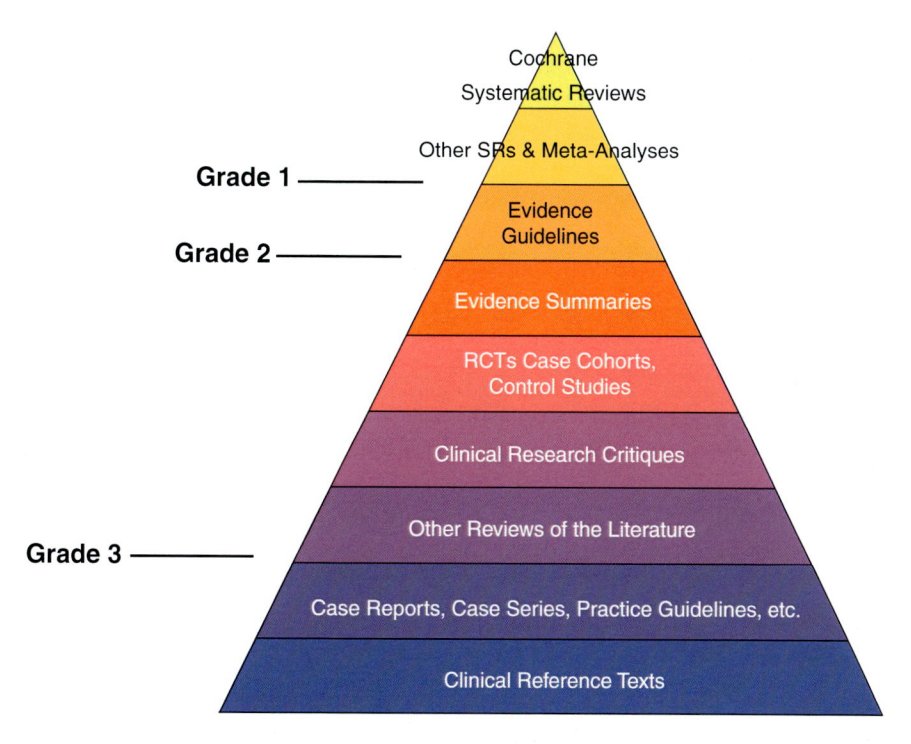

Fig. 8.1 Grades of evidence as per the Cochrane Consumer Network (CCN)

8.3 Why Are Randomized Clinical Trials Needed?

The National Cancer Institute classifies RCTs as a study in which the participants are assigned by chance to separate groups that compare different treatments; neither the researchers nor the participants can choose which group. Using chance to assign people to groups means that the groups will be similar and that the treatments they receive can be compared objectively. At the time of the trial, it is not known which treatment is best. RCTs have been ubiquitous in Phase III settings over the past half century [4]. RCTs serve as the basic clinical research tool for evaluating new interventions or existing methods previously not tested [4]. The methodology for the design, conduct and analysis of clinical trials has evolved greatly but the need has not changed. RCTs today still stand as the most effective way to discriminate the effects of treatments for a given patient population.

Given the variation in clinical trial design, not all RCTs can be defined as equal in terms of their objectivity. Chalmers et al. [5] were among the first to suggest the importance of evaluating the design, implementation, and analysis of RCT. The qualification of RCTs was suggested to be based on four factors: (1) basic descriptive material, (2) the study protocol, (3) the analysis of the data, and (4) data useful for potential combining of several RCT results [5]. By considering these factors in clinical evidence, a clinician is equipped with tools to determine whether new findings in an indication should be considered in the treatment plan of patient population. Table 8.3 offers an overview of intervention RCTs currently conducted in endometrial cancer, which are either complete, actively recruiting or not yet recruiting (search conducted on www.clinicaltrials.gov, accessed 9th October 2017). The outcomes of these studies will guide the future standard of care options for patients with endometrial cancer.

8.4 Primary End-Points in Clinical Trials Matter

There is no single ideal clinical trial end-point for all situations, but there are many new ways to define end-points beyond the classical terms. Given that most cases of endometrial cancer are diagnosed in women who are past menopause and aged in their mid-60s, the primary endpoints which are selected in new RCTs should be carefully matched to the needs of this patient population. In the European context, there has been recent scrutiny over the lack of evidence of benefits on overall survival and quality of life of cancer drugs approved by European Medicines Agency (EMA) since 2009 by a retrospective cohort study [6]. This suggests that more than ever before must clinicians carefully design their trials to incorporate the most favorable outcomes for patients especially in intervention studies. Below is a list of classical primary end-points used as well as some new options that are becoming increasingly more popular in new clinical trial designs.

Overall Survival (OS)—high impact for patients but its relevance can be hampered in elderly patients due to death by other causes and does not include QoL.

8 The Need for Level 1 Clinical Evidence in Daily Practice

Table 8.3 Currently active or complete RCTs in endometrial cancer

Status	Study title	Intervention
Completed	2D Versus 3D Radical Laparoscopic Hysterectomy for Endometrial Cancer: a Prospective Randomized Trial	Procedure: 3D laparoscopy Procedure: standard laparoscopy
Active, not recruiting	Randomized Trial of Radiation Therapy With or Without Chemotherapy for Endometrial Cancer	Radiation: radiation therapy Drug: cisplatin Drug: carboplatin Drug: paclitaxel
Completed	Zoptarelin Doxorubicin (AEZS 108) as Second Line Therapy for Endometrial Cancer	Drug: AEZS-108/zoptarelin doxorubicin Drug: doxorubicin
Completed	Doxorubicin and Cisplatin With or Without Paclitaxel in Treating Patients With Locally Advanced, Metastatic, and/or Relapsed Endometrial Cancer	Drug: cisplatin Drug: doxorubicin hydrochloride Drug: paclitaxel
Completed	Comparison of Two Combination Chemotherapy Regimens Plus Radiation Therapy in Treating Patients With Stage III or Stage IV Endometrial Cancer	Drug: doxorubicin hydrochloride Drug: cisplatin Biological: filgrastim Biological: pegfilgrastim Drug: paclitaxel
Recruiting	Trial of Letrozole + Palbociclib/Placebo in Metastatic Endometrial Cancer	• Drug: palbociclib/placebo • Drug: letrozole
Completed	Combination Chemotherapy With or Without G-CSF in Treating Patients With Stage III, Stage IV, or Recurrent Endometrial Cancer	Biological: filgrastim Drug: cisplatin Drug: doxorubicin hydrochloride Drug: paclitaxel
Recruiting	Trial Between Two Follow up Regimens With Different Test Intensity in Endometrial Cancer Treated Patients	Procedure: intensive/low-risk follow up (IA G1; IA G2) Procedure: intensive/high-risk follow up ($\geq$IA G3) Procedure: minimalist/low-risk follow up (IA G1; IA G2) Procedure: minimalist/high-risk follow up ($\geq$IA G3)
Completed	Radiation Therapy With or Without Chemotherapy in Treating Patients With High-Risk Endometrial Cancer	Drug: cisplatin Drug: doxorubicin hydrochloride Drug: epirubicin hydrochloride Procedure: adjuvant therapy Procedure: conventional surgery Radiation: radiation therapy
Recruiting	Carboplatin-Paclitaxel ± Bevacizumab in Advanced (Stage III–IV) or Recurrent Endometrial Cancer	Drug: bevacizumab Drug: carboplatin AUC 5 + paclitaxel 175 mg/mq q 21 for 6–8 cycles
Completed	Radiation Therapy or Observation Only in Treating Patients With Endometrial Cancer Who Have Undergone Surgery	Radiation: radiation therapy

(continued)

Table 8.3 (continued)

Status	Study title	Intervention
Recruiting	Hormone Receptor Positive endometrIal Carcinoma Treated by Dual mTORC1/mTORC2 Inhibitor and Anastrozole (VICTORIA)	Drug: AZD2014 Drug: anastrozole
Active, not recruiting	Doxorubicin Hydrochloride, Cisplatin, and Paclitaxel or Carboplatin and Paclitaxel in Treating Patients With Stage III–IV or Recurrent Endometrial Cancer	Drug: carboplatin Drug: cisplatin Drug: doxorubicin Hydrochloride Biological: filgrastim Other: laboratory biomarker analysis Drug: paclitaxel Biological: pegfilgrastim
Recruiting	Paclitaxel and Carboplatin With or Without Metformin Hydrochloride in Treating Patients With Stage III, IV, or Recurrent Endometrial Cancer	Drug: carboplatin Other: laboratory biomarker analysis Drug: metformin hydrochloride Drug: paclitaxel Other: placebo
Recruiting	Feasibility Study of Laparoendoscopic Single Site Surgical Staging for Endometrial Cancer	• Procedure: single-port laparoscopic surgical staging • Procedure: four-port laparoscopic surgical staging
Recruiting	Robot Assisted Laparoscopic Hysterectomy vs. Abdominal Hysterectomy in Endometrial Cancer	• Procedure: abdominal total hysterectomy • Procedure: robot assisted laparoscopic hysterectomy
Completed	Temsirolimus With or Without Megestrol Acetate and Tamoxifen Citrate in Treating Patients With Advanced, Persistent, or Recurrent Endometrial Cancer	• Other: laboratory biomarker analysis • Drug: megestrol acetate • Drug: tamoxifen citrate • Drug: temsirolimus
Active, not recruiting	Carboplatin and Paclitaxel With or Without Cisplatin and Radiation Therapy in Treating Patients With Stage I, Stage II, Stage III, or Stage IVA Endometrial Cancer	Drug: carboplatin Drug: cisplatin Radiation: internal radiation therapy Drug: paclitaxel Other: quality-of-life assessment Radiation: radiation therapy
Active, not recruiting	Trametinib With or Without GSK2141795 in Treating Patients With Recurrent or Persistent Endometrial Cancer	• Drug: Akt inhibitor GSK2141795 • Other: laboratory biomarker analysis • Drug: trametinib
Completed Has results	The Study of Oral Steroid Sulphatase Inhibitor BN83495 Versus Megestrol Acetate (MA) in Women With Advanced or Recurrent Endometrial Cancer	• Drug: BN83495 • Drug: megestrol acetate (MA)

Table 8.3 (continued)

Status	Study title	Intervention
Completed	Clinical Trial of Ridaforolimus Compared to Progestin or Chemotherapy for Advanced Endometrial Carcinoma (MK-8669-007 AM6)	• Drug: ridaforolimus • Drug: medroxyprogesterone acetate tablets • OR megestrol acetate • Drug: chemotherapy
Active, not recruiting	Laparoscopic Approach to Cancer of the Endometrium	• Procedure: total abdominal hysterectomy • Procedure: total laparoscopic hysterectomy
Recruiting	Combination Chemotherapy With Nintedanib/Placebo in Endometrial Cancer	Drug: nintedanib or placebo; carboplatin, paclitaxel
Active, not recruiting	Everolimus and Letrozole or Hormonal Therapy to Treat Endometrial Cancer	• Drug: everolimus • Drug: tamoxifen • Drug: letrozole • Drug: medroxyprogesterone acetate
Completed	Tachosil for the Prevention of Symptomatic Lymph Cysts	Drug: tachosil fibrin patch
Recruiting	Evaluation of Sentinel Node Policy in Early Stage Endometrial Carcinomas at Intermediate and High Risk of Recurrence	Drug: pre-operative SN mapping with nanocis Drug: intra-operative SN mapping with patent V blue dye Drug: Intra-operative SN mapping with indocyanin green Procedure: full bilateral laparoscopic lymphadenectomy and hysterectomy Procedure: current initial staging protocols
Completed	Laparoscopic Surgery or Standard Surgery in Treating Patients With Endometrial Cancer or Cancer of the Uterus	• Procedure: laparoscopic surgery • Other: quality-of-life assessment • Procedure: therapeutic conventional surgery
Completed	Radiation Therapy or No Further Treatment Following Surgery in Treating Patients With Cancer of the Uterus	• Radiation: radiation therapy
Completed	A Study Assessing the Safety and Utility of PINPOINT® Near Infrared Fluorescence Imaging in the Identification of Lymph Nodes in Patients With Uterine and Cervical Malignancies Who Are Undergoing Lymph Node Mapping	• Device: PINPOINT
Recruiting	The Efficacy and Safety of the Postoperative Adjuvant Treatment in Patients With High-risk Stage I Endometrial Carcinoma	Drug: paclitaxel Drug: paraplatin (carboplatin injection) Radiation: pelvic radiation Radiation: vaginal brachytherapy 1 Radiation: vaginal brachytherapy 2

(continued)

Table 8.3 (continued)

Status	Study title	Intervention
Completed	Hormone Therapy in Preventing Endometrial Cancer in Patients With a Genetic Risk For Hereditary Nonpolyposis Colon Cancer	• Drug: medroxyprogesterone • Drug: ethinyl estradiol • Drug: norgestrel • Other: laboratory biomarker analysis
Completed	Lifestyle Change and Quality of Life in Obese Patients With Stage I/II Endometrial Cancer in Remission	• Behavioral: behavioral dietary intervention • Other: counseling intervention • Other: educational intervention
Completed	Exercise and Healthy Diet or Standard Care in Patients in Remission From Stage I or Stage II Endometrial Cancer	• Behavioral: behavioral dietary intervention • Behavioral: exercise intervention • Other: counseling intervention
Active, not recruiting	Robotic Versus Abdominal Surgery for Endometrial Cancer	• Procedure: robotic surgery • Procedure: abdominal surgery
Recruiting NEW	A Study of Ketogenic Diet in Newly Diagnosed Overweight or Obese Endometrial Cancer Patients	• Other: ketogenic diet (KD) • Other: standard diet (SD)
Recruiting	Assisted Exercise in Obese Endometrial Cancer Patients	• Behavioral: exercise on stationary recumbent exercise cycle • Behavioral: health education • Behavioral: questionnaires
Active, not recruiting	Evaluation of Carboplatin/Paclitaxel With and Without Trastuzumab (Herceptin) in Uterine Serous Cancer	• Drug: carboplatin/paclitaxel • Drug: trastuzumab
Completed	Surgery With or Without Lymphadenectomy and Radiation Therapy in Treating Patients With Endometrial Cancer	• Procedure: adjuvant therapy • Procedure: conventional surgery • Radiation: brachytherapy • Radiation: radiation therapy
Completed	Comparison of Radiation Therapy With or Without Combination Chemotherapy Following Surgery in Treating Patients With Stage I or Stage II Endometrial Cancer	• Drug: cisplatin • Drug: paclitaxel • Procedure: adjuvant therapy • Radiation: radiation therapy
Recruiting	Chemotherapy or Observation in Stage I–II Intermediate or High Risk Endometrial Cancer	• Drug: carboplatin and paclitaxel • Other: observation
Completed	External-Beam Radiation Therapy Compared With Vaginal Brachytherapy After Surgery for Stage I Endometrial Cancer	• Radiation: external beam radiation therapy • Radiation: vaginal brachytherapy
Recruiting	Phase 2 Study of MLN0128, Combination of MLN0128 With MLN1117, Paclitaxel and Combination of MLN0128 With Paclitaxel in Women With Endometrial Cancer	• Drug: paclitaxel • Drug: MLN0128 • Drug: MLN1117

Table 8.3 (continued)

Status	Study title	Intervention
Recruiting	Radiation Therapy With or Without Cisplatin in Treating Patients With Recurrent Endometrial Cancer	• Radiation: 3-dimensional conformal radiation therapy • Drug: cisplatin • Radiation: intensity-modulated radiation therapy • Radiation: internal radiation therapy
Recruiting	Medroxyprogesterone Acetate With or Without Entinostat Before Surgery in Treating Patients With Endometrioid Endometrial Cancer	• Drug: entinostat • Procedure: hysterectomy • Other: laboratory biomarker analysis • Drug: medroxyprogesterone acetate
Completed	Radiation Therapy Compared With Combination Chemotherapy in Treating Patients With Advanced Endometrial Cancer	• Drug: cisplatin • Drug: doxorubicin hydrochloride • Radiation: low-LET photon therapy
Active, not recruiting	Pelvic Radiation Therapy or Vaginal Implant Radiation Therapy, Paclitaxel, and Carboplatin in Treating Patients With High-Risk Stage I or Stage II Endometrial Cancer	• Radiation: 3-dimensional conformal radiation therapy • Drug: carboplatin • Radiation: intensity-modulated radiation therapy
Active, not recruiting	Standard Versus Intensity-Modulated Pelvic Radiation Therapy in Treating Patients With Endometrial or Cervical Cancer	• Radiation: 3-dimensional conformal radiation therapy • Radiation: intensity-modulated radiation therapy
Completed	Olaparib in Combination With Carboplatin for Refractory or Recurrent Womens Cancers	• Drug: carboplatin • Drug: olaparib
Recruiting	Trial of Cisplatin Plus Radiation Followed by Carbo and Taxol vs. Sandwich Therapy of Carbo and Taxol Followed Radiation Then Further Carbo and Taxol	• Drug: cisplatin • Drug: carboplatin • Drug: paclitaxel • Radiation: radiation therapy
Completed	Surgery With or Without Chemotherapy in Treating Patients With Soft Tissue Sarcoma	Biological: filgrastim Drug: doxorubicin hydrochloride Drug: ifosfamide Drug: isolated perfusion Procedure: adjuvant therapy Procedure: conventional surgery Radiation: radiation therapy
Completed	Endometrial Cancer—LOHP Alone and With 5FU	• Drug: oxaliplatin, 5 FU
Recruiting	Selective Targeting of Adjuvant Therapy for Endometrial Cancer (STATEC)	• Procedure: abdominal surgery • Procedure: lymphadenectomy
Completed Has results	Intravenous Weekly Topotecan In Subjects With Recurrent Or Persistent Endometrial Cancer	• Drug: topotecan

(continued)

Table 8.3 (continued)

Status	Study title	Intervention
Completed	Systematic Pelvic Lymphadenectomy Versus no Lymphadenectomy in Clinical Stage I–II Endometrial Cancer	• Procedure: systematic pelvic lymphadenectomy
Completed	END-1: First Line Chemotherapy for Advanced or Recurrent Endometrial Carcinoma With Carboplatin and Liposomal Doxorubicin	• Drug: liposomal doxorubicin • Drug: carboplatin
Recruiting	Prospective Randomised Phase II Trial Evaluating Adjuvant Pelvic Radiotherapy Using Either IMRT or 3-Dimensional Planning for Endometrial Cancer. ICORG 09-06	Radiation: 45 Gy/25 fractions
Recruiting	A Study of Durvalumab With or Without Tremelimumab in Endometrial Cancer	Drug: durvalumab Drug: tremelimumab
Recruiting	STELLA 2 Trial: Transperitoneal vs. Extraperitoneal Approach for Laparoscopic Staging of Endometrial/Ovarian Cancer	Procedure: extraperitoneal laparoscopic aortic lymphadenectomy Procedure: transperitoneal Laparoscopic aortic lymphadenectomy
Completed	Targeted Disruption to Cancer Metabolism and Growth Through Dietary Macronutrient Modification	Other: ketogenic diet Other: AND diet
Recruiting	Improving the Treatment for Women With Early Stage Cancer of the Uterus	Drug: levonorgestrel Drug: metformin

Disease-specific survival (DSS)—perhaps a better measure but essentially it does not matter to the patient what the cause of death is.

Progression-Free Survival (PFS)—"the length of time during and after the treatment of a disease, such as cancer, that a patient lives with the disease but it does not get worse".

Functional Decline (FD)—a new endpoint which considers if there are new loss of independence in self-care capabilities associated with deterioration in mobility and in the performance of activities of daily living such as dressing, toileting, and bathing. This end-point can be incorporated into elderly patient trials [7].

Overall Treatment Utility (OTU)—at set intervals: was the treatment worthwhile for the patient? Decided by the patient and the clinician.

Good OTU score: satisfied patient, clinician and low toxicity.

Classical endpoints are frequently not suitable for elderly patient populations. Thus, co-primary endpoints are recommended and statisticians often prefer a composite endpoint which can take into account multiple dimensions. A hallmark example of a composite endpoint (overall treatment utility) is illustrated by FOCUS2, a UK phase II randomized trial in which older and frail patients with inoperable colorectal cancer were randomized to receive treatment with infusional fluorouracil/levofolinic acid or capecitabine or either fluoropyrimiide schedule with the addition of oxaliplatin [8]. These drugs were administered at 80% of the standard doses. The composite endpoint included measures of response, toxicity, as well as clinician and patient perception of treatment efficacy. This trial is an exceptional example of how clinical trials can address the needs of the patient population at hand with well-designed and rational clinical end-points.

8.5 Clinical Trials in the New Era of Personalized Medicine

Several terms, including *precision medicine*, *stratified medicine*, *targeted medicine*, and *pharmacogenomics*, are sometimes used interchangeably to describe *personalized medicine* [9]. The European Union describes personalized medicine as "providing the right treatment to the right patient, at the right dose at the right time." The National Cancer Institute extends upon this definition by stating that personalized medicine is "a form of medicine that uses information about a person's genes, proteins, and environment to prevent, diagnose, and treat disease" [9]. In order to fulfill this health delivery ethos, future clinical trial designs must be able to accessibly integrate molecular analysis such as next-generation sequencing in order to profile patient prior to entry into intervention studies. Furthermore, a number of parallel translational research activities must be performed in order to tailor personalized medicine for future patient populations. Endometrial cancer is no exception to the diseases which can be approached with this transformative healthcare approach. Below are some key definitions of relevant clinical trial designs.

Comparative Trials: also known as controlled, clinical trials involve one group of patients who receive the new drug and a control group who receives a placebo or gold standard treatment. Comparative studies are typically conducted as double-blind trials, where neither the physician nor the patient knows which group is receiving the new drug. Double-blind trials help to eliminate any biased results [10].

Open Label Trials: do not attempt to disguise the new drug or treatment, meaning that no standard treatment or placebo is utilized. This leans towards bias, as both the patient and the physician are aware of which groups are receiving what type of treatment [10].

Basket Trials: test the effect of one drug on a single mutation in a variety of tumor types, at the same time. These studies also have the potential to greatly increase the number of patients who are eligible to receive certain drugs relative to other trial designs [11].

Umbrella Trials: have many different treatment arms within one trial and one indication. People are assigned to a particular treatment arm of the trial based on their type of cancer and the specific molecular makeup of their cancer [11].

The phases of clinical trials are described as I, II, and III below [11].

Phase I Clinical Trials: An experimental drug or treatment, which has proven to be safe for use in animals, is tested in a small group of people (15–30) for the first time. Data are collected on the dose, timing, and safety of the treatment. The purpose is to evaluate its safety and identify side effects.

Phase II Clinical Trial: An experimental drug or treatment is tested in a larger group (100 or less) to provide more detailed information about the safety of the treatment, in addition to evaluating how well it works for a broader range of people. Phase II trials usually take about 2 years to complete.

Phase III Clinical Trials: Before an experimental drug or treatment is approved by the FDA and made available to the public, Phase III trials are conducted on a large group of people (from 100 to several thousand). At least two (and often more than two treatment options, including standard of care) are compared to find out whether the new treatment is better, and possibly has fewer side effects, than the current standard treatment. Phase III clinical trials are usually randomized, meaning that patients receive either the investigational drug or treatment or another drug or treatment in a non-ordered way.

Phase IV Clinical Trial: After a drug is approved by the FDA and made available to the public, researchers track its safety, seeking more information about a drug or treatment's risks, benefits, and optimal use. Several hundred to several thousand people participate in Phase IV trials.

Future clinical trial design for endometrial cancer patients must progress with the innovations achieved across other cancer forms such as the inclusion of a translational research aspects across all phases of trials, pre-stratification of patients via next-generation sequencing (NGS), and or immuno-profiling. Evidence-based medicine is an approach to clinical problem-solving which will continue to drive better treatment options for patients with endometrial cancer.

References

1. Guyatt G. Dave Sackett and the ethos of the EBM community. J Clin Epidemiol. 2016;73:75.
2. Sackett DL, Rosenberg WM, Gray JM, Haynes RB, Richardson WS. Evidence based medicine. Br Med J. 1996;313(7050):170.
3. Fletcher RH, Fletcher SW. David Sackett was one of a kind. J Clin Epidemiol. 2016;73:67–72.
4. DeMets DL. Methods for combining randomized clinical trials: strengths and limitations. Stat Med. 1987;6(3):341–8.
5. Chalmers TC, Smith H, Blackburn B, Silverman B, Schroeder B, Reitman D, Ambroz A. A method for assessing the quality of a randomized control trial. Control Clin Trials. 1981;2(1):31–49.
6. Davis C, Naci H, Gurpinar E, Poplavska E, Pinto A, Aggarwal A. Availability of evidence of benefits on overall survival and quality of life of cancer drugs approved by European Medicines Agency: retrospective cohort study of drug approvals 2009-13. Br Med J. 2017;359:j4530.
7. McVey LJ, Becker PM, Saltz CC, Feussner JR, Cohen HJ. Effect of a geriatric consultation team on functional status of elderly hospitalized patients: a randomized, controlled clinical trial. Ann Intern Med. 1989;110:79–84.
8. Ring A, Harari D, Kalsi T, Mansi J, Selby P, editors. Problem solving in older cancer patients: a case-study based reference and learning resource. Oxford: Clinical Publishing; 2016.

9. US Food and Drug Administration. Paving the way for personalized medicine: FDA's role in a new era of medical product development. Silver Spring: US Food and Drug Administration; 2013.
10. Accord Clinical. https://www.accordclinical.com/clinical-study/types-of-clinical-trials/. Accessed 18 Oct 2017.
11. ASCO. https://www.asco.org/research-progress/clinical-trials/clinical-trial-resources/clinical-trial-design-and-methodology#Other%20Types. Accessed 18 Oct 2017.

Summary of Management Guidelines for Endometrial Cancer

9

Ilaria Colombo, Stephanie Lheureux, and Amit M. Oza

Important aspects of endometrial cancer management remain active areas for research to better define how to improve patient outcome. Controversy remains in many areas of clinical management and is the subject of continued research. For example, this includes: the role for extensive lymphadenectomy in early stage endometrial cancer; how to optimally select patients who would benefit most from adjuvant treatment; and how to combine or sequence radiotherapy and chemotherapy in the adjuvant setting. Results from clinical trials are eagerly awaited to address this uncertainty.

Evidence-based guidelines to support physician choices are necessary and need to be updated as new data from clinical trials becomes available. Evidence-based recommendations are usually presented as a final document summarizing the consensus obtained from a multidisciplinary panel of experts in the management of endometrial cancer. Clinicians should follow evidence-based guidelines in daily practice using their judgment to tailor diagnosis and treatment procedures on a patient-to-patient basis.

9.1 Summary of ESMO-ESGO-ESTRO Clinical Practice Guidelines

In December 2014, the first joint consensus conference on endometrial cancer involving the European Society for Medical Oncology (ESMO), the European Society for Radiotherapy and Oncology (ESTRO), and the European Society of Gynecological Oncology (ESMO) experts took place in Milan, Italy. The panel of experts was tasked with answering specific clinically relevant questions on

---

I. Colombo (✉) · S. Lheureux · A. M. Oza
Gynecology and Drug Development Program, Princess Margaret Cancer Centre,
Toronto, ON, Canada
e-mail: ilaria.colombo@uhn.ca

controversial topics. Results have since been published adding details to 2013 ESMO Clinical Practice Guidelines [1, 2]. Notably, a high level of consensus has been reached between the panel members with an agreement of 94–100% on all 12 questions discussed during the consensus conference.

9.1.1 Diagnosis and Staging

The most common symptom of presentation for endometrial cancer is postmenopausal vaginal bleeding. In the past few years there has been a trend in the use of less-invasive techniques for endometrial cancer diagnosis and the 2013 ESMO guidelines having already recognized ultrasound and endometrial biopsy as the preferred exams for diagnosis, replacing the more invasive dilatation and curettage (D&C).

The recent consensus conference has further explored the role of surveillance for women at risk for endometrial cancer in specific settings, underlining the following recommendations:

- Women with average-increased risk for endometrial cancer (unopposed estrogen therapy, late menopause, tamoxifen therapy, nulliparity, infertility or failure to ovulate, obesity, diabetes, or hypertension): routine surveillance is not recommended.
- Women with granulosa cell tumor with no hysterectomy performed: endometrial sampling is recommended. If this does not show malignancies or premalignancies no further screening is required.
- Women with epithelial ovarian cancer undergoing fertility-sparing treatment: endometrial sampling is recommended at the time of diagnosis.
- Women receiving treatment with tamoxifen: routine screening for endometrial cancer is not recommended.
- Women with high risk for endometrial cancer (known carriers of Lynch Syndrome or subjects without genetic test performed but strong cancer family history): surveillance of the endometrium by gynecological examination, transvaginal ultrasound and aspiration biopsy starting from age 35 performed annually until hysterectomy. Prophylactic surgery should be discussed at the age of 40.

In the 2013 ESMO Guidelines authors reported that pre-surgery evaluation may include chest X-ray, clinical and gynecological examination, transvaginal ultrasound, blood counts, liver and renal function profiles, abdominal computed tomography (CT) to exclude the presence of extra pelvic disease, magnetic resonance imaging (MRI) for myometrial invasion definition, and 18F-Fluoro-2-deoxyglucose-positron emission tomography (FDG-PET)/CT to detect distant metastasis. Updated recommendations go on to further define which tests are mandatory and which are optional. For example, the mandatory preoperative work-up includes: family history, assessment of comorbidities, geriatric assessment if appropriate, clinical examination including pelvic exam, transvaginal or trans-rectal ultrasound, complete pathological assessment of endometrial biopsy or curettage specimen with indication of histological subtype and grade. Optional preoperative work-up may include: expert ultrasound or MRI or intraoperative pathological examination of the uterus to assess myometrial invasion in clinical stage I grade 1 and 2; thoracic, abdominal, and pelvic CT scan or MRI or PET scan or ultrasound should be considered to exclude ovarian, peritoneal, nodal, or metastatic disease. There is no indication for serum tumor markers dosing, including CA125.

For the first time during this consensus conference there was a discussion regarding the use of immunohistochemistry (IHC) to distinguish between precancerous or cancerous lesions and benign abnormalities when diagnosis is unclear based only on morphological characteristics.

IHC analysis recommended by the panel are:

- PTEN and PAX-2 to distinguish atypical hyperplasia/endometrial intraepithelial neoplasia from benign mimics. Others could be MLH1 and ARID1a.
- IHC is not recommended to distinguish atypical polypoid adenomyoma from atypical hyperplasia or endometrial intraepithelial neoplasia.
- p53 to distinguish between serous endometrial intraepithelial carcinoma from its mimics.
- ER, vimentin, CEA, and p16 to exclude possible endocervical origin of the tumor.
- For serous tumors WT-1 may help to discriminate ovarian origin.
- Atypical hyperplasia/endometrial intraepithelial neoplasia distinguished by endometrioid endometrial cancer (ECC) by morphology and not IHC.

9.1.2 Treatment

9.1.2.1 Surgical Management

The cornerstone of treatment in endometrial cancer is surgery, consisting of total hysterectomy (TH) and bilateral salpingo-oophorectomy (BSO) with or without lymphadenectomy. Over the last several years, minimally invasive surgical techniques have been accepted as substitute for laparotomy with significant benefit in reduction of hospital stay, fewer complications, less surgery-related pain, and an improvement in patient quality of life. The consensus recommends this technique for low-intermediate risk endometrial cancer and states that this can be considered in the management of high-risk endometrial cancer. For patients with low-risk endometrial cancer unsuitable for standard surgical treatment, vaginal hysterectomy with BSO could be a considerable option. Should surgery be contraindicated for other medical conditions, radiation therapy or hormone therapy could be considered.

One of the main controversial topics in the surgical management of endometrial cancer is the role of lymphadenectomy. Lymphadenectomy should be considered a staging procedure and it is relevant to define the need for adjuvant treatment. The updated guidelines have defined specific indication for lymphadenectomy according to the level of risk and include:

- Low-risk tumors (grade 1 or 2 and myometrial invasion <50%) lymphadenectomy *is not* recommended.
- Intermediate risk (grade 3 or myometrial invasion >50%) lymphadenectomy *can be* considered for staging purposes.
- High-risk (grade 3 and myometrial invasion >50%): lymphadenectomy *should be* recommended.
- High-risk patients who have received incomplete surgery need to complete staging with lymphadenectomy to better address adjuvant therapy.

When lymphadenectomy is considered, removal of pelvic and para-aortic nodes up to the level of the renal veins should be considered. An interesting technique already established in other cancer types is the sentinel lymph node dissection (SLND) that has been shown to be feasible also in endometrial cancer although remains experimental. For that reason, guidelines did not recommend SLND as standard procedure. Surgical recommendations are listed in Table 9.1 below.

For ovarian preservation, the panel recommends that this can be considered for women less than 45 years of age with stage I G1 endometrioid endometrial cancer and less 50% of myometrial invasion and no obvious ovarian or extrauterine disease. In case of ovarian preservation, salpingectomy is recommended. Ovarian preservation is not recommended for patients with cancer family history involving risk for ovarian cancer (e.g. *BRCA* mutation or Lynch Syndrome) and in patients with non-endometrioid histology.

9.1.3 Fertility Preserving Treatment for Grade 1 Endometrioid Tumors

Standard management for endometrial cancer in young women of childbearing age is hysterectomy and bilateral salpingo-oophorectomy (BSO). A conservative approach using oral progestin may be considered for grade 1 tumors; however,

Table 9.1 Surgery recommendation according to tumor stage

Stage		Recommendation	LOE
I	IA G1–2	TH + BSO	I
	IA G3	TH + BSO +/− bilateral pelvic-para-aortic lymphadenectomy	II
	IB	TH + BSO +/− bilateral pelvic-para-aortic lymphadenectomy	II
II		TH + BSO + bilateral pelvic-para-aortic lymphadenectomy Radical hysterectomy considered only if required to obtain free margins	IV
III		Maximal surgical cytoreduction and comprehensive staging Multimodality management to be considered when surgery may impact vaginal function	IV
IV	IVA	Anterior and posterior pelvic exenteration	IV
	IVB	Systemic therapy with consideration for palliative surgery	IV

TH total hysterectomy, *BSO* bilateral salpingo-oophorectomy, *LOE* level of evidence

the panel strongly recommends that patients must be referred to a specialized center and received dilatation and curettage (D&C) for accurate histological diagnosis; pathology results need to be confirmed by a specialized gynecologist pathologist; and a pelvic MRI is required to exclude myometrial invasion. Patients must be informed that fertility-sparing treatment is not a standard treatment and should be willing to accept close follow-up and possible hysterectomy if needed. Recommended treatment options are medroxyprogesterone acetate 400–600 mg/day or megestrol acetate 160–320 mg/day; levonorgestrel intrauterine device with or without gonadotropin-releasing hormone can also be considered. Response to treatment should be assessed after 6 months with imaging and D&C. If no response is documented, standard surgical treatment is warranted. Patients with response will be encouraged to conception followed by hysterectomy. Patients who prefer to delay pregnancy need to be followed every 6 months with hysteroscopy.

9.1.4 Adjuvant Treatment

Endometrial cancer has been divided in risk categories according to clinical and pathological features to identify patients that may benefit more from adjuvant treatment. The recent consensus conference has updated the previously used risk categories adding lymphovascular space invasion (LVSI) as prognostic factor following data from trials and meta-analysis [3–6] (Table 9.2).

Table 9.2 Risk groups to guide adjuvant treatment (ESMO/ESGO/ESTRO)

Risk group	Description	LOE
Low	Stage I[a] endometroid, rade 1–2, <50% myometrial invasion, LVSI negative	I
Intermediate	Stage I endometrioid, grade 1–2, ≥50% myometrial invasion, LVSI neg	I
High-intermediate	– Stage I endometrioid, grade 3, <50% myometrial invasion, regardless of LVSI status	I
	– Stage I endometrioid, grade 1–2, LVSI unequivocally positive, regardless of depth of invasion	II
High	– Stage I endometrioid, grade 3, ≥50% myometrial invasion, regardless of LVSI status	I
	– Stage II	I
	– Stage III endometrioid, no residual disease	I
	– Non-endometrioid (serous or clear cell or undifferentiated carcinoma or carcinosarcoma)	I
Advanced	Stage III residual disease and stage IVA	I
Metastatic	Stage IVB	I

LOE level of evidence, *LVSI* lymphovascular space invasion
[a]Stages are defined according to FIGO 2009

The current recommendations from ESMO/ESGO/ESTRO consensus have updated the previous guidelines according to the more specific definition of risk groups. New details have been added to define indication for adjuvant treatment when surgical staging has not been performed and more importance has been given to histological subtype with specific indication for adjuvant chemotherapy for non-endometrioid tumors. These recommendations are summarized in Table 9.3 below.

9.1.5 Advanced and Recurrent Endometrial Cancer

Standard treatment for loco-regional relapse is dependent upon the site of relapse and previous treatment. In case of vaginal relapse after surgery the standard treatment is external beam radiation therapy combined with brachytherapy. In the case of central pelvic recurrence surgery or radiotherapy are possible options. Regional pelvic recurrence needs to be treated with radiation and if possible with chemotherapy. In the case of previous radiation, retreatment could be considered in highly selected patients using specialized techniques, like IMRT (intensity modulated radiation therapy) and SBRT (stereotactic body radiation therapy).

For local advanced endometrial cancer, complete agreement on the best management has not been reached and usually a combination of surgery, radiation, and chemotherapy is used. When optimal cytoreduction can be achieved, surgical cytoreduction is recommended. When tumor is unresectable or surgery is contraindicated, radiation may be indicated. Palliative surgery and palliative radiation may be considered for symptom control. In the case of oligo-metastases or pelvic or retroperitoneal lymph node relapse, if complete resection could be achieved the surgery must be considered.

Systemic treatment available for relapsed or metastatic endometrioid tumors are hormone therapy and chemotherapy. Hormone therapy is indicated in endometrioid endometrial cancer and is more likely to be effective in grade 1 and 2 tumors without rapidly progressive disease. Hormone receptor status should be determined before hormone therapy is initiated and biopsy of recurrence could be considered as there may be differences between primary and metastatic tumors. Agents to be considered are progestogens, tamoxifen, aromatase inhibitors, and fulvestrant. Standard chemotherapy is represented by six cycles of 3 weekly carboplatin and paclitaxel. No standard of care is available for second-line chemotherapy.

9.1.6 Follow-up

ESMO guidelines suggest follow-up visit every 3–4 months with physical and gynecological examination for the first 2 years after radical treatment and then every 6 months until 5 years. Further investigations with CT, MRI, PET scans or ultrasound could be performed if clinically indicated. There is no role for routinely perform PAP smear to detected vaginal recurrence.

9 Summary of Management Guidelines for Endometrial Cancer

Table 9.3 Adjuvant treatment options (ESMO/ESGO/ESTRO guidelines)

Risk group	Adjuvant treatment	LOE
Low-	– Observation	I
Intermediate	– Adjuvant brachytherapy	I
	– Observation (specially <60 years old)	II
High-intermediate	Surgical node staging performed and negative:	
	– Adjuvant brachytherapy	III
	– Observation	III
	No surgical node staging:	
	– Adjuvant EBRT for LVSI unequivocally positive	III
	– Adjuvant brachytherapy for grade 3 and LVSI negative	III
	Benefit from adjuvant chemotherapy is uncertain	III
High risk	*Stage I*	
	Surgical node staging performed and negative:	
	– EBRT should be considered	I
	– Adjuvant brachytherapy may be considered	III
	– Adjuvant systemic therapy is under investigation	II
	No surgical nodal staging:	
	– Adjuvant EBRT is recommended	III
	– Sequential chemotherapy may be considered	II
	– More evidence for giving chemotherapy and EBRT in combination rather than either treatment alone	II
	Stage II	
	Surgical node staging performed and negative:	
	– If grade 1–2, LVSI neg vaginal brachytherapy	III
	– If grade 3 or LVIS positive:	
	EBRT	III
	Consider brachytherapy boost	IV
	Chemotherapy is under investigation	III
	No surgical node staging:	
	– EBRT is recommended	III
	– Consider brachytherapy boost	IV
	– \For grade 3 or LVSI positive, sequential adjuvant chemotherapy should be considered	III
	Stage III	
	– EBRT	I
	– Chemotherapy	II
	– More evidence to give chemotherapy and EBRT in combination than either alone	II
	Non-endometrioid	
	Serous and clear cell	
	– Consider chemotherapy and encourage clinical trials	III
	– Stage IA, LVSI negative: Consider only vaginal brachytherapy with no chemotherapy	IV
	– Stage ≥IB: EBRT may be considered in addition to chemotherapy specially if nodes positive carcinosarcoma and undifferentiated tumors	III
	– Chemotherapy is recommended	II
	– Consider EBRT, clinical trials are encouraged	III

LOE level of evidence, *EBRT* external beam radiotherapy, *LVSI* lymphovascular space invasion

9.2 Summary of NCCN and SGO Guidelines

The National Comprehensive Cancer Network (NCCN) guidelines have been developed by a multidisciplinary panel of experts from major US oncological centers. These guidelines are strictly evidence-based and are an important tool to guide clinicians in their daily decision-making process. These guidelines are continuously updated considering the increasing availability of data from clinical trials and as such, the guidelines cover the different aspects of cancer management, from diagnosis to treatment. NCCN indications have, unless otherwise specified, level 2A evidence (see Appendix). Level 1 evidence recommendations are not available as consequence of lack of high level evidence from clinical trials. The last updated version is 2.2016 accessible on line at www.nccn.org [7].

The Society of Gynecologic Oncology (SGO) has developed a series of clinical documents to provide evidence-based information on how to better treat women with endometrial cancer. In 2014 the SGO's Clinical Practice Committee created recommendations published in the *Gynecologic Oncology* journal [8, 9] and a Practice Bulletin has also been published on April 2015 in collaboration with The American College of Obstetricians and Gynecologists [10].

9.2.1 Diagnosis and Staging

For women with suspected uterine neoplasm NCCN guidelines recommend initial work-up with history collection, physical examination, complete blood count, endometrial biopsy, and expert pathology review. In case of negative biopsy, dilatation, and curettage under anesthesia needs to be performed and hysteroscopy could be useful. Optional tests may include biochemistry and genetic testing for possible Lynch Syndrome. Immunohistochemistry (IHC) for defective DNA mismatch repair and/or microsatellite instability (MSI) could also be considered to select patients that should undergo genetic testing.

For disease staging, CT scan, MRI, or PET scan may be done as clinically indicated, but are not mandatory. The tumor marker CA125 could be considered and may be helpful in monitoring clinical response, especially in non-endometrioid tumors.

The SGO guidelines are in accordance with NCCN guidelines and highlight the importance to exclude malignancy in each woman presenting with postmenopausal bleeding that needs to be assessed with transvaginal ultrasound and endometrial biopsy. If these are not conclusive, D&C and/or hysteroscopy may be required.

9.2.2 Treatment

NCCN guidelines provide recommendations about which primary treatment is indicated accordingly to disease extension and histological subtypes differentiating endometrioid and non-endometrioid tumors, as reported in Table 9.4.

9 Summary of Management Guidelines for Endometrial Cancer

Table 9.4 Primary treatment according to NCCN guidelines

Endometrioid tumors	
Disease limited to the uterus	*Medically operable*: – TH/BSO and surgical staging
	Not suitable for primary surgery: – RT – In selected patient hormone therapy could be considered
Cervical involvement	*Medically operable*: – TH/BSO and surgical staging or – RT (category 2B) +/− chemotherapy followed by TH/BSO and surgical staging
	Not suitable for primary surgery: – RT +/− chemotherapy followed by surgical resection if become operable or – Chemotherapy (category 2B) followed by surgery if become operable or followed by RT if still not operable
Extrauterine disease	*Intra-abdominal (ascites, omentum, nodes, ovaries, peritoneum)*: – TH/BSO + staging/surgical debulking with the goal to have no measurable disease – Preoperative chemotherapy could be considered
	Initially unresectable extrauterine pelvic disease (vaginal, bladder, bowel, rectum, parametrial invasion): – RT+ brachytherapy +/− chemotherapy or – Chemotherapy followed by radiation or surgery if become operable
	Extra-abdominal or liver metastasis: – Chemotherapy or – RT or – Hormone therapy or – Combinations of these treatments – Palliative TH/BSO may be considered
Non endometrioid (serous, clear cell and carcinosarcoma)	
– Primary treatment may include TH/BSO and surgical staging as for ovarian cancer and effort needs to be done to achieve maximal tumor debulking – In case of extensive disease neoadjuvant chemotherapy may be considered	

TH total hysterectomy, *BSO* bilateral salpingo-oophorectomy, *RT* radiation therapy

9.2.3 Surgical Management

For NCCN guidelines the milestone surgical procedure is total hysterectomy and bilateral-salpingo-oophorectomy with pelvic nodal dissection continuing to be an important element of surgical staging. However, the indication for para-aortic lymph nodes remains controversial. In these recently updated guidelines, the panel recommendation is to reserve full lymphadenectomy for selected patients to avoid overtreatment, considering the lack of data supporting routine use of extensive lymphadenectomy [11]. It is important to note that the possibility to select patients with nodal involvement who could benefit from adjuvant treatment is still the main indication for pelvic and para-aortic node dissection. Preoperative and operative findings may guide the decision to perform lymphadenectomy. Tumors with less than 50% of myometrial invasion, less than 2 cm of dimension, and with well or moderate differentiation may have a low risk of nodes spread and these criteria could be used to identify patients with no benefit from lymphadenectomy, although not confirmed by randomized trials [12]. In conclusion NCCN panel recommends that para-aortic lymphadenectomy should be offered to selected patients with high risk endometrial cancer.

Another element of controversy is the adoption of sentinel lymph node mapping. This may be used for patients with disease confined to the uterus and with low-risk features to avoid morbidity related to extensive lymphadenectomy [13]. The panel suggests that this technique may be considered in centers with high levels of expertise but not routinely applied especially in non-endometrioid histology.

SGO guidelines detail the importance of having surgery performed by high surgical volume centers to reduce complications and improve patients' outcome. As for NCCN panel, also for SGO guidelines indication for comprehensive surgical staging including lymphadenectomy is still under discussion. The importance of surgical staging in define prognostic information to further address adjuvant treatment is still maintained. It is also recognized that low-grade and early-stage tumors may not benefit from extensive surgery that could potentially increase the risk of overtreatment and complications. Sentinel lymph node mapping has shown promising results; although, in the absence of prospective clinical trials this technique cannot be applied routinely. Taken together, SGO consensus defines that the standard surgical management needs to include TH, BSO, pelvic and para-aortic lymphadenectomy, and collection of peritoneal cytology. In accordance with NCCN, SGO guidelines also define the importance of optimal cytoreductive surgery for stage III and IV endometrial carcinoma considering that patients without macroscopic residual disease could achieve a benefit in survival [14].

Surgical technique guidelines describe the trend to move from laparotomy to minimally invasive surgical approaches with laparoscopy and robotic-assisted laparoscopy. Vaginal approach is not acceptable for patients with malignant neoplasm, unless for early stage tumor in patients at high risk of surgical morbidity.

9.2.3.1 Incomplete Surgical Staging

For patients that have not received complete surgery, the NCCN panel recommends surgical restaging with lymph node dissection in patients with high-grade and deeply invasive tumors, as specified below.

- If stage IA, G1–2 and <50% myometrial invasion, no lympho-vascular space invasion (LVSI) and <2 cm tumor: observe, no further surgery.
- If stage IA, G1–2 and <50% myometrial invasion with LVSI or >2 cm or IA, G3 or IB or II and imaging negative for suspicious persistence disease: no indication for further surgery. Indication for adjuvant treatment as will be described after.
- If IA, G1–2 and <50% myometrial invasion with LVSI or >2 cm or IA G3 or IB or II and imaging positive or suspicious for persistence of disease: surgical restaging indicated and then define indication for adjuvant treatment as described after.

- If IA, G1–2 and <50% myometrial invasion with LVSI or >2 cm or IA G3 or IB or II with no images available: consider surgical restaging.

SGO guidelines are concordant with NCCN and suggest that patients incidentally diagnosed with endometrial cancer after hysterectomy planned for other reason, need to be carefully reviewed for complete staging balancing benefit and risks. In the case of G1 or G2 tumors, endometrioid histology, small tumor volume, superficial or no myometrial invasion, further surgery may not be indicated considering the low risk of relapse. Patients with high risk of extrauterine disease, such as patients with high-risk histological subtypes, G3 tumors, or deep myometrial invasion, should be considered for complete surgery.

9.2.3.2 Fertility-Sparing Surgery

According to both NCCN and SGO guidelines, fertility-sparing surgery could be considered if all these criteria are present:

- G1 endometrioid adenocarcinoma on dilatation and curettage
- Disease limited to endometrium as defined by MRI or transvaginal ultrasound
- No metastatic disease on imaging
- No contraindication to medical therapy and pregnancy
- Patients who have received counselling and are made aware that fertility-sparing option is not standard of care

If all of the above criteria are met, the patient could receive progesterone-based treatment and new endometrial sampling needs to be performed every 3–6 months. If after 6 months a complete response is achieved, the patient will be encouraged to get pregnant and have TH/BSO after childbearing. If after 6 months endometrial cancer will still be present, patient will undergo surgery.

9.2.4 Adjuvant Treatment

Indication to adjuvant treatment (chemotherapy, radiation or both) is defined according to the estimated risk of recurrence that is strictly related to presence of risk factors [15]. Risks factors associated with increased risk of recurrence include tumor stage, age, G2 or G3, presence of lympho-vascular space invasion, outer-third myometrial invasion, tumor size, and lower uterine segment involvement. NCCN indications for adjuvant treatment are detailed in Table 9.5 for endometrioid histology and in Table 9.6 for non-endometrioid histology. Of note, NCCN guidelines use TNM seventh edition 2010.

SGO guidelines give essentially the same indication, suggesting the consideration of adjuvant treatment when risk factors are present. The lack of data regarding the best approach for adjuvant treatment has again been highlighted in these guidelines and as such, data from ongoing trials are eagerly awaited to help answer these outstanding questions (single modality treatment versus combination, sequential approach versus

Table 9.5 Adjuvant treatment indication for endometrioid tumors

Stage	Risk factors	Grade	Treatment
IA	No	G1	Observation
		G2	Observation or Vaginal brachytherapy[a]
		G3	Observation or Vaginal brachytherapy
	Yes	G1	Observation or Vaginal brachytherapy
		G2	Observation or Vaginal brachytherapy and/or EBRT (external beam RT, category 2B)
		G3	Observation or Vaginal brachytherapy and/or EBRT (category 2B)
IB	No	G1	Observation or Vaginal brachytherapy
		G2	Observation or Vaginal brachytherapy
		G3	Vaginal brachytherapy and/or EBRT or Observe (category 2B)
	Yes	G1	Observation or Vaginal brachytherapy and/or EBRT
		G2	Observation or Vaginal brachytherapy and/or EBRT
		G3	EBRT and/or vaginal brachytherapy Chemotherapy could be considered (category 2B)
II		G1	Vaginal brachytherapy and/or EBRT
		G2	Vaginal brachytherapy and/or EBRT
		G3	EBRT +/− vaginal brachytherapy +/− chemotherapy (category 2B)
IIIA			Chemotherapy +/− RT or Tumor-directed RT +/− chemotherapy or EBRT +/− vaginal brachytherapy
IIIB			Chemotherapy or Radiotherapy or Chemotherapy + tumor-directed RT
IIIC			Chemotherapy or Radiotherapy or Chemotherapy + tumor-directed RT
IV, with no macroscopic residual disease			Chemotherapy +/− RT

RT radiotherapy, *EBRT* external beam radiotherapy
[a]RT needs to start as soon as the vaginal cuff has healed, no later than 12 weeks from surgery. Standard adjuvant and first-line chemotherapy is represented by combination of carboplatin and paclitaxel

Table 9.6 Adjuvant treatment indication for non-endometrioid tumors

Stage	Treatment
IA	Observation or Chemotherapy +/− vaginal brachytherapy or Tumor-directed RT
IB, II, III, IV	Chemotherapy +/− tumor-directed RT

RT radiotherapy

sandwich). The SGO panel specifies that in stage I and II, radiation can reduce the relapse rate but will not influence the overall survival [6]. Patients with early-stage disease can receive brachytherapy instead of whole pelvic radiation with same efficacy but less toxicity [16]. Moreover, these guidelines do not recommend the use of adjuvant chemotherapy for stage I and II as there is no evidence from randomized trials.

9.2.5 Treatment at Relapse

The NCCN panel has defined possible treatment options for relapsed endometrial cancer according to the site of relapse: loco-regional relapse, isolated metastasis, and disseminated metastasis.

9.2.5.1 Loco-regional Relapse
Optimal treatment depends on previous management and specific site of local relapse:

- No previous radiation (RT): RT and brachytherapy or surgery, if feasible.
- Previous brachytherapy:
  o disease confined to vagina: tumor-directed RT +/− brachytherapy +/− chemotherapy,
  o disease in pelvic lymph nodes: tumor-directed RT +/− brachytherapy +/− chemotherapy,
  o disease in para-aortic or common iliac lymph nodes: tumor-directed RT +/− chemotherapy.
- Previous external beam BRT: surgical resection +/− IORT (intraoperative radiotherapy, category 3 for IORT) or hormone therapy or chemotherapy.

9.2.5.2 Isolated Metastases
If amenable of local treatment, resection and/or RT or ablative therapy (category 2B) or chemotherapy (category 3) may be considered. If local treatment is not feasible or there is further relapse after local treatment, the patient needs to be treated as having disseminated disease.

9.2.5.3 Disseminated Metastases
In the case of low-grade tumor, asymptomatic progression or expression of estrogen/progestin receptors hormone therapy is recommended. If disease is symptomatic, the

tumor is moderate-poor differentiated or large burden of disease is present, recommendation is for chemotherapy with or without palliative RT for symptoms control. When possible, enrollment in clinical trials must be considered specially for second or more advanced line of treatment.

First-line chemotherapy is represented by a combination of carboplatin and paclitaxel and has shown same efficacy but less toxicity compared to triple agents combination [17]. No defined standard second-line chemotherapy is available. Chemotherapy agents most commonly used for second or more advanced lines are doxorubicin, weekly paclitaxel, topotecan, cisplatin, and carboplatin. As hormone treatment, megestrol, tamoxifen, or aromatase inhibitors can be administered.

9.2.6 Follow-up

According to NCCN and SGO guidelines, follow-up of patients with endometrial cancer that have received radical treatment needs to include:

- Physical exam every 3–6 months for 2–3 years then every 6 months for other 2–3 years then annually.
- CA125 is optional.
- Imaging as clinically indicated for suspicious disease relapse.
- Consider genetic counseling/testing for patients less than 50 years old and those with a significant family history of endometrial and/or colorectal cancer or with IHC on their tumors showing mismatch repair system deficiency.
- Patient education about symptoms of recurrence and importance of healthy lifestyle.

9.3 Conclusions

The guidelines described in this chapter have attempted to provide evidence-based recommendations for diagnosis, treatment, and follow-up of endometrial cancer. There remains significant uncertainty around several therapeutic topics because there is little to no level 1 evidence. Trial heterogeneity is one of the limitations of data available for endometrial cancer today, translating into varying approaches in real-life practice that are often dependent on the center or physician preference. Examples of this include:

- the indication and extension of lymphadenectomy for intermediate risk endometrial cancer;
- when to offer adjuvant treatment to patient that had radical surgery and the choice between mono- or multimodality approaches for adjuvant treatment;
- how to combine adjuvant chemotherapy and radiotherapy or which is the best second line of treatment.

The different guidelines can also express some discordance in the opinion of the panel of experts, notably the approach related to lymphadenectomy.

Regarding indication for adjuvant treatment, the main difference between those guidelines is the definition of risk groups. ESMO guidelines have proposed a division of endometrial cancer in six risk groups: low, intermediate, high-intermediate, high, advanced, and metastatic. The indication for adjuvant treatment is defined according to the risk group but also the presence or absence of surgical node staging. NCCN guidelines do not include surgical staging as a factor to guide adjuvant treatment and have not created groups of risk. Furthermore, grade 1 and 2 tumors are considered separately for adjuvant treatment indication in NCCN but not in ESMO recommendations.

Future clinical trials are needed to address areas of uncertainty to define optimal clinical practice for patients.

Appendix

NCCN categories of evidence

Category	Definition
1	Based upon high-level evidence, there is uniform NCCN consensus that intervention is appropriate
2A	Based upon lower-level evidence, there is uniform NCCN consensus that the intervention is appropriate
2B	Based upon lower-level evidence, there is NCCN consensus that the intervention is appropriate
3	Based upon any level of evidence, there is major NCCN disagreement that the intervention is appropriate

Levels of evidence and grades of recommendations used in ESMO guidelines[a]

Levels of evidence	
I	Evidence from at least one large randomized controlled trial of good methodological quality (low potential for bias) or meta-analyses of well-conducted, randomized trials without heterogeneity
II	Small randomized trials or large randomized trials with a suspicion of bias (lower methodological quality) or meta-analyses of such trials or of trials with demonstrated heterogeneity
III	Prospective cohort studies
IV	Retrospective cohort studies or case-control studies
V	Studies without control group, case reports, expert opinions

Grades of recommendation	
A	Strong evidence for efficacy with a substantial clinical benefit
B	Strong or moderate evidence for efficacy but with a limited clinical benefit, generally recommended

Grades of recommendation	
C	Insufficient evidence for efficacy or benefit does not outweigh the risk or the disadvantages (adverse events, cost,…), optional
D	Moderate evidence against efficacy or for adverse outcome, generally not recommended
E	Strong evidence against efficacy or for adverse outcome, never recommended

[a]Adapted version of the "Infectious Disease Society of America-United States Public Health Service Grading System

References

1. Colombo N, Creutzberg C, Amant F, et al. ESMO-ESGO-ESTRO consensus conference on endometrial cancer: diagnosis, treatment and follow-up. Ann Oncol. 2016;27:16–41.
2. Colombo N, Preti E, Landoni F, et al. Endometrial cancer: ESMO clinical practice guidelines for diagnosis, treatment and follow-up. Ann Oncol. 2013;24(Supplement 6):vi33–8.
3. Blake P, Swart AM, Orton J, et al. Adjuvant external beam radiotherapy in the treatment of endometrial cancer (MRC ASTEC and NCIC CTG EN.5 randomized trials): pooled trial results, systematic review, and meta-analysis. Lancet. 2009;373:137–46.
4. Creutzberg CL, Van Putten WL, Koper PC, et al. Surgery and postoperative radiotherapy versus surgery alone for patients with stage-1 endometrial carcinoma: multicentre randomized trial. PORTEC Study Group. Post operative radiation therapy in endometrial carcinoma. Lancet. 2000;355:1404–11.
5. Keys HM, Roberts JA, Brunetto VL, et al. A phase III trial of surgery with or without adjunctive external pelvic radiation therapy in intermediate risk endometrial adenocarcinoma: a Gynecologic Oncology Group study. Gynecol Oncol. 2004;92:744–51.
6. Kong A, Johnson N, Kitchener HC, et al. Adjuvant radiotherapy for stage I endometrial cancer: an update Cochrane systematic review and meta-analysis. J Natl Cancer Inst. 2012;104:1625–34.
7. Koh WJ, Abu-Rustum NR, Bean S, et al. Uterine neoplasms, Version 1.2018, NCCN clinical practice guidelines in oncology. J Natl Compr Canc Netw. 2018;16(2):170–99. https://doi.org/10.6004/jnccn.2018.0006.
8. SGO Clinical Practice Endometrial Cancer Working Group, Burke WM, Orr J, Leitao M, et al. Endometrial cancer: a review and current management strategies. Part 1. Gynecology. Oncology. 2014;134:385–92.
9. SGO Clinical Practice Endometrial Cancer Working Group, Burke WM, Orr J, Leitao M, et al. Endometrial cancer: a review and current management strategies. Part 2. Gynecology. Oncology. 2014;134:385–92.
10. Practice Bulletin. Clinical management guidelines for obstetrician-gynecologist. Society of Gynecologic Oncology and the American College of Obstetricians and Gynecologists. Number 149, April 2015.
11. Kumar S, Mariani A, Bakkum-Gamez JN, et al. Risk factors that mitigate the role of paraaortic lymphadenectomy in uterine endometrioid cancer. Gynecol Oncol. 2013;130:441–5.
12. Milam MR, Java J, Walker JL, et al. Nodal metastasis risk in endometroid endometrial cancer. Obstet Gynecol. 2012;119:286–92.
13. Khoury-Collado F, Murray MP, Hensley ML, et al. Sentinel lymph node mapping for endometrial cancer improves the detection of metastatic disease to regional lymph nodes. Gynecol Oncol. 2011;122:251–4.
14. Shih KK, Yun E, Gardner GJ, et al. Surgical cytoreduction in stage IV endometrioid endometrial carcinoma. Gynecol Oncol. 2011;122:608–11.

15. Creutzberg CL, van Stiphout RG, Nout RA, et al. Nomograms for prediction of outcome with or without adjuvant radiation therapy for patients with endometrial cancer: a pooled analysis of PORTEC-1 and PORTEC-2 trials. Int J Radiat Oncol Biol Phys. 2015;91:530–9.
16. Nout RA, Smith VT, Putter H, et al. Vaginal brachytherapy versus pelvic external beam radiotherapy for patients with endometrial cancer of high-intermediate risk (PORTEC-2): an open-label, non inferiority, randomized trial. Lancet. 2010;375(9717):816–23.
17. Miller D, Filiaci V, Fleming G, et al. Randomized phase III noninferiority trial of first line chemotherapy for metastatic or recurrent endometrial carcinoma: a Gynecologic Oncology Group study. Gynecol Oncol. 2012;125:771.

Part IV
Surgical Management of Endometrial Cancer

Surgical Principles of Endometrial Cancer

10

Anne Gauthier, Martin Koskas, and Frederic Amant

10.1 Introduction

Worldwide, endometrial cancer (EC) is the sixth most common malignant disorder with approximately 290,000 new cases annually. In Europe it is the fourth common woman cancer in terms of incidence [1].

Prognostic factors identified are histological type (endometrioid or not), stage (Table 10.1), grade, lymphovascular space invasion, the depth of myometrial invasion, and lymph node involvement.

Preoperative data (estimation of the depth of myometrial invasion, cervical involvement, lymph node enlargement on magnetic resonance imaging (MRI) and histology defined on the endometrial biopsy) allow to assess a priori the stage and the EC risk of recurrence for stages FIGO I in four groups (ESMO classification, Table 10.2) [2].

For early stage EC, a hysterectomy with bilateral salpingo oophorectomy is the cornerstone of treatment. The decision to perform a lymphadenectomy depends on the local practice and the risk of nodal disease (determined a priori by the preoperative or intraoperative data).

A. Gauthier
Department of Gynecology and Obstetrics, Bichat University Hospital, Paris Diderot University, Paris, France

M. Koskas
Department of Gynecology and Obstetrics, Bichat University Hospital, Paris Diderot University, Paris, France

Department of Oncology, Catholic University of Leuven, Leuven, Belgium

F. Amant (✉)
Department of Oncology, Catholic University of Leuven, Leuven, Belgium

Center for Gynecologic Oncology, Netherlands Cancer Institute and Amsterdam University Medical Centers, Amsterdam, The Netherlands
e-mail: frederic.amant@uzleuven.be

Table 10.1 Revised 2009 FIGO staging for endometrial cancer

Stage I—limited to the body of the uterus
Ia—no or less than half myometrial invasion
Ib—invasion equal to or more than half of the myometrium
Stage II—cervical stromal involvement (endocervical glandular involvement only is stage I)
Stage III—local and/or regional spread of the tumor
IIIa—tumor invades the serosa of the body of the uterus and/or adnexa
IIIb—vaginal involvement and/or parametrial involvement
IIIc—pelvic or para-aortic lymphadenopathy
IIIc1v—positive pelvic nodes
IIIc2—positive para-aortic nodes with or without positive pelvic nodes
Stage IV—involvement of rectum and/or bladder mucosa and/or distant metastasis
IVa—bladder or rectal mucosal involvement
IVb—distant metastases, malignant ascites, peritoneal involvement

Table 10.2 Définition des groupes à risque de récidive sur la base des données histologiques définitives selon les recommandations ESMO- ESGO-ESTRO 2016

Critères	Groupe à risque de récidive
Type 1/stade FIGO IA/grade 1-2/sans emboles lymphovasculaires	Faible
Type 1/stade FIGO IB/grade 1-2/sans emboles lymphovasculaires	Intermédiaire
Type 1/stade FIGO IA/grade 3 avec ou sans emboles lymphovasculaires Type 1/stade FIGO IA-IB/grade 1-2/avec emboles lymphovasculaires	Intermédiaire- élevé
Type 1/ stade FIGO IB de grade 3 avec ou sans emboles lymphovasculaires Tumeurs de type 2 Stades FIGO II ou III sans reliquat tumoral	Élevé

Colombo N, Creutzberg C, Amant F, Bosse T, Gonzalez-Martin A, Ledermann J, et al. ESMO-ESGO-ESTRO consensus conference on endometrial cancer: diagnosis, treatment and follow-up. Ann Oncol 2016;27(1):16–41

Although the stage can be presumed preoperatively, EC is by definition surgically staged.

10.2 Principles

Surgery for cancer of the uterus is based on several basic principles:

10.2.1 No Morcellation

The specimen must be handled carefully to avoid any release of tumor cells and fragmentation is prohibited.

10.2.2 Surgical Approach

10.2.2.1 Rational

Whereas there is no difference in terms of major complications between abdominal hysterectomy and laparoscopically assisted vaginal hysterectomy or total laparoscopic hysterectomy, the laparoscopic approach is associated with a significantly shorter hospital stay, less pain, and quicker resumption of daily activities [3, 4], without clear difference between robotic-assisted surgery and conventional laparoscopy [5, 6].

Early-stage EC can be treated effectively with either total laparoscopic hysterectomy (TLH) or laparoscopy-assisted vaginal hysterectomy (LAVH) [5, 6]. Both LAVH and TLH can be performed in early-stage EC, with similar surgical outcomes [7].

Moreover, in obese patients, it has been suggested that robotic-assisted surgery reduces operating time, blood loss, and increases the number of lymph nodes removed compared to the conventional laparoscopy [8]. Obesity therefore appears to be good indication for robot-assisted surgery since it has been reported to be a common cause of laparoconversion. However, the experience of the surgeon also needs to be taken into consideration indicating that a good laparoscopist has little benefit by transforming to robotic system.

Moreover, obese patients may benefit more from TLH than from LAVH in terms of shorter operating time [7].

10.2.2.2 Recommendations

Since the oncological safety of the laparoscopic approach has now been demonstrated in several randomized studies [9, 10], hysterectomy and bilateral salpingo-oophorectomy should be performed by laparoscopy in patients with no contraindications to laparoscopy (e.g. large-volume uterus, insufficient mobility, significant myometrial invasion of the tumor) to avoid the risk of uterine rupture [11].

10.2.3 Type of Hysterectomy

The main goal of surgery is therapeutic by removal of the tumor. In addition, uterine resection allows determination of prognostic factors and hence decisions on the adjuvant treatment.

Hysterectomy must be:

- total, because of the risk of cervical invasion,
- extrafascial, because of the presence of myometrial fibers in the uterine fascia making extension possible at this level,
- nonconservative, even if the tubes and ovaries appear normal, as they may contain micro metastases. However, in young patients with grade 1 intramucous endometrial adenocarcinoma, ovarian preservation is not associated with an increase in cancer-related mortality.

10.2.4 Lymphadenectomy

10.2.4.1 Rational

Lymphadenectomy is historically recommended to ensure proper individual staging.

The major lymphatic trunks are the utero-ovarian (infundibulopelvic), parametrial, and pre sacral trunks that drain into the hypogastric, external iliac, common iliac, presacral, and para-aortic nodes. Complete lymphatic exploration then comprises of pelvic and para-aortic lymphadenectomy.

Randomized studies have been published suggesting that pelvic lymphadenectomy has no impact on overall and disease-free survival in patients with early stage EC. An Italian randomized trial of pelvic (and in 30% para-aortic) lymphadenectomy versus no lymphadenectomy in 540 women also did not show any difference in rates of relapse or survival [12]. In the UK, the MRC ASTEC trial, which randomized 1400 women undergoing surgery for presumed Stage I endometrial cancer to pelvic lymphadenectomy or no lymphadenectomy, showed no therapeutic benefit [13]. Both studies have been criticized because of a limited effort with respect to the extent of dissection and lymph node evaluation, because of the high proportion of low-risk patients, and because of no direct decision on adjuvant therapy based on lymphadenectomy result.

However, these results have been discussed in light of studies demonstrating that para-aortic lymphadenectomy associated with pelvic lymphadenectomy is associated with longer overall survival for patients with intermediate- or high-risk EC when compared with pelvic lymphadenectomy alone [14]. But again, this was a retrospective study and prospective data are awaited for. In addition, adjuvant therapy was not comparable in the two groups. In patients who underwent both pelvic and para-aortic lymphadenectomy, 77% received chemotherapy, whereas this was given in 45% of patients who underwent pelvic lymphadenectomy alone. This suggests that undergoing both pelvic and para-aortic lymphadenectomy is beneficial in comparison with patients who will undergo pelvic lymphadenectomy alone; it does not imply that extensive lymphadenectomy improves survival in comparison with no lymphadenectomy.

However, since low-risk tumors (well differentiated and <1/2 myometrial invasion) have positive nodes in less than 5% of cases, it is now well accepted that these patients do not require full surgical staging [15]. Lymphadenectomy should be considered in women with intermediate or high-risk factors. Although a direct survival benefit of lymphadenectomy has not been clearly documented, the procedure identifies node-positive patients that may benefit from adjuvant treatment [16]. Preoperative exploration aims at identifying risk factors supporting lymphadenectomy. Deciding lymphadenectomy is also possible during surgery. Intraoperative assessment mainly involves assessment of myometrial invasion. Grading on frozen section is possible, though suboptimal compared with postoperative grading.

10.2.4.2 Recommendations

As a minimal approach, any enlarged or suspicious lymph node should be removed.

For high-risk patients pelvic lymphadenectomy is recommended due to a high rate of lymph node involvement and its positive impact on survival [14, 17]. Outside clinical trials, lymphadenectomy is mainly performed for staging purposes in high-risk cases. There is little evidence to support a therapeutic benefit, but it should be used to select women with positive nodes who may benefit from adjuvant therapy. An international trial of the role of lymphadenectomy to direct adjuvant therapy for high-risk endometrial cancer (STATEC) is planned. The ongoing ENGOT-EN2-DGCG/EORCT 55102 trial aims to answer this question by comparing survival in patients with stage I–II grade 3 endometrioid EC or type 2 EC without metastatic node after randomization to adjuvant chemotherapy or no further treatment.

For patients with low or intermediate risk, lymphadenectomy is not recommended based on ASTEC and Italian trials [12, 13].

10.2.5 Sentinel Lymph Nodes

10.2.5.1 Rational

The lymphatic drainage pathways of the myometrium are:

- for isthmus and mid-corpus (drainage is similar to the cervix): lymphatics following the uterine vessels in broad ligament to the pelvic ganglia (and more particularly those in external iliac subvein position),
- for fundal and cornual areas: drainage pathways follow the lumbosacral ovarian pedicle (in the infudibulo-pelvic ligament) to drain into the para-aortic nodes above the inferior mesenteric artery and below the left renal vein and rarely to the iliac nodes [18].

Burke et al. first described in 1996 the sentinel lymph node (SLN) biopsy applied in patients with EC [19]. The potential interest of the technique of SLN in EC is to reduce morbidity of complete lymphadenectomy (lymphedema, seroma), but also allow for node ultrastaging (search for micrometastases) on a limited number of nodes.

Three routes of administration have been described:

- subserosal intraoperative injection as originally described,
- cervical injection (pre- and/or intraoperative): most reproducible but main criticism is that this approach reflects the drainage of the cervix and not the tumor,
- hysteroscopic intraoperative submucosal injection: in close proximity to the tumor; some authors emphasize the potential risk of tumor cell dissemination in connection with intracavitary hypertension (tubal dissemination) and cervical dilation (lymphatic dissemination), but it should be noted that the pressure used during hysteroscopy for the injection of the tracer is very low. So there would be no increase in the incidence of positive peritoneal washings after diagnostic hysteroscopy.

There are several techniques to detect the SLN:

- colored detection (patent blue or indocyanine green (ICG), with a better detection rate),
- isotopic detection (technetium) with lymphoscintigraphy,

– combined detection (colored and isotopic).

Detection may be preoperative (by lymphoscintigraphy or SEPCT, real-time 3-dimensional single-photon emission computed tomographic) or intraoperative (color (blue channels and sentinel nodes) and/or isotope (hot sentinel node)).

Ultra-staging can identify micro-metastasis (between 0.2 and 2 mm) and isolated tumor cells ($\leq$0.2 mm).

10.2.5.2 Recommendations
While the accuracy of the SLN procedure has been validated in patients with early-stage EC at low and intermediate risk of recurrence, its low accuracy for high-risk EC makes SLN unsuitable in such cases [20]. Based on those findings, SLN biopsy could be a trade-off between systematic lymphadenectomy and no dissection at all in patients with EC of low or intermediate risk, avoiding the morbidity of full dissection and the under treatment of node-positive patients.

Besides, considering aberrant drainage territories, SLN biopsy could be useful in current management of patients with early-stage EC. However, its safety should be confirmed and expert experience is needed before implementation in routine practice is recommended.

10.3 Techniques

10.3.1 Hysterectomy

Since 1988, the classification of EC established by the FIGO is based on the pathological findings after primary surgery.

10.3.1.1 Prerequisites
Laparoscopy is the standard surgical approach for early stage EC with a normal sized uterus [21]. It can be a TLH or a LAVH in which the laparoscopic time can be limited to the first dissections or go to the dissection-section of the uterine artery.

Instrumentation for Laparoscopy
In addition to the standard instrumentation for any operative laparoscopy, a uterine manipulator is useful for uterine mobilization, valves for the exposition of the cul-de-sac, and vaginal occlusion to avoid gas leakage.

The American Association of Gynecologic Laparoscopists (AAGL) has developed a classification of laparoscopic hysterectomy [22]. The abbreviated classification describes five types of laparoscopic hysterectomies:

Type 0 Laparoscopic-directed preparation for vaginal hysterectomy.
Type I Occlusion and division of at least one ovarian pedicle, but not including uterine artery(ies).

10 Surgical Principles of Endometrial Cancer

Type II Type I plus occlusion and division of the uterine artery, unilateral or bilateral.
Type III Type II plus a portion of the cardinal-uterosacral ligament complex, unilateral or bilateral.
Type IV Complete detachment of cardinal-uterosacral ligament complex, unilateral or bilateral, with or without entry into the vagina.

Positioning

Ideally, the patient lies in the following position: supine position, Trendelenburg position with a 15t entry into the vaginasation, valves for the exposition of the cul-de-sac and vaginal tions, or go to the dissection-section of the uterine arteries recommending access to the vagina and buttocks protruding generously over the edge of the table to allow manipulation of the uterus using a manipulator. The patient is supported by spacers over the shoulders to prevent slippage due to the Trendelenburg position. Skin and vaginal disinfections are the first step.

The chief surgeon stands to the patient's left. The patient is lying on her back in the Trendelenburg position, at an angle of 15 degrees, with her legs slightly apart to allow the use of valves for exposure of the cul-de-sac. An endo-uterine manipulator is placed after possible cervical dilation. To reduce the risk of uterine perforation, the endo-uterine manipulator can be put under laparoscopic control. Some have advised for tubal occlusion before placing the uterine manipulator considering the potential risk of transtubal dissemination using such device [23].

Initial Steps

A pneumoperitoneum is established by the use of Palmer needle or through an open-technique laparoscopy. Two 5-mm lateral trocars and one 10- to 12-mm midline trocar are inserted. The two lateral trocars should be placed on a line joining the anteroposterior iliac spines, two or three fingers through the inside of them, outside the epigastric vessels and the midline trocar on the midline midway between the pubis symphysis and the umbilicus. For ergonomic purposes, the mid-trocar is ideally positioned above the level of the lateral trocars. Repositioning of trocars during the surgery should be avoided to limit the risk of parietal metastases. A balloon trocar reduces the incidence of unintended extraction of the trocar (and hence the repositioning). If the uterus is oversized, the trocars should be placed higher. The second assistant positioned between the legs must push the fundus upward and always on the side opposite that of the dissection.

Visual exploration should pay particular attention to:

- gastric area, diaphragmatic dome, liver capsule,
- retroperitoneal reflection next to the para-aortic axis,
- pelvic peritoneum including pouch of Douglas,
- Uterine serosa, adnexa.

This exploration should look for carcinomatosis or secondary lesions. Any tumoral protruding through the uterine serosa constitutes a contraindication for laparoscopic approach. Biopsy of any suspicious lesion is recommended and if the surgical management is modified, intraoperative pathological examination is performed. Peritoneal cytology is not recommended anymore.

The patient is placed in Trendelenburg position in order to allow better exposure of the pelvis with regression of the intestines.

10.3.1.2 Simple Hysterectomy: Total Extrafascial Nonconservative Hysterectomy [21]

This technique is considered in stage I disease and involves several steps:

Coagulation and Section of the Round Ligament

The round ligament must be put under traction by opposite tractions, and with intrauterine manipulator help. Coagulation and section must be middle, after locating the triangle formed by the uterine side, the round ligament, and the extern iliac vessels.

Opening of the Anterior Leaflet of the Broad Ligament

The entire section of the round ligament results in the intrusion of carbon dioxide between the two peritoneal layers. The incision of the anterior leaflet of the broad ligament is followed by coagulation-section to the right edge of vesicouterine peritoneal reflection.

Fenestration of the Broad Ligaments and Coagulation/Section of the Infundibulopelvic Ligament

In depth the front of the posterior leaflet of the broad ligament, the triangular avascular area is perforated. The window thus formed is then enlarged by opposite traction. This action, carried out in a safe area, causes isolation of the infundibulopelvic ligament, facilitating its coagulation and sectioning.

Posterior Dissection and Vesicouterine Dissection

The dissection of the posterior leaflet of the broad ligament peritoneum is then continued until proximity of the uterosacral ligaments. The uterosacral ligaments should not be sectioned yet and only the peritoneum is incised. This is the prime time for spotting the right ureter if it has not been spotted in the section of the infundibulopelvic ligament.

Then, the vesicouterine fold must be opened until a lower limit defined by the movable valve cannulator and dissected in an avascular plane: uterus must be pushed to the promontory and anterior valve of the intrauterine manipulator inserted in the vesicouterine cul-de-sac. Laterally, the vesicouterine detachment continues in the front opening of the broad ligament.

Uterine Vessels Dissection (with Ureter Identification) and Coagulation of the Uterine Vessels

A careful coagulation and section of the uterine vessels perpendicularly, at distance from the ureter, is executed. The cervico-vaginal vessels, lower in the parametrium, should not be forgotten.

Opening of the Vagina: Circular Colpotomy

Mobile cannulator valve is maintained in the vagina into the previous cul-de-sac where it protrudes. Vaginal section is carried out using the monopolar energy. The movable valve acts as a block on which the closed monopolar scissors cut the vaginal wall. Back, dissecting the peritoneum next to the upper union of the utero-sacral ligaments (torus uterinum) has the effect of distancing the uterosacral ligaments. These are preserved while opening the posterior vaginal cul-de-sac.

Uterine Extraction and Vaginal Closure

When the uterus is externalized vaginally, the cannulator secures the uterus. Oncological rules prohibit fragmentation, thus only the additional traction by Museux or Pozzi forceps are tolerated. A sterile glove placed intravaginally ensures the seal and prevent leakage of carbon dioxide.

Closure of the circular colpotomy can be performed by laparoscopy. However, the vaginal route is fastest and has been suggested to reduce the risk of vaginal dehiscence [24]. Special attention should be paid to the corners in order firstly to achieve hemostasis and also not to include in the ureter which can be identified upstream of this step. Vaginal suture can be secured by a thread overedge No. 0 braided absorbable.

In case of LAVH, the laparoscopic time is more or less limited before moving to vaginal time. The various steps that can be performed vaginally are here described.

Colpotom

The use of valves allows a good exposure. To perform the vaginal cuff, vaginal section is carried out using Kocher forceps and cold scalpel by pulling on the cervix.

Vesicouterine Dissection

Then vesicovaginal dissection until vesicouterine cul-de-sac is performed in an avascular plane.

The cervix is pulled down and the front valve exerts counterpressure towards the vaginal vault.

Vaginal bank is seized with toothed forceps and towed up. Scissors are oriented at 45 al vault.e. out using Kocher forceps and cold scalpel by pulling on the cervix. ided absorbable.l attention should be paid to the corners in order firstly to the seal ace created by dissection. The anterior peritoneal cul-de-sac is viewable as a thin transverse white edging and can be opened with scissors.

Posterior Dissection

Then posterior dissection until Douglas cul-de-sac is performed in an avascular plane.

The cervix is pulled up and the posterior valve exerts counter pressure towards the vaginal vault.

Vaginal bank is seized with toothed forceps and towed down to visualize the fibrous tract dissecting then the cul-de-sac of Douglas. The opening is done with scissors and the by introducing finger to open the Douglas and to place the posterior leaflet that will protect the rectum.

The anterior and posterior valves assigned to aid define the base settings on each side. A lateral valve can be placed in the lateral side.

Uterine Vessels Ligation and Section and Coagulation/Section of the Infundibulopelvic Ligament

Usually, this time is laparoscopic.

Verification of Hemostasis and Closure

The vagina is closed be an over edge with 2 X points in the corners.

10.3.1.3 Radical Hysterectomy

It is considered in cases where overt cervical extension is present or suspected.

The radical hysterectomy involves removal of the uterus, the parametria, and the vaginal vault.

The Querleu classification [25] which is used for patients with cervical cancer defines four main categories based on anatomical landmark (ureter, internal iliac vessels, pelvic wall), according to extent of removal of paracervix.

- *The type A* consists in a paracervical resection medial to the ureter but lateral to the cervix (halfway) (cervix removed in toto). It is an extrafascial hysterectomy in which the position of the ureter is determined by palpation or direct vision after opening the ureteral tunnels without freeing the ureters from their beds. The bladder and rectal pillar are not transected.
- *The type B* consists in a paracervical resection at the level of the ureter. The ureter is unroofed and rolled laterally. The neural component of the paracervix is not transected; there is only a resection of the fibrous component. The bladder and rectal pillars are resected at a distance from the uterus. There are subcategories: *B1*, as described; and *B2* with additional lateral paracervical lymph node dissection.
- *The type C* consists in a paracervical resection at the level of the hypogastric vessels (resection of entire paracervix). The ureter is completely mobilized, and the rectal and bladder pillars are resected. There are two subcategories: *C1*, dissection with nerve sparing (Vagina: at least 15–20 mm) and *C2* without nerve sparing dissection (the paracervix is transsected lower than the deep uterine vein).
- *The type D* consists in a paracervix resection at the level of the pelvic sidewall (exenterative procedures). There are two subcategories: *D1*, resection of the entire paracervix at the pelvic sidewall along with the hypogastric vessels exposing the roots of the sciatic nerve; *D2*, D1 + adjacent fascial or muscular structures.

10.3.1.4 The Radical Hysterectomy Involves Several Steps [26]

Opening of Spaces

Lateral Peritoneum
The incision of the peritoneum is performed just above the external iliac vessels, from the paracolic fossa to the round ligament of the uterus, which is sectioned.

Pelvic Ureter
The adnexa must be pulled medially with an atraumatic grasper. The pelvic ureter is identified on the deep surface of the peritoneum. The ureter is not dissected at this stage of the procedure.

Paravesical Fossa
The umbilical artery is dissected and then pulled medially with an atraumatic grasper. The paravesical space is opened using simple divergent traction of the graspers, one toward the external iliac vessels and the other toward the umbilical artery. This plan is usually easy to find. The dissection requires no cauterization, as it is performed in a bloodless plane. It is pursued until the latero-vesical pelvic wall, the plane of the levator ani muscles and overlying pectineal ligament. This step can be facilitated by placing the uterine fundus under tension by retracting it cranially, anteriorly and toward the opposite side with the uterine manipulator. Posteriorly, dissection of the umbilical artery is pursued down to its origin on the internal iliac artery.

Pararectal Fossa
This opening is facilitated by the identification of the iliac arterial bifurcation. The dissection begins medially to the limits of the internal iliac artery, which is followed to the floor of the levator ani muscles. Cauterization of the small arteries arising directly from the internal iliac artery is sometimes required. As for the opening of the paravesical fossa, this step can be facilitated by placing the uterine fundus under tension by retracting it toward the opposite side with the uterine manipulator.

Parametrium Treatment

Uterine Artery Division
The uterine fundus is retracted cranially, anteriorly, and toward the opposite side. At the superior limit of the parametrium, the uterine artery is identified. It is clipped or cauterized at its origin, and then sectioned.

Division of the Parametrium: According to the Categories of Querleu Classification
Type B consists in sectioning the parameter plumb with the ureter. Its advantage is essentially the preservation of the bladder innervation.

Type C: the parametrium is individualized between paravesical fossa forward and outside pararectal fossa and back and within. The base of the parameter is then coagulated against the pelvic wall with the bipolar forceps before being severed so that the paravesical and pararectal fossa are not separated.

Freeing Pelvic Ureter: According to the Categories of Querleu Classification

Dissection of the Bladder
The uterine fundus is placed in median and posterior position. The vesicouterine space is opened (as for simple hysterectomy), identifies the external bladder pillar and divides it. The anterior border of the parametrium is thereby freed from the bladder wall.

Parametrial Ureter
The uterine fundus is retracted cranially, anteriorly, and toward the opposite side. The parametrial ureter is first freed laterally, and is then freed from its attachments to the parametrium. This requires careful coagulation-section of ureteric vessels from the uterine vessels. The section of the tissue adjacent to the uterine artery plumb with the ureter allows dissection and the section of dissected parameter within the ureter (Type B).

Juxtavesical Ureter
The ureter is dissected down to its entry into the bladder. The internal bladder pillar is identified and divided. The release of the ureters before they enter into the bladder provides completely individualization of the parametria and the paravagina forward.

Posterior Step: According to the Categories of Querleu Classification

Rectovaginal Space
This step involves opening the rectovaginal space and laterally freeing the uterosacral ligaments on each side at a distance from the uterus. It enables the surgeon to cauterize and section the paravaginal attachments.

Uterosacral Ligaments
The uterosacral ligaments are then sectioned 2 cm from the posterior surface of the uterus.

Vaginal Step/Closure

Colpotomy
The vaginal incision is performed laparoscopically or transvaginally more than 2 cm from the cervix or the tumor. It allows the one-piece removal of the uterus and parameters.

Vaginal Suture
Vaginal suture is secured by a thread overedge No. 0 braided absorbable.

The Radical LAVH [27]

The preliminary laparoscopic surgical time of the LAVH is a time for exploration, pelvic lymphadenectomy. Similarly, laparoscopic identification of uterine arteries and their coagulation-section, coagulation-section of round and infundibulopelvic ligaments is performed.

The use of valves allows to drive back the vaginal walls and expose the bottom of the vagina and cervix.

Achievement of Vaginal Cuff

A cuff of about 2 cm is usually carried out in a circular manner with Kocher forceps. The vaginal incision is circular and done with a cold scalpel, slightly upstream of Kocher forceps.

Anterior Steps

The clamps are pulled down to open the space between the anterior vaginal wall and the posterior surface of the bladder. Vesicovaginal dissection must be done in an avascular plane to vesicouterine cul-de-sac, without penetrating intrafascial.

After the dissection, the pillars of the bladder will be cut with identification and dissection of the ureter. The pillars are individualized between the vesicovaginal space and paravesical fossa. The opening of the paravesical fossa is in contact with the vaginal wall tensioned by clamps. The detachment is then expanded to put in place a valve in this space. Similarly, a valve will lift the bladder base. The bladder pillar which is located between the vesicovaginal space and the paravesical space is tensioned.

Once identified the ureter, the bladder pillar is cut, mid-distance between the surgical specimen and the bladder base. The sheath of the ureter is opened, and the ureter is dissected to push it up.

It remains only to treat the uterine artery. The operative time was often initially prepared by laparoscopy. We can then, by simple traction, bringing the artery in the operative field.

If laparoscopic preparation was not done, we will bind and cut the uterine artery to its crossing with the ureter. This crossing is identified in the portion of the inner pillar next to the ureter. It is at this level that is the afferent limb of the arch of the uterine artery that can quite easily pick a dissector. The vessel is then doubly bonded and then cut. The uterine artery to be sectioned as high as possible.

Once released, the uterine artery, bladder, and ureter base terminal are distant frankly, and the front surface of the parameter completely unobstructed.

Posterior Steps

Back, dissection begins at the midline to open the cul-de-sac. The perirectal fatty tissue acts as a guide on the orientation of the section plane. After opening Douglas, this opening is enlarged in order to put in place a valve to rule out the rectum. Tensioning by the valve allows to visualize the start of opening of pararectal fossa. Opening pararectal fossa made in the same manner as that of paravesical fossa with a dissector moved into contact with the vaginal wall. The opening of this fossa is generally easy and bloodless. Then we can individualize between the Douglas cul-de-sac and pararectal fossa, the recto-uterine ligaments. These are cut from the bottom up to the level of their insertion on the surgical specimen. The posterior surface of parameter is thus released.

Parameter Treatment
The parameter section is adapted to the degree of radicality of the hysterectomy. Vaginally, we can go up to type B.

After parameter section, the surgical specimen is no longer retained by the broad ligament, the peritoneum vesicouterine cul-de-sac.

End of the Procedure
The broad ligament is sectioned.

The specimen is then extracted. Radicality of resection and hemostasis is checked.

Vaginal vault is closed by a circular hemostatic continuous suture made on the vaginal section, leaving a small central opening for spontaneously draining the operating area.

The final stage surgery is laparoscopic.

10.3.1.5 Complications

Hemorrhagic
It is essential to achieve complete hemostasis, especially at the level of the uterine artery and vaginal vault.

Urinary
The presence of hemorrhagic urine is a warning sign that may indicate bladder lesions. A bladder lesion is detected by the blue test. The proximity of the ureter with the uterine pedicle and with the infundibulopelvic ligament constitutes a good reason to always identify the ureter during the dissection and check its integrity. In the presence of a serious cautery of the ureter, it may be intact though cause a fistula when necrosis at the cautery level occurs.

For radical hysterectomy, postoperative morbidity mainly includes ureterovaginal fistula (1–3%) and vesicovaginal and voiding disorders [28]. Fistulas can occur early after surgery, due to direct trauma of the organ or later, secondary to necrosis.

In immediate postoperative phase, retention due to nerve trauma is common, but almost always spontaneously reversible. It is less common after Type B and if the paravaginal resection is limited down.

Digestive
The reposition of bowel loops out of the surgery field in early surgery should be done with caution and bowel handling should always be done de visu.

Parietal
Eventration on trocar orifice is possible, especially in obese patients.

10.3.2 Lymphadenectomy [29]

10.3.2.1 Pelvic Nodes
The pelvic lymphadenectomy is a technique to remove lymph nodes located between the iliac bifurcation above, the inguinal ring to bottom, the depth obturator nerve, the external iliac artery laterally, the umbilical artery medially.

This procedure can be performed if patient conditions allow transperitoneal laparoscopy. Alternatively, median or extended Pfannenstiehl laparotomy can be decided.

Peritoneal incision is made at the round ligament and is then extended along the round ligament and along the infundibulopelvic ligament. The external iliac artery and vein are identified as well as the psoas muscle with genitofemoral nerve laterally. Then the umbilical artery must be dissected until the internal iliac artery.

The common iliac arterial bifurcation is identified and crosses the ureter, left medially. The obturator nerve is then spotted deep in the paravesical fossa. Lymph node chain located between these limits is removed avoiding fragmentation to limit the risk of seepage and dissemination.

10.3.2.2 Para-aortic Lymphadenectomy
The para-aortic dissection is a technique to remove lymph node tissue laterocaval, precaval, inter-aorto-caval, pre-aortic, latero-aortic, and at the bifurcatio aortae. This procedure can be performed if the specific conditions of the patient permit by laparoscopy extra- or transperitoneal or by median laparotomy.

The limits of the dissection area are: lumbar ureters laterally, aortic bifurcation caudally, and the left renal vein cranially. Removal of retrovascular nodes does not belong to a standard para-aortic lymphadenectomy.

The dissection must be sus- and sub-mesenteric.

Transperitonal Route
One approach can consist in incising the peritoneum just above the aorta after mobilization of the bowels. Alternatively, the different steps of another approach are:

Pelling Right Colic
The incision is made in the crossing between the right colon and the wall; it bypasses the cecum and rises along the ascending colon to the transverse.

Kocher Maneuver
The Kocher maneuver is performed to expose the retroperitoneum behind the duodenum and pancreas. The small intestine and colon are externalized protected by wet fields and maintained by valves.

Ligation of Right Gonadal Vein
The right pedicle infundibulopelvic is released over its entire height, separated from the ureter which is pushed outside. The right ovarian vein is tied and severed without damaging the arch of the lumbar azygo.

Dissection of Latero-caval Area, Pre-caval Area, and Inter-aorto-caval Areas
After opening the sheath of the vena cava, lymphatic tissue located along the right edge and its front face is resected. Excision of inter-aorto-caval lymph nodes is done from the bottom up. A retractor Papin can be helpful to push aside the large vessels. The upper part of this plate contains the chylous trunks. The metal clips are used to identify the upper limit of dissection and ensure proper lymphostasis. Inter-aorto-caval blade is separated from the prevertebral fascia without injuring the lumbar vessels.

Dissection of Latero-aortic Area and Pre-aortic Area
The origin of the inferior mesenteric artery must be first dissected, 3–4 cm above the aortic bifurcation on the left side of the aorta. After identifying the ureter, the left infundibulopelvic ligament is resected.

The lymphatic tissue located along the left edge and front face of aorta is resected. Posterior plan is muscle (Psoas).

Removal of the Lymph Nodes of the Promontory
Lymphatic tissue below the aortic bifurcation (in front of the sacrum and cava bifurcation) is resected taking care to presacral veins and cava bifurcation located a little lower but almost on the same plane.

Bilateral Common Iliac Lymphadenectomy
This blade is continuous with the external iliac nodes already taken, forward and outside the common iliac artery and into the ureter. The procedure ends without peritonization.

Extraperitoneal Route [29, 30]
The laparoscopic route for patients with EC is accompanied by unique challenges given its known association with obesity. According to the series published by the Mayo clinic [30], extra-peritoneal laparoscopy has advantages over transperitoneal laparoscopy for assessment of the para-aortic lymph nodes in patients with EC, particularly in patients with BMI higher than 35.

A 2 cm incision is made two finger-breadths medial to and three fingerbreadths superior to the left anterior superior iliac spine. The fibers of the underlying obliques and transversalis muscles are then split until the peritoneum itself is identified. The retroperitoneal space beneath the transversalis muscle is developed posteriorly until the left psoas muscle is palpated. A 10-mm trocar is then positioned in the left flank and the retroperitoneal space insufflated. Additional blunt dissection is then performed using the index finger in the first incision and the laparoscope within the port until the psoas muscle is readily visualized and until identify beyond the left ureter, the left gonadal vessels and common iliac artery. A 5-mm subcostal trocar is then placed under direct visualization and a 10-mm third trocar placed in the initial incision. Improper placement will handicap the ability of the surgeon by reducing the operating area, or else result in perforation of the peritoneum, making this approach difficult or impossible.

Initial insufflation pressures (10 mm Hg) and flow rates (3 L/min) are low in order to minimize the risk of peritoneal perforation, and theoretically reduce the risk of pneumothorax and hypercapnia. If additional exposure is necessary the pressure can be gradually increased, although 15 mm Hg is rarely necessary. Emphysema is commonly noted in the mesentery of the sigmoid colon. However, when the lower most left flank trocar is converted to an intraperitoneal position for transperitoneal pelvic lymphadenectomy, this emphysema rapidly dissipates and does not interfere with subsequent intraperitoneal procedures.

The left ureter and adjacent infundibulopelvic ligament are readily identified just medial to the psoas muscle and allowed to retract anteriorly and out of the field by the pressure of insufflation. The dissection is pursued medially until the left common iliac artery and aorta are identified. The gonadal vein is followed superiorly into the left renal vein. The gonadal vessels are ligated and resected. At this point all critical anatomy has been identified and the para-aortic nodes between the aortic bifurcation and left renal vein are removed after identifying the inferior mesenteric artery. To remove the right para-aortic nodes, the dissection is continued medially over the aorta and down to the inferior vena cava. The right ureter can be identified just lateral to the dissection. Once isolated from the underlying inferior vena cava, the right para-aortic nodes are then stripped from the anterior peritoneum. After the nodes are removed in endoscopic bags, the lowermost trocar may be converted to an intraperitoneal position (achieved simply by advancing this trocar through the peritoneum) to be used for the transperitoneal pelvic lymphadenectomy.

10.3.2.3 Complications

Hemorrhagic
- They may be due to anatomical variations such as the presence of an anterior obturator vein accompanying the nerve. The pelvic arteries can be tortuous due to the presence of atheroma. Lethal bleeding may occur when the corona mortis, located below the obturator nerve, is harmed.
- Small wounds of the aorta or the vena cava are common. They must therefore be controlled through simple gestures of vascular surgery. Anatomical variations are frequent. They can be sources of vascular wounds. This risk can be reduced by careful study of the preoperative scanner and careful dissection.

The most common anatomical variations are: inferior polar renal arteries, renal arteries ectopic, double vena cava, retroaortic left renal vein, lower right renal artery as the left renal artery or urinary tract malformations.

The renovascular azygo lumbar arch can come from the left renal vein, the left ovarian vein or may not be displayed in the field. In case of a laceration, it can be very difficult to control.

Postoperative bleeding associated with a vascular ligation failure are rare.

Lymphatic

Lymphorrhoea is constant when dissected nodes, hence the usefulness of a good lymphostasis. Para-aortic level, it is increased when approaching the renal vein since the chylous trunks are located above. The high inter-aortocaval region and the left renal vein area are places of important collectors and lymphostasis must be particularly careful and checked.

The lymphocele are the most common postoperative complications (5–10%). The peritoneal incision must be left wide open. Peritoneal lymphocele seems more common after extra-peritoneal route, despite the peritoneal marsupialization. Drains have been reported to be useless to reduce lymphocyst formation [31].

Digestive

Direct digestive wounds by burn or instruments is possible. The risk of sigmoid necrosis by section of the inferior mesenteric artery is low.

Urinary

The risk of ureteral damage is reduced by careful handling and continuous identification of the ureters.

Parietal

Eventration on the trocar orifice is possible, especially after a transperitoneal approach in obese patients. The transplant of tumor to the trocar orifice is rare and can be limited by avoidance of fragmentation and using endoscopic bags.

Nerve

Genito-femoral nerve injury leads to hypoesthesia of the inner face of the thigh and labium majus. Obturator nerve injury can compromise thigh adduction and lateral rotation and can lead to hypoesthesia of the anteromedial face of the thigh.

Moreover, sympathetic disorders occur when sympathetic nerves are injured.

10.3.3 Sentinel Lymph Nodes [32]

For direct cervical injection, there are two different options: 4-quadrant option and 2-sided option (at 3 and 9 o 'clock) ent nerves are injured. thigh and labium majus. Obturator nerve injury can compromise thigh adduction and lateral rotation and can lead to hypoesthesia of the inner thigh.

For isotopic detection, cervical injections of radiolabeled colloids, like unfiltered technetium sulfur colloid, are administered the day before or morning before surgery. Scintigraphic images are obtained 2 h after the injections and then every 30 min to detect the SLN. Then optional lymphoscintigraphy or SPEC-CT can be performed.

The other technique using hysteroscopy consists of a peritumoral colored dye injection (5 mg) during operative hysteroscopy. Laparoscopic inspection is performed using a laparoscopic fluorescence imaging system if the ICG was used.

For subserosal injection, the detection rate appears directly related to the number of injection points.

10.4 Recurrent Endometrial Cancer

Overall, about 75% of recurrences are symptomatic and 25% asymptomatic, and neither recurrence-free nor overall survival are improved in asymptomatic cases compared with those detected at clinical presentation. Most (65–85%) recurrences are diagnosed within 3 years of primary treatment, and 40% of recurrences were local [33].

The treatment of recurrent endometrial cancer depends on the tumor biology (referring to the disease-free interval), number of lesions, resectability and the general condition of the patient.

Isolated recurrences in the vaginal vault, pelvis and para-aortic area in nonirradiated patients still have a chance to be cured [34]. These patients deserve maximal–combined-treatment. In contrast, the outcome of widespread recurrent EC with a short disease free interval, in the range of few months or 1 year, is dismal. Here, surgery has no chance to alter the course of the disease and improve the chances of the patient. Only palliative surgery may in some cases relieve symptoms.

The number of lesions at recurrence, the location and the disease-free interval determine the treatment modalities.

In fact, isolated vaginal recurrences of endometrial cancer can be treated with radiotherapy and have an excellent prognosis (81–88% survival) [34–36]. However, survival is lower when high-grade lesions cause the relapse [37]. Therefore, for vaginal or pelvic nodal recurrence, chemotherapy with RT could be considered in patients with high-risk features for systemic relapse [34].

Isolated para aortic recurrences can be treated with surgery followed by radiotherapy. In order to avoid spilling and trocar metastasis, an open procedure is preferred. This approach also allows to explore the abdominal cavity. Individual case experience shows that this approach can cure patients.

For bulky lesions (>4 cm diameter), surgical resection or chemotherapy prior to radiotherapy may improve local control [34].

Some endometrial cancers, typically low-grade tumors, have a tendency towards a more indolent behavior with late (systemic) recurrences and more isolated disease. When the patient is fit enough and when complete resection is possible without extensive surgery and its associated side effects, resection till no residual disease is a reasonable approach. Robust evidence however on a survival benefit does not exist. But, the resection will allow determination of biomarkers such as the presence of hormonal receptors and remove cell clones harboring new genomic changes that may alter the tumor biology to a higher-grade disease.

Patients with isolated pelvic recurrences in irradiated field may survive thanks to exenterative surgery. Even when systemic disease is excluded and when the recurrence is centrally not invading the pelvic wall, the chance for cure is around 20–40% [38, 39].

10.5 Conclusion

The surgical management of EC aims to be adapted to each stage and histological type. We are moving towards a de-escalation therapy on early stages. However, preoperative staging could be further improved, to avoid over- or under-treatment and their consequences. The technique of sentinel node, of which the assessment remains ongoing, deserves further study.

Minimal invasive surgery also reduces the rate of complications, especially in obese patients, and should be implemented as much as possible.

References

1. Ferlay J, Steliarova-Foucher E, Lortet-Tieulent J, Rosso S, Coebergh JW, Comber H, et al. Cancer incidence and mortality patterns in Europe: estimates for 40 countries in 2012. Eur J Cancer. 2013;49:1374–403.
2. Colombo N, Creutzberg C, Amant F, Bosse T, Gonzalez-Martin A, Ledermann J, et al. ESMO-ESGO-ESTRO consensus conference on endometrial cancer: diagnosis, treatment and follow-up. Ann Oncol. 2016;27(1):16–41.
3. Walker JL, Piedmonte MR, Spirtos NM, Eisenkop SM, Schlaerth JB, Mannel RS, et al. Laparoscopy compared with laparotomy for comprehensive surgical staging of uterine cancer: Gynecologic Oncology Group Study LAP2. J Clin Oncol Off J Am Soc Clin Oncol. 2009;27:5331–6.
4. Galaal K, Bryant A, Fisher AD, Al-Khaduri M, Kew F, Lopes AD. Laparoscopy versus laparotomy for the management of early stage endometrial cancer. Cochrane Database Syst Rev. 2012;9:CD006655.
5. Magrina JF, Kho RM, Weaver AL, Montero RP, Magtibay PM. Robotic radical hysterectomy: comparison with laparoscopy and laparotomy. Gynecol Oncol. 2008;109:86–91.
6. Coronado PJ, Herraiz MA, Magrina JF, Fasero M, Vidart JA. Comparison of perioperative outcomes and cost of robotic-assisted laparoscopy, laparoscopy and laparotomy for endometrial cancer. Eur J Obstet Gynecol Reprod Biol. 2012;165:289–94.
7. Ghezzi F, Cromi A, Bergamini V, Uccella S, Beretta P, Franchi M, Bolis P. Laparoscopic management of endometrial cancer in nonobese and obese women: A consecutive series. J Minim Invasive Gynecol. 2006;13(4):269–75.
8. Gehrig PA, Cantrell LA, Shafer A, Abaid LN, Mendivil A, Boggess JF. What is the optimal minimally invasive surgical procedure for endometrial cancer staging in the obese and morbidly obese woman? Gynecol Oncol. 2008;111:41–5.
9. Lu Q, Liu H, Liu C, Wang S, Li S, Guo S, et al. Comparison of laparoscopy and laparotomy for management of endometrial carcinoma: a prospective randomized study with 11-year experience. J Cancer Res Clin Oncol. 2013;139:1853–9.
10. Mourits MJ, Bijen CB, Arts HJ, ter Brugge HG, van der Sijde R, Paulsen L, et al. Safety of laparoscopy versus laparotomy in early-stage endometrial cancer: a randomised trial. Lancet Oncol. 2010;11:763–71.
11. Occelli B, Samouelian V, Narducci F, Leblanc E, Querleu D. The choice of approach in the surgical management of endometrial carcinoma: a retrospective serie of 155 cases. Bull Cancer. 2003;90:347–55.
12. Benedetti Panici P, Basile S, Maneschi F, Alberto Lissoni A, Signorelli M, Scambia G, et al. Systematic pelvic lymphadenectomy vs. no lymphadenectomy in early-stage endometrial carcinoma: randomized clinical trial. J Natl Cancer Inst. 2008;100:1707–16.
13. Kitchener H, Swart AM, Qian Q, Amos C, Parmar MK. Efficacy of systematic pelvic lymphadenectomy in endometrial cancer (MRC ASTEC trial): a randomised study. Lancet. 2009;373:125–36.

14. Todo Y, Kato H, Kaneuchi M, Watari H, Takeda M, Sakuragi N. Survival effect of para-aortic lymphadenectomy in endometrial cancer (SEPAL study): a retrospective cohort analysis. Lancet. 2010;375:1165–72.
15. Colombo N, Preti E, Landoni F, Carinelli S, Colombo A, Marini C, et al. Endometrial cancer: ESMO Clinical Practice Guidelines for diagnosis, treatment and follow-up. Ann Oncol. 2013;24(Suppl 6):vi33–8.
16. Randall ME, Filiaci VL, Muss H, Spirtos NM, Mannel RS, Fowler J, Thigpen T, Benda JA. Randomized phase III trial of whole-abdominal irradiation versus doxorubicin and cisplatin chemotherapy in advanced endometrial carcinoma: a Gynecologic Oncology Group study. J Clin Oncol. 2006;24(1):36–44. https://doi.org/10.1200/JCO.2004.00.7617.
17. Aalders JG, Thomas G. Endometrial cancer—revisiting the importance of pelvic and para aortic lymph nodes. Gynecol Oncol. 2007;104(1):222–31. https://doi.org/10.1016/j.ygyno.2006.10.013.
18. Alay I, Turan T, Ureyen I, Karalok A, Tasci T, Ozfuttu A, et al. Lymphadenectomy should be performed up to the renal vein in patients with intermediate-high risk endometrial cancer. Pathol Oncol Res. 2015;21:803–10.
19. Burke TW, Levenback C, Tornos C, Morris M, Wharton JT, Gershenson DM. Intraabdominal lymphatic mapping to direct selective pelvic and paraaortic lymphadenectomy in women with high-risk endometrial cancer: results of a pilot study. Gynecol Oncol. 1996;62:169–73.
20. Ballester M, Dubernard G, Lecuru F, Heitz D, Mathevet P, Marret H, et al. Detection rate and diagnostic accuracy of sentinel-node biopsy in early stage endometrial cancer: a prospective multicentre study (SENTI-ENDO). Lancet Oncol. 2011;12:469–76.
21. Poilblanc M, Catala L, Lefebvre-Lacoeuille C, Sentilhes L, Descamps P. Technique chirurgicale du traitement des cancers de l'endomètre par laparoscopie (à l'exception de la lymphadénectomie). EMC - Techniques chirurgicales - Gynécologie. 2009:1–10. [Article 41-725].
22. Olive DL, Parker WH, Cooper JM, Levine RL. The AAGL classification system for laparoscopic hysterectomy. Classification committee of the American Association of Gynecologic Laparoscopists. J Am Assoc Gynecol Laparosc. 2000;7(1):9–15.
23. Sonoda Y, Zerbe M, Smith A, Lin O, Barakat RR, Hoskins WJ. High incidence of positive peritoneal cytology in low-risk endometrial cancer treated by laparoscopically assisted vaginal hysterectomy. Gynecol Oncol. 2001;80:378–82.
24. Uccella S, Ceccaroni M, Cromi A, Malzoni M, Berretta R, De Iaco P, et al. Vaginal cuff dehiscence in a series of 12,398 hysterectomies: effect of different types of colpotomy and vaginal closure. Obstet Gynecol. 2012;120:516–23.
25. Uccella S, Ceccaroni M, Cromi A, Malzoni M, Berretta R, De Iaco P, Roviglione G, Bogani G, Minelli L, Ghezzi F. Vaginal cuff dehiscence in a series of 12,398 hysterectomies: effect of different types of colpotomy and vaginal closure. Obstet Gynecol. 2012;120:516–23.
26. Pomel C, Rouzier R. Colpohystérectomie élargie par laparoscopie. Technique et difficultés opératoires. Hystérectomie radicale. EMC - Techniques Chirurgicales - Gynécologie. 2006;1(1):1–8.
27. Mathevet P, Dargent D. Hystérectomie élargie par voie basse ou opération de Schauta-Stoeckel. EMC - Techniques chirurgicales - Gynécologie. 2006;1(1):1–11. https://doi.org/10.1016/S1624-5857(05)41013-3.
28. Likic IS, Kadija S, Ladjevic NG, Stefanovic A, Jeremic K, Petkovic S, et al. Analysis of urologic complications after radical hysterectomy. Am J Obstet Gynecol. 2008;199:644 e1–3.
29. Leblanc E, Narducci F, Gouy S, Morice P, Ferron G, Querleu D. Lymphadénectomies laparoscopiques dans les cancers gynécologiques. EMC - Techniques Chirurgicales - Gynécologie. 2013;8(1):1–15. Article 41-734.
30. Dowdy SC, Aletti G, Cliby WA, Podratz KC, Mariani A. Extra-peritoneal laparoscopic paraaortic lymphadenectomy—a prospective cohort study of 293 patients with endometrial cancer. Gynecol Oncol. 2008;111:418–24.
31. Franchi M, Trimbos JB, Zanaboni F. Randomised trial of drains versus no drains following radical hysterectomy and pelvic lymph node dissection: a European Organisation for Research and Treatment of Cancer-Gynaecological Cancer Group (EORTC-GCG) study in 234 patients. Eur J Cancer. 2007;43(8):1265.

32. Abu-Rustum NR. Update on sentinel node mapping in uterine cancer: 10-year experience at memorial sloan-kettering cancer center. J Obstet Gynaecol Res. 2014;40(2):327–34.
33. Amant F, Mirza MR, Koskas M, Creutzberg CL. Cancer of the corpus uteri. Int J Gynaecol Obstet. 2015;131(Suppl 2):S96–104.
34. Colombo N, Creutzberg C, Amant F, Bosse T, González-Martín A, Ledermann J, Marth C, Nout R, Querleu D, Mirza MR, Sessa C, ESMO-ESGO-ESTRO Endometrial Consensus Conference Working Group. ESMO-ESGO-ESTRO consensus conference on endometrial cancer: diagnosis, treatment and follow-up. Int J Gynecol Cancer. 2016;26(1):2–30.
35. Poulsen HK, Jacobsen M, Bertelsen K, Andersen JE, Ahrons S, Bock J, Bostofte E, Engelholm SA, Hølund B, Jakobsen A, Kiær H, Nyland M, Pedersen PH, Strøyer I, from the Danish Endometrial Cancer Group (DEMCA). Adjuvant radiation therapy is not necessary in the management of endometrial carcinoma stage I, low-risk cases. Int J Gynecol Cancer. 1996;6:38–43.
36. Huh WK, Straughn JM, Mariani A. Salvage of isolated vag. Int J Gynecol Cancer. 2007;17:886–9.
37. Lin LL, Grigsby PW, Powell MA, Mutch DG. Definitive radiotherapy in the management of isolated vaginal recurrences of endometrial cancer. Int J Radiat Oncol Biol Phys. 2005;63(2):500–4.
38. Barakat RR, Goldman NA, Patel DA, Venkatraman ES, Curtin JP. Pelvic exenteration for recurrent endometrial cancer. Gynecol Oncol. 1999;75:99–102.
39. Bradford LS, Rauh-Hain JA, Schorge J, Birrer MJ, Dizon DS. Advances in the management of recurrent endometrial cancer. Am J Clin Oncol. 2015;38:206–12.

Surgical Principles in Endometrial Cancer

11

Andrea Mariani and Francesco Multinu

For decades, the standard of treatment for endometrial cancer has been total abdominal hysterectomy with bilateral salpingo-oophorectomy, and the surgical assessment of lymph nodes was reported for the first time in the 1960s [1]. In 1988 the International Federation of Gynecology and Obstetrics (FIGO), following the recommendation of a seminal Gynecologic Oncology Group (GOG) study [2], replaced the clinical staging adopted in 1971 and introduced the concept of surgical staging for endometrial cancer [3]. Comprehensive surgical staging includes hysterectomy, bilateral salpingo-oophorectomy, pelvic and para-aortic lymphadenectomy, and pelvic washing [4]. Pelvic lymphadenectomy consists of the removal of iliac nodes, including common iliac, external iliac, and internal iliac, and obturator lymph nodes. Para-aortic lymphadenectomy consists of the removal of lymph nodes above and below the inferior mesenteric artery, and up to the renal vessels [5]. The current guidelines of the American College of Obstetricians and Gynecologists [4] and the Society of Gynecological Oncology [4] recommend that "the initial management of endometrial cancer should include comprehensive surgical staging." However, after more than 25 years, the role of lymphadenectomy is still debated and the treatment of endometrial cancer varies largely across practitioners [6–9].

The potential diagnostic and therapeutic benefits of lymphadenectomy are numerous. The diagnostic role is to define the extent of disease, thus targeting adjuvant therapy and identifying patients who may not need postsurgical treatment. The potential therapeutic role is to eradicate existing disease in the nodal tissue. By

A. Mariani (✉)
Division of Gynecologic Surgery, Department of Obstetrics and Gynecology,
Mayo Clinic, Rochester, MN, USA
e-mail: Mariani.Andrea@mayo.edu

F. Multinu
Division of Gynecologic Surgery, Department of Obstetrics and Gynecology,
Mayo Clinic, Rochester, MN, USA

Department of Gynecology, IEO, European Institute of Oncology IRCSS, Milan, Italy

© Springer Nature Switzerland AG 2020
M. R. Mirza (ed.), *Management of Endometrial Cancer*,
https://doi.org/10.1007/978-3-319-64513-1_11

contrast, comprehensive surgical staging is associated with an increase in morbidities and cost [10], and the gynecological oncological community has to find a balance between risks and benefits.

The overall incidence rate of pelvic and para-aortic lymph node metastasis in patients with endometrial cancer has been estimated between 9–17% and 6–12%, respectively [2, 11].

According to the 26th Annual Report of the FIGO on carcinoma of the corpus uteri, 48.7% of the patients were FIGO stage IA (tumor confined to the corpus uteri and myometrial invasion <50%), with an overall 5-year survival higher than 92% [12, 13]. However, approximately 10% of patients supposedly at stage I present with lymph node involvement at the time of diagnosis [14]. Considering the lack of standardized accurate preoperative tests to determine lymph node metastasis, surgical staging remains the gold standard to identify extrauterine dissemination.

11.1 Pre- and Intraoperative Identification of the Population at Risk of Lymph Node Involvement

Preoperative and intraoperative identification of patients at low risk for lymph node dissemination is of paramount importance, and may reduce morbidity and the cost related to unnecessary postsurgical treatment, while preserving oncologic outcome.

Stage alone, as defined by the revised FIGO staging in 2009, is not accurate at differentiating patients at low risk from patients at high risk [10].

Risk factors associated with lymph node metastasis are tumor diameter, depth of myometrial invasion, FIGO grade, lymphovascular invasion, cervical stromal invasion, adnexal involvement, positive peritoneal cytology, and subtype [2, 14, 15].

A study by Schink et al. reported that, among 142 patients with clinical stage I, only 4% of patients with tumor diameter ≤2 cm had lymph node metastasis, compared with 15% of patients with tumors >2 cm in diameter [16].

In the seminal GOG study, which drove the change of the FIGO staging from clinical staging to surgical staging in 1988, Creasman et al. demonstrated risk of lymph node metastasis in patients with stage I endometrial carcinoma is positively related with an increase in tumor grade and depth of myometrial invasion. They identified patients with absent myometrial invasion or grade 1 histology with superficial myometrial invasion (excluding clear cell and papillary serous cases) as low risk (<5%) for pelvic lymph node metastasis, and patients with grade 3 or myometrial invasion >33% as high risk (>10%). All other cases were identified as moderate risk (5–10%) for pelvic lymph node metastasis [2, 17] (Table 11.1).

Table 11.1 Frequency of Pelvic and Para-aortic Nodal disease by histologic grade and depth of invasion (adapted from Creasman et al. [2])

Depth of Invasion	Grade		
	Grade I ($n = 180$)	Grade II ($n = 288$)	Grade III ($n = 153$)
Endometrial only ($n = 86$)	0%/0%	3%/3%	0%/0%
Inner one-third ($n = 281$)	3%/1%	5%/4%	9%/4%
Middle one-third ($n = 115$)	0%/5%	9%/0%	4%/0%
Outer one-third ($n = 139$)	11%/6%	19%/14%	34%/23%

In 2000, Mariani et al. proposed a stratification system (later defined as the "Mayo criteria") able to identify patients at low risk who can be adequately treated with hysterectomy and bilateral oophorectomy alone, while preserving oncologic outcomes. This algorithm, which relies entirely on intraoperative frozen section, considers patients with the following characteristics to have low-risk disease: (1) type 1, (2) grade 1 or 2, (3) myometrial invasion <50%, and (4) primary tumor diameter ≤ 2 cm. Results showed that no patients with primary tumor diameter ≤ 2 cm had positive lymph nodes or died of disease. By contrast, node involvement was detected in 7% of patients with primary tumor diameter ≥ 2 cm [18]. Subsequently, these findings have been prospectively validated by the same group [10] and other groups [19, 20]. In the validation cohort of 1393 patients with endometrial cancer surgically managed at Mayo Clinic, the low-risk group accounted for 27.6% of the entire cohort and 34.1% of the endometrioid type, with a prevalence of lymph node metastasis of 1/385 (0.3%) [10]. Based on this very low prevalence of lymph node involvement, and a cause-specific survival of 98.6%, the lymphadenectomy in this low-risk population is not justifiable. Therefore, using the Mayo criteria, approximately 76% of patients with endometrial cancer require complete surgical staging [10].

Selective lymphadenectomy based on Mayo criteria has been criticized due to lack of accurate intraoperative frozen section in the majority of hospitals worldwide [21, 22]. In fact, although high accuracy rates of intraoperative frozen section (agreement between frozen section findings and final pathology reports) in the assessment of histologic grade and myometrial invasion has been reported by different groups [23–25], several reports showed a poor correlation of intraoperative frozen section with permanent section analysis [21, 22, 26]. Unfortunately, the lack of homogeneous quality of frozen sections remains an obstacle to individualized lymphadenectomy on a wider scale. Therefore, Al Hilli et al. recently demonstrated that, when an accurate frozen section is not available, patients with endometrial cancer can be effectively stratified into risk categories (low, intermediate, high) on the basis of (1) preoperative biopsy (which is usually available), (2) intraoperative tumor diameter (easily measured on fresh tissue), and (3) presence/absence of macroscopic extrauterine disease. They observed that patients at low risk (type 1 endometrial cancer with grade 1 and 2, primary tumor diameter <2 cm, and no gross extrauterine disease) have <1% risk of lymph node metastasis or lymph node recurrence. By contrast, patients at intermediate risk (type 1 endometrial cancer with grade 1 and 2, primary tumor diameter >2 cm, no gross extrauterine disease) and high-risk (type 1 endometrial cancer with grade 3 or type 2 endometrial cancer, or presence of gross metastatic disease) have a higher risk of lymph node involvement (11% and 27%, respectively), and may benefit from lymphadenectomy [27].

Imaging modalities, such as magnetic resonance imaging (MRI), computed tomography (CT), positron emission tomography (PET)/CT, and ultrasound, have been proposed in the preoperative identification of lymph node metastasis [28–31]. A prospective study comparing MRI, PET/CT, and transvaginal two-dimensional ultrasound (2D-US) showed that PET/CT was the most reliable of the three techniques in predicting lymph node dissemination [29]. Unfortunately, due to their low-moderate sensitivity, imaging modalities alone cannot replace surgical staging and can be useful only in patients who are poor candidates for lymphadenectomy. However, higher sensitivity in the identification of lymph node dissemination is achieved when imaging modalities are associated with other preoperative variables. Several groups have proposed different risk prediction models to identify patients at low risk for lymph node dissemination using preoperative imaging [32, 33]. The Korean Gynecologic Oncology Group (KGOG), using serum CA-125 levels and MRI to assess myometrial invasion, lymph node enlargement, and extension of disease beyond the uterus, developed and externally validated a model able to identify 43% of patients at low risk for lymph node metastasis, with a false negative rate of 1.4% [32]. Subsequently, the ability of KGOG criteria in identifying patients at low risk has been confirmed in two Japanese cohorts [34]. Further, Todo et al. showed that serum CA-125 levels, histology, grade, and MRI (to assess myometrial invasion and volume index) can predict retroperitoneal lymph node dissemination in the preoperative setting [33]. However, both the high cost associated with MRI and the lack of demonstrated clinical benefit for the use of these preoperative risk prediction models do not allow us to support their systematic use in clinical practice.

Other authors have proposed risk scoring systems that can be used to predict lymph node metastasis and identify patients who can benefit from secondary surgical staging after incomplete surgical staging, due to either incidental diagnosis of endometrial cancer or to discrepancy between pre- or intraoperative and final histology [14, 35]. Interestingly, Al Hilli developed and internally validated a nomogram, using a set of five variables; lymphovascular space invasion, myometrial invasion, tumor diameter, cervical stromal invasion, and FIGO grade, which provide an accurate estimate of the risk of lymphatic dissemination and can facilitate postsurgical counseling [14]. Recently, Bendifallah et al. externally validated the nomogram developed by Al Hilli et al. [36].

Alternatively, investigators have proposed the use of molecular and serum biomarkers to identify patients at high risk of lymph node metastasis [37]. Serum levels of human epididymis protein 4 (HE4) have shown to be elevated in a high proportion of endometrial cancer patients, when compared with matched controls without a history of cancer [38]. Furthermore, HE4 showed higher sensitivity than CA-125, and a high correlation with tumor diameter and myometrial invasion [38]. Future studies are needed to confirm HE4's role in risk stratification and screening for patients with endometrial cancer. DNA ploidy in curettage specimens has been recently demonstrated as an independent predictor of lymph node metastasis among patients without distant metastasis at diagnosis [39]. Stathmin overexpression, detected both in curettage and hysterectomy specimens, has been linked to aggressive endometrial cancer and identifies endometrial cancer with lymph node metastasis and poor survival [40]. These findings had been already suggested in the study by Mariani et al., which determined the utility of histologic and molecular analysis on pretreatment curettage specimens in the prediction of lymph node status [41]. Furthermore, a multicenter prospective trial has recently recognized double negative hormone receptor status (ER/PR loss) in preoperative endometrial carcinoma biopsies as an independent predictor of lymph node dissemination and poor survival [42]. However, further prospective multicenter studies are needed to validate and integrate these promising biomarkers in standard clinical practice. This process will allow us to better identify patients at risk of lymph node metastasis, thus tailoring individualized surgical and adjuvant treatment.

11.2 Pattern of Lymph Node Metastasis

The lymphatic circulation draining the uterus is complex and involves both pelvic and para-aortic nodes [43]. In fact, in contrast to cervical cancer, which tends to have a more orderly dissemination, the pattern of dissemination of endometrial cancer is less predictable with more routes of spread available [44]. Understanding the patterns of lymphatic dissemination of endometrial cancer is imperative and provides essential information on the extent of lymphadenectomy required.

An investigation to determine the lymphatic dissemination of endometrial cancer included 188 randomly selected cases of endometrial cancer ranging from stage I to IV at necropsy. Pelvic and para-aortic lymph nodes were reported positive in 62% and 18%, respectively [44].

The overall incidence rate of pelvic and para-aortic lymph node metastasis in patients with early-stage endometrial cancer has been estimated between 5–9% and 3–6%, respectively [2, 45]. However, among patients with positive pelvic lymph nodes, the incidence of positive para-aortic lymph nodes increases to approximately 50% [11]. Moreover, when pelvic lymph nodes are positive bilaterally, para-aortic nodes are positive in approximately 60% of patients, compared to 24% when pelvic lymph nodes are positive unilaterally [46]. In addition to positive pelvic lymph nodes, other risk factors for para-aortic involvement include lymphovascular space invasion, advanced stage, FIGO grade, myometrial invasion >50%, and cervical involvement [47, 48]. Recently, Todo et al. reported that ultrastaging (defined as assessment of the presence of isolated tumor cells and micrometastasis with immunohistochemistry (IHC) using anti-cytokeratin AE1:AE3) of para-aortic lymph nodes in patients with stage IIIC can frequently identify occult para-aortic lymph node metastasis (11/15 patients = 73%) [49]. Although some studies on breast cancer report a poor prognostic value of micrometastasis [50], the impact on survival of isolated tumor cells (≤0.2 mm) and micrometastasis (>0.2 mm but ≤2 mm) in endometrial cancer has not yet been adequately studied. In fact, only limited series have been reported in the literature [49, 51, 52]. This suggests a possible role of micrometastases as a poor prognosticator in patients with high-risk endometrial cancer and "negative" lymph nodes, when analyzed with traditional pathology techniques.

Performed at Mayo Clinic, a study evaluating the different patterns of lymphatic spread among 112 patients with pelvic and para-aortic lymph node metastasis showed that the external iliac lymph nodes were the most frequently involved site of metastasis. They were also determined as the most common site harboring an isolated metastasis [53].

Recently, Odagiri et al. retrospectively evaluated the precise mapping of lymph node metastasis among 266 patients with endometrial cancer treated with systematic pelvic and para-aortic lymphadenectomy. After analyzing the anatomical location of positive lymph nodes among 42 (15.8%) patients with lymph node metastasis, the most prevalent site of positive lymph nodes was found to be the para-aortic area (9.8%, 26/266), followed by obturator nodes (9.4%, 25/266), and internal iliac nodes (7.1%, 19/266). Interestingly, the involvement of the deep inguinal nodes [namely, circumflex iliac nodes distal to the external iliac nodes (CINDEIN) and circumflex iliac nodes distal to obturator nodes] was extremely rare (1/266, 0.38%) [54]. Moreover, Abu-Rustum et al. [55] and Hareyama et al. [56] previously reported that the removal of CINDEIN increased the incidence of lower limb lymphedema in patients treated for endometrial cancer. Taken together, these findings suggest that CINDEIN could be preserved.

11.3 Extent of Lymphadenectomy

The extent of lymphadenectomy varies among practitioners, reflecting the current controversies on surgical staging. Among SGO members who were asked about their surgical management of endometrial cancer, respectively 66% and 90% of respondents perform both pelvic and para-aortic lymph node dissection in grade 2 and grade 3 endometrial cancer. Furthermore, when performing para-aortic lymphadenectomy, 50% of gynecologic oncologists carry the dissection to the level of the inferior mesenteric artery (IMA), whereas only 11% extend the lymphadenectomy up to the renal vessels [57].

A prospective assessment of lymphatic dissemination in 422 patients with endometrial cancer was performed at Mayo Clinic. Among 310 (73%) patients with endometrial cancer deemed at high risk of lymph node dissemination based on Mayo Criteria, 281 underwent systematic pelvic and para-aortic lymphadenectomy, resulting in 63 (22%) patients with lymphatic dissemination. After stratifying the prevalence by histologic type, lymph node dissemination among endometrioid type and non-endometrioid type was documented in 34 (16%) and 29 (40%) patients, respectively. Evaluation of the pattern of spread in the 63 patients with lymph node involvement showed that 53 cases (84%) had positive pelvic nodes and 39 cases (62%) had positive para-aortic nodes. In particular, 24 cases (38%) had only positive pelvic nodes, 10 cases (16%) had only positive para-aortic nodes, and 29 (46%) had both pelvic and para-aortic node involvement [5]. Moreover, Kumar et al. demonstrated that the majority of the patients with involvement of the para-aortic nodes have metastasis above the IMA. Thirty-five percent of these patients were declared free of metastatic disease in the ipsilateral nodes below the IMA [11]. However, considering this group accounts for only 4% of patients at risk for lymph node metastasis, extending the lymphadenectomy up to the IMA in all patients at risk for lymph node metastasis is controversial. Table 11.2 shows the prevalence of para-aortic lymph node metastasis and their location.

Para-aortic lymph node dissemination is uncommon, occurring in 6% of patients with clinical stage I endometrial cancer [2]. In addition, a systematic infrarenal lymphadenectomy is associated with significant morbidity [10]. With the aim of defining a subgroup of patients at negligible risk of para-aortic metastasis, who may

11 Surgical Principles in Endometrial Cancer

Table 11.2 Summary of the probability of lymph node metastasis in the para-aortic area and their location in different subgroups of patients (adapted from Kumar et al. [11])

Subgroup	% with PA LNM	% with high PA LNM	% with high PA LNM with negative low PA nodes
Total "at-risk" population	12%	9%	4%
Patients with negative pelvic nodes	3%	3%	2%
Patients with positive pelvic nodes	51%	46%	12%
Patients with positive para-aortic nodes	100%	88%	35%

LNM Lymph Node Metastases, *PA* Para-aortic

potentially forego para-aortic lymphadenectomy, Kumar et al. assessed the risk of para-aortic dissemination in a cohort of 946 patients treated at Mayo Clinic. Para-aortic metastasis (among patients who underwent para-aortic lymphadenectomy) or para-aortic recurrence within 2 years (among patients without para-aortic lymphadenectomy, or with negative para-aortic lymph nodes when an inadequate [<5 nodes] para-aortic lymphadenectomy was performed) were observed in 4% (36/946) of patients. Also, they found that involvement of para-aortic dissemination is strongly related with (1) positive pelvic lymph nodes, (2) lymphovascular space invasion, and (3) deep myometrial invasion (>50%). Using these criteria, they predicted that when all three factors are absent (77% of cases in their cohort) the PA lymphadenectomy may be omitted with a probability of PA metastasis or PA recurrence of 0.6%, obtaining a reduction in surgical morbidity and cost in the majority of patients [48].

11.4 Therapeutic Role of Lymphadenectomy

The therapeutic role of lymphadenectomy is one of the most debated issues in the management of patients with endometrial cancer. The main criticisms are based on the results of two randomized controlled trials that assessed the role of lymphadenectomy in early-stage endometrial cancer [58, 59]. Both trials showed pelvic lymphadenectomy to have no benefit on overall or recurrence-free survival. However, these studies have been criticized due to several limitations in the study design [60–64]. In particular, the ASTEC study has been criticized for the following reasons. First, the number of lymph nodes harvested was inadequate in many patients. Although patients who had more than 11 pelvic lymph nodes removed had better overall and progression-free survival [45], only 65% of patients had ten or more nodes removed (median 12). Second, one of the potential benefits of comprehensive surgical staging is the utility of nodal status in modulating adjuvant therapy. The study design does not consent to evaluate this hypothesis. Third, since para-aortic metastases are detected in 67% of endometrial cancer patients with positive nodes [5], in order to remove metastatic nodal disease the lymphadenectomy must be extended bilaterally up to the renal vessels. However, the study did not include systematic para-aortic lymphadenectomy, and para-aortic node sampling was performed at the discretion of the surgeon. Fourth, the high rate of patients at low risk included in the study (44.7% of all cases had stage IA-IB, with grade 1 or 2 disease) decreased the possibility of identifying a therapeutic effect of lymphadenectomy in the high-risk group.

The most relevant data on the therapeutic role of para-aortic lymphadenectomy comes from the SEPAL (survival effect of para-aortic lymphadenectomy in endometrial cancer) study [65]. In response to two randomized trials that failed to demonstrate therapeutic value from pelvic lymphadenectomy, Todo et al. conducted a retrospective study to establish the role of comprehensive surgical staging in patients at intermediate and high risk of recurrence. They demonstrated that, among a subgroup of patients at intermediate or high risk of recurrence, overall, disease-specific, and recurrence-free survival were significantly higher in the group of patients who underwent pelvic and para-aortic lymphadenectomy when compared with the group of patients who underwent only pelvic lymphadenectomy. The authors concluded that both pelvic and para-aortic lymphadenectomy are recommended for patients with endometrial carcinoma at intermediate or high risk of recurrence. Furthermore, no significant benefits were recorded between the treatment groups for overall, disease-specific, and recurrence-free survival for patients at low risk of recurrence (stage IA-IB with grade 1–2 endometrioid subtype and no lymphovascular space invasion) [65]. The SEPAL study has, however, been criticized because the use of adjuvant therapy was different between the two groups. In fact, patients in the systematic pelvic and para-aortic group received chemotherapy or radiotherapy in 77% and 1% respectively, compared with 45% and 39% received by the patients who underwent only pelvic lymphadenectomy. Furthermore, only 8% of patients enrolled had type 2 endometrial cancer which prevents generalization of the results to patients with type 2 endometrial cancer [65].

Other groups evaluated the therapeutic role of lymphadenectomy [66–69]. Chan et al., using the Surveillance, Epidemiology, and End Results (SEER) database, demonstrated that patients with intermediate or high-risk endometrioid uterine cancer have survival benefit from an extensive lymphadenectomy. This result was not confirmed in patients with low-risk endometrioid uterine cancer [67]. In addition, when the survival of patients who underwent lymphadenotomy with patients was compared with those who did not undergo lymphadenectomy, results showed that lymphadenectomy is associated with better survival in patients with stage I grade 3 and more advanced stage disease [69]. However, several limitations may affect the interpretations of these results [67, 69].

11.5 Morbidity and Costs of Lymphadenectomy

Given the lack of standardized surgical treatment in patients with endometrial cancer, the assessment of lymphadenectomy-related complications has important relevance in guiding the surgical decision. Further, the increased morbidity and costs associated with lymphadenectomy are probably among the main reasons for which the debate on the role of lymphadenectomy is still open. The evaluation of the morbidity directly attributable to lymphadenectomy is challenging. Many confounders such as the presence of comorbidities (e.g. diabetes, obesity, etc.) and the administration of adjuvant therapy should be taken into account in the assessment of lymphadenectomy-related complications. Due to these limitations, studies addressing the complications associated with lymphadenectomy have varied and contradictory results have been reported [10, 70–72].

In particular, the clinical trial evaluating the role of pelvic lymphadenectomy conducted by Benedetti Panici et al. showed a statistically significant increase in both early and late postoperative complications among the lymphadenectomy arm when compared with the no-lymphadenectomy arm. The difference was largely attributable to lymphocysts and lymphedema [59]. Moreover, the ASTEC trial reported that, despite the low risk of major complications in both arms, the lymphadenectomy group experienced longer median operative time and a higher number of specific complications such as ileus, deep vein thrombosis, lymphocyst, and major wound dehiscence [58].

By contrast, two studies published in the early 1990s reported that lymphadenectomy does not significantly increase the morbidity from hysterectomy [71, 72].

At Mayo Clinic, we analyzed 30-day complications and cost associated with pelvic and para-aortic lymphadenectomy in 1369 patients treated for endometrial cancer at our institution. Results showed that patients who underwent pelvic and para-aortic lymphadenectomy experienced more than double the risk (OR = 2.3) of grade 2 or higher complications (categorized according to the Expanded Accordion Classification [73]). Further to this, compared with patients who underwent hysterectomy alone, patients who underwent pelvic lymphadenectomy and pelvic plus para-aortic lymphadenectomy incurred a 25% and 56% higher 30-day cost, respectively ($P < 0.01$) [70]. When the analysis focused only on patients with low-risk endometrial cancer (as defined by the Mayo criteria), lymphadenectomy significantly impacted operating time, length of hospital stay, blood loss, and 30-day morbidity, without survival advantages [10].

Lymphedema has been reported as the most frequent and disabling complication by several studies [74–76]. A study performed at Mayo Clinic estimated the prevalence of lower-extremity lymphedema among patients surgically treated for endometrial cancer using a validated 13-item questionnaire. Interestingly, nearly half of the 591 responders were affected by lower extremity lymphedema. Lymphadenectomy was also independently associated with lymphedema with an attributable risk of 23% [76, 77]. Whether the introduction of sentinel lymph node (SLN) mapping will reduce the rate of lymphedema among women with endometrial cancer remains to be determined. Studies addressing the overall complication rate related to SLN mapping are needed and will be the subject of future investigation.

References

1. Gray LA. Lymph node excision in the treatment of gynecologic malignancies. Am J Surg. 1964;108:660–3.
2. Creasman WT, et al. Surgical pathologic spread patterns of endometrial cancer. A Gynecologic Oncology Group Study. Cancer. 1987;60(8 Suppl):2035–41.
3. FIGO Cancer Committee. Announcements. Gynecol Oncol. 1989;35(1):125–7.
4. ACOG S. Practice bulletin no. 149: endometrial cancer. Obstet Gynecol. 2015;125(4):1006–26.
5. Mariani A, et al. Prospective assessment of lymphatic dissemination in endometrial cancer: a paradigm shift in surgical staging. Gynecol Oncol. 2008;109(1):11–8.
6. Bogani G, et al. Role of pelvic and para-aortic lymphadenectomy in endometrial cancer: current evidence. J Obstet Gynaecol Res. 2014;40(2):301–11.
7. Koskas M, Rouzier R, Amant F. Staging for endometrial cancer: the controversy around lymphadenectomy – can this be resolved? Best Pract Res Clin Obstet Gynaecol. 2015;29(6):845–57.
8. AlHilli MM, Mariani A. The role of para-aortic lymphadenectomy in endometrial cancer. Int J Clin Oncol. 2013;18(2):193–9.
9. Casarin J, Multinu F, Abu-Rustum N, et al. Factors influencing the adoption of the sentinel lymph node technique for endometrial cancer staging: an international survey of gynecologic oncologists. Int J Gynecol Cancer. 2019;29:60–7.
10. Dowdy SC, et al. Prospective assessment of survival, morbidity, and cost associated with lymphadenectomy in low-risk endometrial cancer. Gynecol Oncol. 2012;127(1):5–10.
11. Kumar S, et al. Prospective assessment of the prevalence of pelvic, paraaortic and high para-aortic lymph node metastasis in endometrial cancer. Gynecol Oncol. 2014;132(1):38–43.
12. Creasman WT, et al. Carcinoma of the corpus uteri. Int J Gynecol Obstet. 2006;95:S105–43.
13. Pecorelli S. Revised FIGO staging for carcinoma of the vulva, cervix, and endometrium. Int J Gynecol Obstet. 2009;105(2):103–4.
14. AlHilli MM, et al. Risk-scoring system for the individualized prediction of lymphatic dissemination in patients with endometrioid endometrial cancer. Gynecol Oncol. 2013;131(1):103–8.
15. Mariani A, et al. Predictors of lymphatic failure in endometrial cancer. Gynecol Oncol. 2002;84(3):437–42.
16. Schink JC, et al. Tumor size in endometrial cancer. Cancer. 1991;67(11):2791–4.
17. Creasman WT, Miller DS. Adenocarcinoma of the uterine corpus. In: Clinical gynecologic oncology. 8th ed; 2012. p. 141–74.
18. Mariani A, et al. Low-risk corpus cancer: is lymphadenectomy or radiotherapy necessary? Am J Obstet Gynecol. 2000;182(6):1506–19.
19. Convery PA, et al. Retrospective review of an intraoperative algorithm to predict lymph node metastasis in low-grade endometrial adenocarcinoma. Gynecol Oncol. 2011;123(1):65–70.
20. Vargas R, et al. Tumor size, depth of invasion, and histologic grade as prognostic factors of lymph node involvement in endometrial cancer: a SEER analysis. Gynecol Oncol. 2014;133(2):216–20.
21. Papadia A, et al. Frozen section underestimates the need for surgical staging in endometrial cancer patients. Int J Gynecol Cancer. 2009;19(9):1570–3.
22. Frumovitz M, et al. Frozen section analyses as predictors of lymphatic spread in patients with early-stage uterine cancer. J Am Coll Surg. 2004;199(3):388–93.
23. Kucera E, et al. Accuracy of intraoperative frozen section during laparoscopic management of early endometrial cancer. Eur J Gynaecol Oncol. 2009;30(4):408–11.
24. Noumoff JS, et al. The ability to evaluate prognostic variables on frozen section in hysterectomies performed for endometrial carcinoma. Gynecol Oncol. 1991;42(3):202–8.
25. Kumar S, et al. A prospective assessment of the reliability of frozen section to direct intraoperative decision making in endometrial cancer. Gynecol Oncol. 2012;127(3):525–31.
26. Case AS, et al. A prospective blinded evaluation of the accuracy of frozen section for the surgical management of endometrial cancer. Obstet Gynecol. 2006;108(6):1375–9.
27. AlHilli MM, et al. Preoperative biopsy and intraoperative tumor diameter predict lymph node dissemination in endometrial cancer. Gynecol Oncol. 2013;128(2):294–9.

28. Crivellaro C, et al. Tailoring systematic lymphadenectomy in high-risk clinical early stage endometrial cancer: the role of 18F-FDG PET/CT. Gynecol Oncol. 2013;130(2):306–11.
29. Antonsen SL, et al. MRI, PET/CT and ultrasound in the preoperative staging of endometrial cancer — a multicenter prospective comparative study. Gynecol Oncol. 2013;128(2):300–8.
30. Chang M-C, et al. 18F-FDG PET or PET/CT for detection of metastatic lymph nodes in patients with endometrial cancer: a systematic review and meta-analysis. Eur J Radiol. 2012;81(11):3511–7.
31. Horowitz NS, et al. Prospective evaluation of FDG-PET for detecting pelvic and para-aortic lymph node metastasis in uterine corpus cancer. Gynecol Oncol. 2004;95(3):546–51.
32. Kang S, et al. Preoperative identification of a low-risk group for lymph node metastasis in endometrial cancer: a Korean Gynecologic Oncology Group Study. J Clin Oncol. 2012;30(12):1329–34.
33. Todo Y, et al. Combined use of magnetic resonance imaging, CA 125 assay, histologic type, and histologic grade in the prediction of lymph node metastasis in endometrial carcinoma. Am J Obstet Gynecol. 2003;188(5):1265–72.
34. Kang S, et al. A low-risk group for lymph node metastasis is accurately identified by Korean gynecologic oncology group criteria in two Japanese cohorts with endometrial cancer. Gynecol Oncol. 2013;129(1):33–7.
35. Bendifallah S, et al. French multicenter study evaluating the risk of lymph node metastases in early-stage endometrial cancer: contribution of a risk scoring system. Ann Surg Oncol. 2015;22(8):2722–8.
36. Bendifallah S, et al. External validation of nomograms designed to predict lymphatic dissemination in patients with early-stage endometrioid endometrial cancer: a multicenter study. Am J Obstet Gynecol. 2015;212(1):56.e1–7.
37. Salvesen HB, Haldorsen IS, Trovik J. Markers for individualised therapy in endometrial carcinoma. Lancet Oncol. 2012;13(8):e353–61.
38. Kalogera E, et al. Correlation of serum HE4 with tumor size and myometrial invasion in endometrial cancer. Gynecol Oncol. 2012;124(2):270–5.
39. Njølstad TS, et al. DNA ploidy in curettage specimens identifies high-risk patients and lymph node metastasis in endometrial cancer. Br J Cancer. 2015;112(10):1656–64.
40. Trovik J, et al. Stathmin overexpression identifies high-risk patients and lymph node metastasis in endometrial cancer. Clin Cancer Res. 2011;17(10):3368–77.
41. Mariani A, et al. Endometrial cancer: can nodal status be predicted with curettage? Gynecol Oncol. 2005;96(3):594–600.
42. Trovik J, et al. Hormone receptor loss in endometrial carcinoma curettage predicts lymph node metastasis and poor outcome in prospective multicentre trial. Eur J Cancer. 2013;49(16):3431–41.
43. Burke TW, et al. Intraabdominal lymphatic mapping to direct selective pelvic and paraaortic lymphadenectomy in women with high-risk endometrial cancer: results of a pilot study. Gynecol Oncol. 1996;62(2):169–73.
44. Henriksen E. The lymphatic dissemination in endometrial carcinoma: A study of 188 necropsies. Am J Obstet Gynecol. 1975;123(6):570–6.
45. Cragun JM. Retrospective analysis of selective lymphadenectomy in apparent early-stage endometrial cancer. J Clin Oncol. 2005;23(16):3668–75.
46. Hirahatake K, et al. A clinical and pathologic study on para-aortic lymph node metastasis in endometrial carcinoma. J Surg Oncol. 1997;65(2):82–7.
47. Mariani A, et al. Endometrial carcinoma: paraaortic dissemination. Gynecol Oncol. 2004;92(3):833–8.
48. Kumar S, et al. Risk factors that mitigate the role of paraaortic lymphadenectomy in uterine endometrioid cancer. Gynecol Oncol. 2013;130(3):441–5.
49. Todo Y, et al. Isolated tumor cells and micrometastases in regional lymph nodes in FIGO stage I to II endometrial cancer. J Gynecol Oncol. 2015;17:17.
50. de Boer M, et al. Micrometastases or isolated tumor cells and the outcome of breast cancer. N Engl J Med. 2009;361(7):653–63.

51. Yabushita H, et al. Occult lymph node metastases detected by cytokeratin immunohistochemistry predict recurrence in node-negative endometrial cancer. Gynecol Oncol. 2001;80(2):139–44.
52. Gonzalez Bosquet J, et al. Cytokeratin staining of resected lymph nodes may improve the sensitivity of surgical staging for endometrial cancer. Gynecol Oncol. 2003;91(3):518–25.
53. Mariani A, et al. Routes of lymphatic spread: a study of 112 consecutive patients with endometrial cancer. Gynecol Oncol. 2001;81(1):100–4.
54. Odagiri T, et al. Distribution of lymph node metastasis sites in endometrial cancer undergoing systematic pelvic and para-aortic lymphadenectomy: a proposal of optimal lymphadenectomy for future clinical trials. Ann Surg Oncol. 2014;21(8):2755–61.
55. Abu-Rustum NR, Barakat RR. Observations on the role of circumflex iliac node resection and the etiology of lower extremity lymphedema following pelvic lymphadenectomy for gynecologic malignancy. Gynecol Oncol. 2007;106(1):4–5.
56. Hareyama H, et al. Reduction/prevention of lower extremity lymphedema after pelvic and para-aortic lymphadenectomy for patients with gynecologic malignancies. Ann Surg Oncol. 2011;19(1):268–73.
57. Soliman PT, et al. Lymphadenectomy during endometrial cancer staging: practice patterns among gynecologic oncologists. Gynecol Oncol. 2010;119(2):291–4.
58. Kitchener H, et al. Efficacy of systematic pelvic lymphadenectomy in endometrial cancer (MRC ASTEC trial): a randomised study. Lancet. 2009;373(9658):125–36.
59. Panici PB, et al. Systematic pelvic lymphadenectomy vs no lymphadenectomy in early-stage endometrial carcinoma: randomized clinical trial. J Natl Cancer Inst. 2008;100(23):1707–16.
60. Amant F, Neven P, Vergote I. Lymphadenectomy in endometrial cancer. Lancet. 2009;373(9670):1169–70.
61. Hakmi A. Lymphadenectomy in endometrial cancer. Lancet. 2009;373(9670):1169.
62. Mourits ME, Bijen CBM, de Bock GH. Lymphadenectomy in endometrial cancer. Lancet. 2009;373(9670):1169.
63. Uccella S, et al. Lymphadenectomy in endometrial cancer. Lancet. 2009;373(9670):1170.
64. Uccella S, et al. Re: systematic pelvic lymphadenectomy vs no lymphadenectomy in early-stage endometrial carcinoma: randomized clinical trial. J Natl Cancer Inst. 2009;101(12):897–8.
65. Todo Y, et al. Survival effect of para-aortic lymphadenectomy in endometrial cancer (SEPAL study): a retrospective cohort analysis. Lancet. 2010;375(9721):1165–72.
66. Abu-Rustum NR, et al. Is there a therapeutic impact to regional lymphadenectomy in the surgical treatment of endometrial carcinoma? Am J Obstet Gynecol. 2008;198(4):457.e1–6.
67. Chan JK, et al. Therapeutic role of lymph node resection in endometrioid corpus cancer. Cancer. 2006;107(8):1823–30.
68. Mariani A, et al. Potential therapeutic role of para-aortic lymphadenectomy in node-positive endometrial cancer. Gynecol Oncol. 2000;76(3):348–56.
69. Chan JK, et al. The outcomes of 27,063 women with unstaged endometrioid uterine cancer. Gynecol Oncol. 2007;106(2):282–8.
70. Dowdy SC, et al. Factors predictive of postoperative morbidity and cost in patients with endometrial cancer. Obstet Gynecol. 2012;120(6):1419–27.
71. Homesley HD, et al. Selective pelvic and periaortic lymphadenectomy does not increase morbidity in surgical staging of endometrial carcinoma. Am J Obstet Gynecol. 1992;167(5):1225–30.
72. Larson DM, Johnson K, Olson KA. Pelvic and para-aortic lymphadenectomy for surgical staging of endometrial cancer: morbidity and mortality. Obstet Gynecol. 1992;79(6):998–1001.
73. Strasberg SM, Linehan DC, Hawkins WG. The accordion severity grading system of surgical complications. Ann Surg. 2009;250(2):177–86.
74. Beesley VL, et al. Incidence, risk factors and estimates of a woman's risk of developing secondary lower limb lymphedema and lymphedema-specific supportive care needs in women treated for endometrial cancer. Gynecol Oncol. 2015;136(1):87–93.
75. Finnane A, et al. Quality of life of women with lower-limb lymphedema following gynecological cancer. Expert Rev Pharmacoecon Outcomes Res. 2011;11(3):287–97.
76. Yost KJ, et al. Lymphedema after surgery for endometrial cancer: prevalence, risk factors, and quality of life. Obstet Gynecol. 2014;124(2 Pt 1):307–15.
77. Yost KJ, et al. Development and validation of a self-report lower-extremity lymphedema screening questionnaire in women. Phys Ther. 2013;93(5):694–703.

The Role of Sentinel Node Dissection

12

Petra Zusterzeel, Annemijn Aarts, Jenneke Kasiu, and Tineke Vergeldt

Hysterectomy with bilateral salpingo-oophorectomy and complete surgical staging by lymph node dissection has been recommended as the standard of care for apparent early-stage endometrial cancer in many national guidelines since 1985 [1]. Other, mainly European, guidelines include neither a lymph node dissection nor lymph node sampling. Whether to perform a lymph node dissection has been one of the most controversial areas in the management of endometrial cancer. Moreover, the extent of the lymph node dissection is of ongoing debate, such as pelvic versus pelvic and para-aortic; below versus above the inferior mesenteric artery; complete lymphadenectomy versus lymph node sampling.

Lymph node status is the most important predictor of survival. Surgical staging with lymphadenectomy defines recurrence risk and guides postoperative treatment planning [2, 3]. Proper surgical staging provides information on the actual extent of disease rather than on perceived risks based on uterine factors, such as grade, histology, and depth of myometrium invasion. However, two randomized controlled prospective European trials evaluating the role of lymph node dissection in early-stage endometrial cancer demonstrated no impact on survival [2, 4, 5].

The ASTEC (A Study in the Treatment of Endometrial Cancer) trial was a multicentre prospective study in which 1308 patients with clinical stage 1 disease were randomized to either a hysterectomy with bilateral salpingo-oophorectomy or standard treatment with lymph node dissection. After a median follow-up of 37 months no differences in disease-free and overall survival were noted between the two arms.

There is increasing awareness of the long-term side effects of lymphadenectomy such as lymphocyst formation, neurovascular injury, and leg lymphedema. Furthermore, complete pelvic and para-aortic lymphadenectomy can be technically

---

P. Zusterzeel (✉) · A. Aarts · J. Kasiu · T. Vergeldt
Department of Gynecological Oncology, Radboud University Medical Center, Nijmegen, The Netherlands
e-mail: Petra.Zusterzeel@radboudumc.nl

© Springer Nature Switzerland AG 2020
M. R. Mirza (ed.), *Management of Endometrial Cancer*,
https://doi.org/10.1007/978-3-319-64513-1_12

challenging, time-consuming, contributes to peri-operative bloodloss, and is not feasible in a significant number of patients because of body habitus and comorbidities. On the other side, when surgical staging is inadequately or not performed at all, patients can be subjected to unnecessary adjuvant treatment, such as pelvic radiation therapy, and its associated side effects [6].

Based on the current standard of treatment, surgeons are faced with the dilemma of "understaging" versus "overtreating."

The use of sentinel lymph node (SLN) mapping in endometrial cancer may be an acceptable solution, providing a middle ground between complete lymphadenectomy and no nodal evaluation.

Although initially described by Gould et al. in 1960 [7], lymphatic mapping did not garner much attention over the ensuing decades in endometrial cancer. SLN mapping is an image-guided procedure that is well established in the treatment of cancers, such as melanoma, breast, and vulva [7–9]. A SLN is defined as the first node to receive drainage from a primary tumour and is most likely to harbor metastases in cancers with lymphatic spread. If the SLN is negative for metastasis, then the ensuing lymph nodes should also be negative. SLN mapping may also detect aberrant lymphatic drainage that would be missed on routine lymph node dissection. A recent study showed that SLN in endometrial cancer patients are three times more likely than non-SLN to harbor metastatic disease [10].

12.1 SLN Mapping Technique: Where to Inject

If SLN biopsy is introduced to the standard clinical care in early-stage endometrial cancer, a consensus should be reached on the most accurate method to perform this procedure. At this time, however, several different techniques have been described and used, including a variety of injection sites and tracers.

One of the main discussion points concerning the procedure is the injection site. In tumors in which SLN biopsy is already frequently used, such as melanoma, breast, and vulva, the tracer is injected around the tumor itself, to access the lymphatic channels draining the tumor. The major obstacle in endometrial cancer is the fact that the uterine corpus is an internal structure and that the tumor is encased within this smooth-muscle organ. This makes peritumoral injection more difficult.

There are three injection sites described in the lymphatic mapping of endometrial cancer: the uterine corpus (subserosal/myometrial), the cervix, and the endometrium via hysteroscopy. By injecting the uterine cervix or the fundus, the lymphatic channels of the organ and not specifically that of the tumor are detected [11]. It remains unclear if cervical injection leads to the identification of the SLN that is representative of the location of the endometrial tumor [12]. Some investigators have injected the fundus to look for the lymphatic channels that follow the ovarian vessels and have routinely found sentinel nodes (SN) along the aorta up to the level of the renal vessels. Nonetheless, this fundal injection approach ignores the important cervical channels that also drain a primary endometrial cancer [13]. By using a hysteroscope to visualize the actual tumor, tracers can be injected peritumorally. In a study using this technique, SN in both the pelvis and the para-aortic region were found [14], but with a low detection rate [15]. Besides that, one of the theoretical concerns when performing hysteroscopic injection in patients with endometrial cancer is the risk of disseminating malignant cells through the fallopian tubes [16].

Although there has been a concern that the nodal spread patterns are different between different injection sites, a meta-analysis published in 2011 showed that cervical injection was not inferior to other methods. Subserosal injection as the only injection site was not advised because it may decrease sensitivity of SLN biopsy [17]. Reasons to choose cervical injection is the accessibility and the fact that the cervix is rarely distorted by anatomic variations, such as myomas, in women with endometrial cancer. A combined superficial (1–3 mm) and deep (1–2 cm) cervical injection has been described as adequate [18].

12.2 SN Mapping Technique: Which Tracer to Use

There are three methods described for the detection of SLN: colorimetric blue dye, radioactive isotopes, and fluorescent indocyanine green (ICG) dye.

Commonly used blue dyes include isosulfan blue, blue violet, and methylene blue. The blue dye is injected in the operating room while the patient is under anesthesia. Visualization of blue-stained lymphatic channels and lymph nodes follows shortly after injection in normal white light. The interval from injection to detectable SLN is approximately 10–20 min. Extended delay between injection and dissection of SLN may result in more diffuse staining of the lymphatic bed and thus increased difficulties in detecting SLNs [19].

Radioactive tracers contain technetium-99m (Tc-99m) radioisotope bound to nanoparticles like colloidal Sulfur or human albumin. This is injected on the day of or 1 day prior to surgery. For detection of the SLN a preoperative scintigraphy can be made and/or an intra-operative handheld gamma probe can be used. In contrast to blue dye, radioisotopes are costly and require more logistic efforts and preparation [16].

More recently, the feasibility of a new near infrared (NIR) fluorescence imaging system using ICG has been described for the purpose of SLN mapping. ICG dye is injected in a similar fashion to that of blue dye but is visualized with a NIR imaging camera. The SLN detection rates with ICG and the bilateral SLN detection rates appear comparable or better than those of blue dye only or Tc-99 m [18, 20].

Studies combining dye with radioactive tracers in endometrial cancer have shown variable results. In a prospective study in 2017, the addition of ICG and NIR imaging to blue dye detected significantly more SLN and detected more metastases than the use of blue dye alone [21]. The combination of blue dye and ICG with NIR

Fig. 12.1 SN procedure with ICG

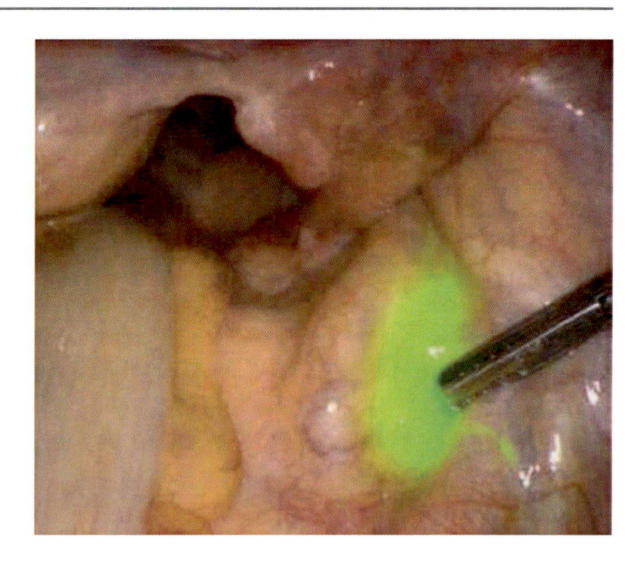

Table 12.1 Detection rate of different tracers in studies including >100 patients

Tracer	Overall detection rate	Bilateral detection rate
Blue dye alone	71% [How]	43% [How]
	84% [Khoury-Collado]	67% [Khoury-Collado]
	81% [Barlin]	
	86% [Desai]	52% [Desai]
Tc-99 alone	88% [How]	71% [How]
ICG alone	87% [How]	65% [How]
	95% [Jewell]	79% [Jewell]
Blue dye + Tc-99	88% [Naoura]	63% [Naoura]
	75% [Frati]	37% [Frati]
Blue dye + ICG	No data	84% [Holloway]
Tc-99 + ICG	No data	No data

imaging had high sensitivity for the detection of lymph node metastasis, and conversely, a low false-negative rate, with no safety issues related to the use of ICG dye or the NIR imaging system (Fig. 12.1).

The detection rates of different tracers described in studies including more than 100 patients is shown in Table 12.1.

12.3 Where to Find the SLN

12.3.1 Lymphatic Drainage of the Uterus

The ideal SLN approach must be based on lymphatic anatomy. Three possible uterine lymphatic pathways are identified so far: the upper paracervical pathway (UPP), the lower paracervical pathway (LPP), and the infundibulo-pelvic pathway (IPP) [22] (Fig. 12.2).

Fig. 12.2 The most common SLN position per lymphatic pathway in endometrial cancer patients [22]

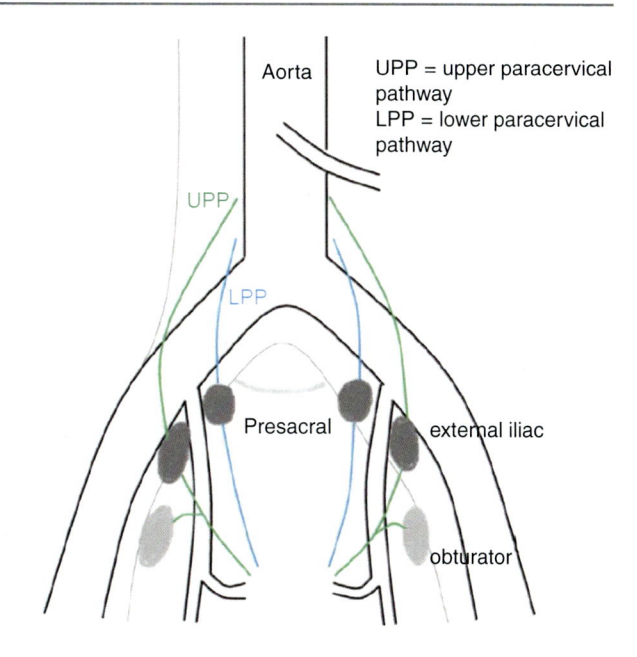

The UPP runs along the uterine artery to drain—whether or not via the obturator lymph nodes—in the external iliac lymph node region. From the external iliac artery, the drainage route continues laterally via the common iliac artery to the precaval and para-aortic regions. The second pathway, the LPP, courses along the upper rim of the sacrouterine ligament towards the hypogastric and presacral region medial of the internal iliac artery. Via the internal iliac artery or presacral region, the drainage route continues medial to the common iliac artery and the precaval and para-aortic regions. The UPP and LPP seem to only be connected via fine lymphatic vessels in the cardinal ligament and function as separate, noncommunicating pathways from there onwards. In addition to the most common, pelvic pathways, the third pathway, the IPP, is the drainage route along the fallopian tube and the upper broad ligament via the infundibulo-pelvic ligament directly to the para-aortic lymph node region. As the UPP and LPP drain via the pelvis towards the lower para-aortic and precaval lymph node regions, it is suggested that a lower inframesenteric para-aortic dye positive lymph node can only be interpreted as the sole SLN in case no pelvic SLN are detected.

It remains undetermined if the uterine lymph drainage is effectuated by one SLN per hemi-pelvis or one SLN per hemi-pelvic drainage pathway. Moreover, anatomical variance between patients is probably a factor that influences the lymphatic pathway and thereby the SLN location(s).

12.3.2 SLN Location

Most SLN are located in the pelvis. Over one half of the SLN were found to be detected along the upper paracervical pathway, in the external iliac and obturator lymph node region [23, 24] (Fig. 12.3).

Fig. 12.3 Distribution of removed blue SLNs [24]

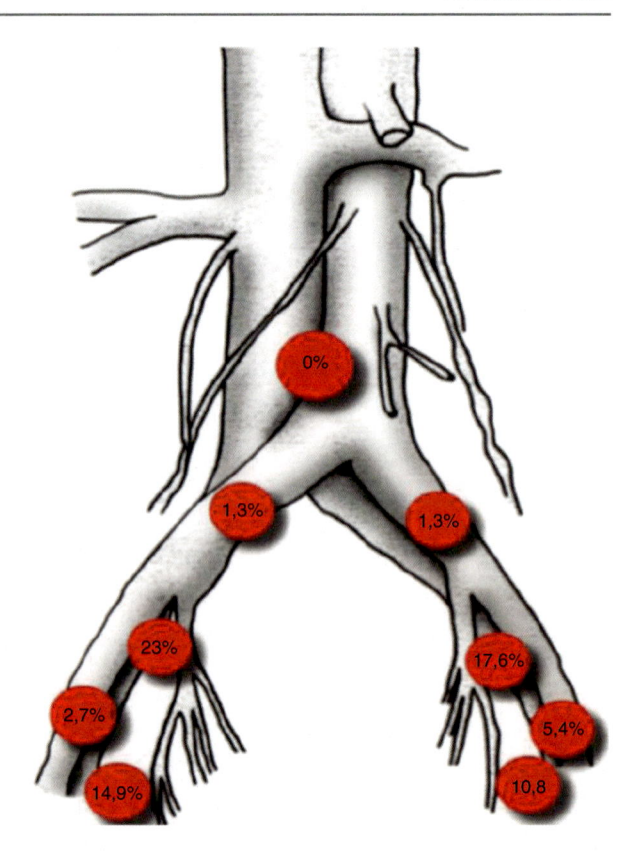

12.3.3 SLN Detection Rate

Data on the percentage of patients in whom one or more SLN are detected varies widely. Defined as the detection of at least one SLN per patient, the overall detection rate was described to be 81% (95% CI 77–84%) [19]. The bilateral detection rate, defined as the detection of at least one SLN on each hemi-pelvis of one patient was reported to be 50% (95% CI 44–55%). Finally, the detection rate of precaval or para-aortic SLNs, defined as the percentage of patients in whom at least one precaval or para-aortic SLN was detected, was found to be lowest, 17% (95% CI 11–23%).

Factors that were found to affect the SLN detection rate were the injection site and the used dye [19]. Patient characteristics such as BMI or surgical approach and tumor characteristics such as type of histology and grade did not significantly influence the SLN detection rate.

12.3.4 The Algorithm

To generate a reproducible, practical, and oncological safe SLN mapping approach, a SLN algorithm was developed by the Memorial Sloan-Kettering Cancer Center. The algorithm was first described in 2012 and extents the removal of dye positive

Fig. 12.4 SLN mapping algorithm [18]. *LND* lymph node dissection

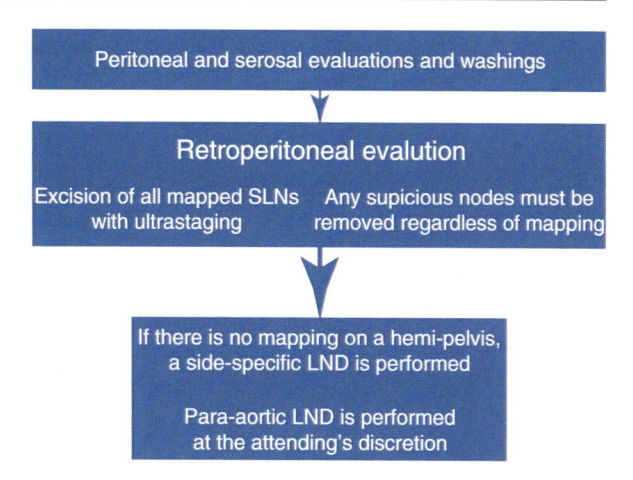

Peritoneal and serosal evaluations and washings

↓

Retroperitoneal evalution

Excision of all mapped SLNs with ultrastaging   Any supicious nodes must be removed regardless of mapping

↓

If there is no mapping on a hemi-pelvis, a side-specific LND is performed

Para-aortic LND is performed at the attending's discretion

lymph nodes [25]. The algorithm includes three main steps as shown in Fig. 12.4. First, the peritoneal and serosal surfaces need to be evaluated and washed. Second, the retroperitoneum must be evaluated. The dye positive lymph nodes need to be removed, as well as all other suspicious nodes, even if these lymph nodes are dye negative. Third, in case no SLNs are detected, a full lymph node dissection needs to be executed of the side-specific hemi-pelvis. The algorithm does not account the performance of a precaval and para-aortal lymph node dissection, which could be interpreted as an algorithm limitation in the rare occasion of isolated precaval or para-aortal lymph node metastases.

12.3.5 The Diagnostic Accuracy of SLN Mapping and the Effect of the Algorithm

To determine the diagnostic accuracy of a SLN procedure the histology of the SLN is assessed in relation to the histology of a pelvic lymph node dissection, whether or not combined with precaval and para-aortal lymph node dissection. The diagnostic accuracy can be calculated by three different approaches. First, the patients in whom the SLN cannot be identified can be categorized as false-negative. As the detection rate represents part of these data, this approach is least used. Second, without application of the algorithm, a hemi-pelvis in which the SLN cannot be found but a suspected lymph node contains the metastasis is accounted for as false-negative. According to the third approach, with use of the algorithm, the same hemi-pelvis will be accounted for as true positive as the suspected lymph node would have been dissected. Therefore, the diagnostic accuracy of a SLN procedure differs, mainly depending on the usage of the algorithm or not.

Without application of the algorithm, the sensitivity of SLN mapping is defined as the percentage of patients with at least one positive SLN divided by the patients with successful SLN mapping and lymph node metastases. This was reported to be 96% (95% CI 93–98%) [19]. The negative predictive value was 99.7%. Moreover, the SLN turned out to be the only lymph node containing metastasis in 60–66% of all cases [19, 23]. The specificity of the SLN will always be 100% as a false-positive SLN is not possible.

The algorithm-specific sensitivity is defined as percentage of patients with at least one positive lymph node dissected according to the rules of the algorithm divided by the patients with lymph node metastases. Barlin et al. reported the first data on the effect of the algorithm on the diagnostic accuracy of the SLN procedure [25]. In 401 of the 498 patients at least one SLN was detected. The accuracy of the SLN mapping was assessed according to the two different approaches: sole removal of the SLN or removal of the lymph nodes by the rules of the algorithm. The sensitivity, negative predictive value, and false-negative rate were 85.1%, 98.1%, 14.9% and 98.1%, 99.8%, 1.9%, respectively. An increase in the diagnostic accuracy of SLN mapping using the algorithm has been confirmed by many other authors, even up to a sensitivity of 100% [26].

Specific attention has been given to detection of a SLN in the precaval or para-aortic lymph node regions in absence of SLNs in the pelvic regions [26]. Overall, two-third of the articles mentioning this topic reported that these isolated para-aortic SLN never occurred. The incidence in the remainder rated generally <5%. Moreover, the incidence of lymph node metastases in high-risk patients were found to be isolated to the precaval or para-aortic lymph node regions in 16% [27].

12.4 Role of Pathologic Ultrastaging

In SN procedures the pathologic technique plays an important role, as the SLN is the main and only tissue evaluated for metastasis. In addition, detection of micrometastasis (MMs) has appeared to be an important prognostic factor in different types of cancer [28, 29] and accounts presumably also for endometrial cancer [30]. There is significant evidence that micrometastases in lymph nodes are associated with recurrence of endometrial cancer [31]. Consequently, the pathologic technique used in SN procedures needs to have high detection rates and low false-negative rates. Pathological ultrastaging of lymph nodes is the most sensitive technique to meet the aforementioned requirements. This technique, using serial sectioning and immunohistochemistry (IHC), is therefore a main focus of the SN concept.

Definitions
- Macrometastasis—tumor cells larger than 2.0 mm.
- Micrometastasis—MMs—metastatic carcinoma in the form of microscopic clusters and single cells, measuring larger than 0.2–2 mm or less.
- Isolated tumor cells—ITCs—metastatic carcinoma in the form of microscopic clusters and single cells, measuring ≤ 0.2 mm.

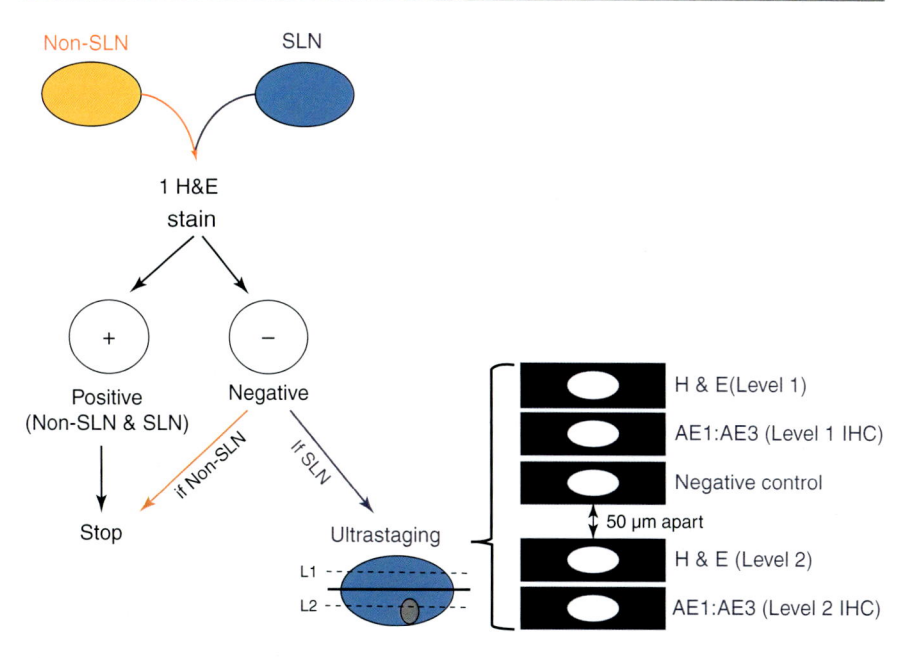

Fig. 12.5 Memorial Sloan-Kettering Cancer Center's pathologic ultrastaging algorithm for SLN. Source: International Journal of Gynecological Cancer 2013; 23(5):964–970

12.4.1 The Technique

Ultrastaging increases the ability to detect low-volume tumor cells as it reevaluates a presumed negative SLN at two additional levels with additional IHC stains. Ultrastaging protocols vary. Results depend on factors including the technique of serial sectioning and the antibodies used for IHC [31, 32]. In most studies assessing the sentinel procedure as part of operative staging of endometrial cancer, the following validated pathologic work up was used [32]. The ultrastaging algorithm is schematically depicted in Fig. 12.5. Only in case a SLN is negative, ultrastaging is applied. It is performed by dissecting the SLNs longitudinally in 4–5 μm section, 40–50 μm apart, perpendicular to the long axis of the node. These sections are stained with H&E and an additional section taken between the third and fourth levels are stained with IHC using the mouse monoclonal anti-AE1/AE3 cytokeratin [29, 33].

12.4.2 Sensitivity and Specificity of Ultrastaging

A meta-analysis of 17 trials with cervical cancer patients reported a 93% detection rate with H&E and IHC compared to 89.4% with H&E alone. This translates into a 96% NPV and 90% sensitivity [34]. For endometrial cancer, in the study by Kim et al. [33] almost half of patients with positive SLNs had occult metastases, including MMs, which were not detected by conventional histology. More specifically, almost 13% of the 508 patients had positive nodes: routine H&E detected 35 patients (7%), ultrastaging detected an additional 23 patients (4.5%) who would have otherwise been missed. Six patients (1.2%) had metastatic disease in their non-SLNs. A 2008 patient series [35] found in almost 25% (10/46) of patients metastatic lymph nodes. In this study, three of the ten metastases corresponded to macrometastases and seven MMs. All the three cases of macrometastases and the three additional MMs were detected by H&E while three MMs were diagnosed by serial sectioning and IHC. A 2010 review, including six studies, showed that the rate of detection of MMs varied from 0 to 15% with a combination of H&E, serial sectioning, and IHC [31]. From 238 patients, 20% had lymph node metastases, including 6% with MMs.

In conclusion, in the performance of SN procedure for endometrial cancer ultrastaging leads to a higher detection and lower false-negative rate of macrometastases and MMs. This means that if the initial H&E staining is negative, then it is of major importance to also perform IHC.

12.5 Clinical Relevance of MMs and Isolated Tumor Cells

The SN procedure including pathologic ultrastaging seems beneficial because of the increased detection of MMs and isolated tumor cells in pelvic and para-aortic lymph nodes. However, it depends on the clinical relevance with respect to prognosis of these positive nodes in order to decide whether adjuvant therapy is needed.

In breast cancer patients with nodal MMs, detected by SN procedures, it was repeatedly shown that recurrences occurred significantly more often than in patients without MMs [36]. The role of ITCs seems to point into the same direction. It is therefore suggested in most studies to adjust adjuvant therapy strategies for these patients. In early cervical cancer MMs also seem to play a role in risk of recurrence. For instance, a retrospective case series with 292 patients, treated by radical hysterectomy, included a group of patients who recurred in a median time of 37 months and a matched control group with no recurrences after 122 months.

MMs occurred tenfold more often in the group of patients who recurred (11/26 and 1/26 respectively). The relative risk was 2.44 (1.58–3.78) [37].

For vulvar cancer the clinical relevance and implications of finding MMs and ITCs is less clear and needs more research [38].

The relevance of MMs in endometrial cancer has not been determined yet. Two studies showed that MMs removal was associated with significant increase in recurrence-free survival (RFS) [39, 40]. Hundred percent of patients without MMs had a RFS of 36 months, while this was only 71% of patients with MMs ($p = 0.0004$). Both RFS and overall survival were statistically significantly inferior for patients having MMs. On the contrary, another study found no evidence of increased recurrence of endometrial cancer in patients with positive MMs [41]. All three studies had small sample sizes and combined low-, moderate and high-risk groups of patients. Particularly in the low and moderate risk groups more research is needed to facilitate decision-making regarding the adjuvant therapy strategy. To date, the clinical relevance of ITCs in endometrial cancer is unknown.SENTI-ENDO study

Some observational retrospective studies evaluated whether the finding of MMs or ITCs during SN procedures impacted choice of adjuvant therapy. In the follow-up of the SENTI-ENDO study 30% of the patients with negative SLN received adjuvant pelvic radiation and 12.5% chemotherapy, compared to 79% receiving pelvic radiation and 50% chemotherapy for those with a positive SLN, including MMs. There was no difference in RFS among groups. Another small study found no impact on RFS when treating MMS with external beam radiation and those with negative SLN with vaginal cuff brachytherapy [42].

In conclusion, at present the clinical relevance of detecting MMs and ITCs in endometrial cancer is uncertain. Future studies should seek for clarification and the possible consequences for choice of adjuvant therapy.

References

1. Creasman WT, Odicino F, Maisonneuve P, Quinn MA, Beller U, Benedet JL, Heintz AP, Ngan HY, Pecorelli S. Carcinoma of the corpus uteri. FIGO 26th annual report on the results of treatment in gynecological cancer. Int J Gynaecol Obstet. 2006;95(Suppl 1):S105–43.
2. Benedetti Panici P, Basile S, Maneschi F, Alberto Lissoni A, Signorelli M, Scambia G, Angioli R, Tateo S, Mangili G, Katsaros D, Garozzo G, Campagnutta E, Donadello N, Greggi S, Melpignano M, Raspagliesi F, Ragni N, Cormio G, Grassi R, Franchi M, Giannarelli D, Fossati R, Torri V, Amoroso M, Crocè C, Mangioni C. Systematic pelvic lymphadenectomy vs. no lymphadenectomy in early-stage endometrial carcinoma: randomized clinical trial. J Natl Cancer Inst. 2008;100(23):1707–16.
3. Sharma C, Deutsch I, Lewin SN, Burke WM, Qiao Y, Sun X, Chao CK, Herzog TJ, Wright JD. Lymphadenectomy influences the utilization of adjuvant radiation treatment for endometrial cancer. Am J Obstet Gynecol. 2011;205(6):562.
4. ASTEC Study Group, Kitchener H, Swart AM, Qian Q, Amos C, Parmar MK. Efficacy of systematic pelvic lymphadenectomy in endometrial cancer (MRC ASTEC trial): a randomised study. Lancet. 2009;373(9658):125–36.
5. Frost JA, Webster KE, Bryant A, Morrison J. Lymphadenectomy for the management of endometrial cancer. Cochrane Database Syst Rev. 2015;9:CD007585.
6. Barakat RR, Lev G, Hummer AJ, Sonoda Y, Chi DS, Alektiar KM, Abu-Rustum NR. Twelve-year experience in the management of endometrial cancer: a change in surgical and postoperative radiation approaches. Gynecol Oncol. 2007;105(1):150–6.
7. Gould EA, Winship T, Philbin PH, Kerr HH. Observations on a "sentinel node" in cancer of the parotid. Cancer. 1960;13:77–8.
8. Cody HS. Sentinel lymph node mapping in breast cancer. Breast Cancer. 1999;6(1):13–22.
9. Morton DL, Wen DR, Wong JH, Economou JS, Cagle LA, Storm FK, Foshag LJ, Cochran AJ. Technical details of intraoperative lymphatic mapping for early stage melanoma. Arch Surg. 1992;127(4):392–9.
10. Khoury-Collado F, Murray MP, Hensley ML, Sonoda Y, Alektiar KM, Levine DA, Leitao MM, Chi DS, Barakat RR, Abu-Rustum NR. Sentinel lymph node mapping for endometrial cancer improves the detection of metastatic disease to regional lymph nodes. Gynecol Oncol. 2011;122(2):251–4.
11. Frumovitz M, Levenback CF. Is lymphatic mapping in uterine cancer feasible? Ann Surg Oncol. 2008;15:1815.
12. Robison K, Holman LL, Moore RG. Update on sentinel lymph node evaluation in gynecologic malignancies. Curr Opin Obstet Gynecol. 2011;23:8.

13. Burke TW, Levenback C, Tornos C, et al. Intraabdominal lymphatic mapping to direct selective pelvic and paraaortic lymphadenectomy in women with high-risk endometrial cancer: results of a pilot study. Gynecol Oncol. 1996;62:169–73.
14. Niikura H, Okamura C, Utsunomiya H, et al. Sentinel lymph node detection in patients with endometrial cancer. Gynecol Oncol. 2004;92:669–74.
15. Clement D, Bats AS, Ghazzar-Pierquet N, Le Frere Belda MA, Larousserie F, Nos C, Lecuru F. Sentinel lymph nodes in endometrial cancer: is hysteroscopic injection valid? Eur J Gynaecol Oncol. 2008;29(3):239–41.
16. Zivanovic O, Khoury-Collado F, Abu-Rustum NR, Gemignani ML. Sentinel lymph node biopsy in the management of vulvar carcinoma, cervical cancer, and endometrial cancer. Oncologist. 2009;14(7):695–705. https://doi.org/10.1634/theoncologist.2009-0075. Epub 2009 Jul 16.
17. Kang S, Yoo HJ, Hwang JH, et al. Sentinel lymph node biopsy in endometrial cancer: meta-analysis of 26 studies. Gynecol Oncol. 2011;123:522.
18. Abu-Rustum NR. Sentinel lymph node mapping for endometrial cancer: a modern approach to surgical staging. J Natl Compr Cancer Netw. 2014;12(2):288–97.
19. Bodurtha Smith AJ, Fader AN, Tanner EJ. Sentinel lymph node assessment in endometrial cancer: a systematic review and meta-analysis. Am J Obstet Gynecol. 2017;216:459–476.e10.
20. Plante M, Touhami O, Trinh XB, Renaud MC, Sebastianelli A, Grondin K, Gregoire J. Sentinel node mapping with indocyanine green and endoscopic near-infrared fluorescence imaging in endometrial cancer. A pilot study and review of the literature. Gynecol Oncol. 2015;137(3):443–7.
21. Holloway RW, Ahmad S, Kendrick JE, Bigsby GE, Brudie LA, Ghurani GB, Stavitzski NM, Gise JL, Ingersoll SB, Pepe JW. A prospective cohort study comparing colorimetric and fluorescent imaging for sentinel lymph node mapping in endometrial cancer. Ann Surg Oncol. 2017;24:1972. https://doi.org/10.1245/s10434-017-5825-3.
22. Geppert B, Lonnerfors C, Bollino M, Arechvo A, Persson J. A study on uterine lymphatic anatomy for standardization of pelvic sentinel lymph node detection in endometrial cancer. Gynecol Oncol. 2017;145:256.
23. Rossi EC, Kowalski LD, Scalici J, Cantrell L, Schuler K, Hanna RK, Method M, Ade M, Ivanova A, Boggess JF. A comparison of sentinel lymph node biopsy to lymphadenectomy for endometrial cancer staging (FIRES trial): a multicentre, prospective, cohort study. Lancet Oncol. 2017;18(3):384–92.
24. Vidal F, Leguevaque P, Motton S, Delotte J, Ferron G, Querleu D, Rafii A. Evaluation of the sentinel lymph node algorithm with blue dye labeling for early-stage endometrial cancer in a multicentric setting. Int J Gynecol Cancer. 2013;23(7):1237–43.
25. Barlin JN, Khoury-Collado F, Kim CH, Leitao MM Jr, Chi DS, Sonoda Y, Alektiar K, DeLair DF, Barakat RR, Abu-Rustum NR. The importance of applying a sentinel lymph node mapping algorithm in endometrial cancer staging: beyond removal of blue nodes. Gynecol Oncol. 2012;125(3):531–5.
26. Cormier B, Rozenholc AT, Gotlieb W, Plante M, Giede C, Communities of Practice (CoP) Group of Society of Gynecologic Oncology of Canada (GOC). Sentinel lymph node procedure in endometrial cancer: a systematic review and proposal for standardization of future research. Gynecol Oncol. 2015;138(2):478–85.
27. Mariani A, Dowdy SC, Cliby WA, Gostout BS, Jones MB, Wilson TO, Podratz KC. Prospective assessment of lymphatic dissemination in endometrial cancer: a paradigm shift in surgical staging. Gynecol Oncol. 2008;109(1):11–8.
28. Cote RJ, Peterson HF, Chaiwun B, et al. Role of immunohistochemical detection of lymph-node metastases in management of breast cancer. International Breast Cancer Study Group. Lancet. 1999;354:896–900.
29. Roy M, Bouchard-Fortier G, Popa I, Grégoire J, Renaud MC, Têtu B, Plante M. Value of sentinel node mapping in cancer of the cervix. Gynecol Oncol. 2011;122(2):269–74.
30. Abu-Rustum NR. The increasing credibility of sentinel lymph node mapping in endometrial cancer. Ann Surg Oncol. 2013;20(2):353–4.

31. Bezu C, Coutant C, Ballester M, et al. Ultrastaging of lymph node in uterine cancers. J Exp Clin Cancer Res. 2010;29:5.
32. Delpech Y, Cortez A, Coutant C, et al. The sentinel node concept in endometrial cancer: histopathologic validation by serial section and immunohistochemistry. Ann Oncol. 2007;18:1799–803.
33. Kim CH, et al. Sentinel lymph node mapping with pathologic ultrastaging: a valuable tool for assessing nodal metastasis in low-grade endometrial cancer with superficial myoinvasion. Gynecol Oncol. 2013;131(3):714.
34. Wu Y, Li Z, Wu H, et al. Sentinel lymph node biopsy in cervical cancer: a meta-analysis. Mol Clin Oncol. 2013;1:1025–30.
35. Ballester M, Dubernard G, Rouzier R, Barranger E, Darai E. Use of the sentinel node procedure to stage endometrial cancer. Ann Surg Oncol. 2008;15(5):1523–9.
36. Tjan-Heijnen VC, Pepels MJ, de Boer M. Prognostic impact of isolated tumor cells and micrometastases in axillary lymph nodes of breast cancer patients. Breast Dis. 2010;31:107–13.
37. Marchiole P, Buenerd A, Benchaib M, Nezhat K, Dargent D, Mathevet P. Clinical significance of lympho vascular space involvement and lymph node micrometastases in early-stage cervical cancer: a retrospective case-control surgico-pathological study. Gynecol Oncol. 2005;97:727–32.
38. Oonk MH, Hollema H, van der Zee AG. Sentinel node biopsy in vulvar cancer: implications for staging. Best Pract Res Clin Obstet Gynaecol. 2015;29(6):812–21.
39. Erkanli S, Bolat F, Seydaoglu G. Detection and importance of micrometastasis in histologically negative lymph nodes in endometrial carcinoma. Eur J Gynaecol Oncol. 2011;32(6):619–25.
40. Yabushita H, Shimazu M, Yamada H, et al. Occult lymph node metastases detected by cytokeratin immunohistochemistry predict recurrence in node-negative endometrial cancer. Gynecol Oncol. 2001;80:139–44.
41. McCoy A, Finan MA, Boudreaux FT, Tucker JA, Lazarchick JJ, Donnell RM, Rocconi RP. The incidence and clinical significance of lymph node micrometastases determined by immunohistochemical staining in stage I—lymph node negative endometrial cancer. Histol Histopathol. 2012;27(2):181–5.
42. Raimond E, et al. Impact of sentinel lymph node biopsy on the therapeutic management of early-stage endometrial cancer: results of a retrospective multicenter study. Gynecol Oncol. 2014;133:506–11.

Fertility-Sparing Treatment in Early-Stage Endometrial Cancer

13

Stefano Greggi, Francesca Falcone, and Giuseppe Laurelli

Endometrial cancer (EC) in women of childbearing age is rare. It is estimated that only 4% of EC patients are younger than 40 years of age [1]. The median age at first delivery, however, is constantly rising in developed countries, due to the trend to postpone parenting for social reasons. Thus, the incidence of EC diagnosed before completion of the reproductive pathway is increasing [2]. Young women are usually diagnosed with low-grade, early-stage disease, and have excellent prognosis with 5- and 10-year disease-free survival (DFS) of up to 99.2 and 98%, respectively [3, 4]. The standard treatment (hysterectomy, bilateral salpingo-oophorectomy, and eventually pelvic and aortic lymphadenectomy) precludes future fertility and may thus be undesirable by women wishing to maintain their reproductive potential. Given the excellent oncologic outcomes associated with early-stage EC, the importance of improving quality of life and preserving fertility has been recognized. Fertility-sparing options for EC management have increasingly been investigated, but a contemporary consensus standardizing a conservative approach has not yet been defined.

Accurate patient selection for fertility preservation is of utmost importance, and candidates for conservative management are generally considered women younger than 40 years of age with intramucous, well-differentiated, endometrioid EC, with no evidence of extrauterine spread, who are highly motivated to maintain their reproductive function [2, 3].

Dilation and curettage (D&C) shows a lower rate (8.7%) of histological undergrading, if compared with pipelle biopsy (17.4%), and it is still considered by some

S. Greggi (✉) · F. Falcone · G. Laurelli
Gynecologic Oncology Surgery, Istituto Nazionale Tumori "Fondazione G. Pascale" – IRCCS, Naples, Italy
e-mail: s.greggi@istitutotumori.na.it

authors the optimal method of diagnosis in a fertility-sparing setting [3, 5, 6]. In the last two decades, however, hysteroscopic biopsy has been increasingly used for the diagnosis of EC. A potential increased risk of peritoneal spread during hysteroscopy caused by the use of liquid distension medium has been raised [7]. In a recent meta-analysis including approximately 3000 patients, although preoperative hysteroscopy resulted in a significantly higher rate of positive peritoneal cytology, this was not confirmed in an early-stage setting, and preoperative hysteroscopy had no impact on prognosis [8].

Few studies have reported the outcomes of fertility-sparing treatment in patients with higher than G1 intramucous EC [9, 10]. In the study of Park et al., the complete response rate in the 17 patients with intramucous G2–3 EC was not significantly lower than that observed in G1 patients (76.5% vs. 77.7%), nor was the recurrence rate higher (23.1% vs. 30.4%) [9]. These encouraging results, however, are based on very limited numbers, and we believe that conservative management of moderate-high-grade disease should still be considered with caution.

Contrast-enhanced magnetic resonance (MR) is the most accurate method to preoperatively diagnose myometrial involvement [11]. Transvaginal ultrasonography (TVS) has also yielded promising results when performed by experienced and dedicated sonographers [12].

Young women diagnosed with EC are potentially (5–10%) harboring a germ-line mutation in DNA mismatch repair (MMR) genes (Lynch II/hereditary non-polyposis colorectal cancer (HNPCC) syndrome), characterized by increased lifetime risk for EC and ovarian cancer (OC) (up to 60% and 24%, respectively) [13, 14]. Current guidelines suggest that EC patients younger than 50 years should be routinely evaluated for Lynch II syndrome [13], and it is debatable whether an EC young patient with an MMR or a BRCA mutation should not be offered a conservative management in the framework of a study protocol at a comprehensive cancer center. EC conservative management should not be considered as a definitive treatment, and it should be followed by total abdominal hysterectomy and bilateral salpingo-oophorectomy (TAH-BSO) after childbearing completion. In this perspective, fertility-sparing treatment may be also offered to patients at genetic high risk after appropriate counseling to be included in the pretreatment workup even in the absence of a positive family history.

Based on small series [15, 16], the risk of a synchronous OC (11–29%) in young EC patients has been likely overestimated. In fact, lower incidence rates ranging from 3 to 4.5% have been more recently reported [17, 18]. To exclude extrauterine spread, a pretreatment laparoscopy has been suggested due to the limited sensitivity of imaging techniques and serum CA125 to detect subclinical synchronous lesions [19]. The usefulness of this approach, however, seems to be questionable, as the presence of occult ovarian malignancy in the setting of intraoperatively benign-appearing ovaries has been reported to vary from 4 to 25% [16, 19].

Current fertility-sparing treatment modalities mainly comprise hormonal therapies involving oral progestins, progestin-releasing intrauterine devices, natural progesterone, oral contraceptives, selective estrogen receptor modulators, gonadotropin-releasing hormone agonist, and aromatase inhibitors.

Of these treatments, oral progestin therapy is the most commonly used, and its efficacy is well-known compared with other treatment modalities. There is no consensus, however, regarding the ideal progestin agent, dose, or duration of treatment. The two most common regimens are medroxyprogesterone acetate (MPA) at 500–600 mg daily and megestrol acetate (MA) at 160 mg daily. The potency of these two drugs (in terms of endometrial response) has been reported to be similar [20]. In general, the most contemporary studies on exclusive oral progestin therapy report a mean complete response rates ranging from 55 to 78% [20–22].

High doses of progestins, however, carry the risks of side effects and complications, with a high likelihood of noncompliance. The choice of progestin, dose, and route of administration should be individualized to minimize risks such as thrombophlebitis, weight gain, headaches, sleep disorders, mood and libido changes, and leg cramps.

The LNG-IUD delivers progesterone locally at a much higher concentration than do oral formulations, avoiding the risks of side effects and complications associated with high doses of oral progestins. Despite LNG-IUD has not been as well studied as oral progestins, preliminary reports have documented that the use of LNG-IUD is equally effective compared to oral progestins in terms of response in patients with early EC [23]. An important additional benefit of LNG-IUD includes the efficacious drug delivery for up to 5 years. This appears very useful for women not planning to attempt pregnancy immediately after achieving complete response. In this setting, maintenance treatment with low-dose cyclic progestin or an LNG-IUD has been shown to lower the risk of recurrence [20].

Due to the heterogeneity of treatment protocols used, it is quite difficult to agree on the optimal duration of treatment with progestins. The minimum duration of treatment needed to achieve a complete regression appears to be 3 months. If the patient shows disease progression at this time point, definitive surgical management should be considered as mandatory. Instead, if the patient has persistent disease without progression at this time point, further treatment with progestin can be performed as some instances of a complete response after 9–12 months of treatment have been reported [5, 20, 24]. Most of the patients, however, will respond within 6 months of treatment, with only a small additional benefit for prolongation of treatment [24]. Patients with persistent disease after 6–9 months of therapy should be counseled about a more definitive approach.

Close surveillance is mandatory after achieving a complete response and should include a 3–6 monthly general and pelvic examination, endometrial sampling, serum CA125, and TVS or computed tomography (CT) to obtain a thorough evaluation of the adnexa. It is important to recognize that conservative treatment is a temporizing measure. Recurrence rates after fertility-sparing therapy justify the main goal of conservative treatment: delaying any definitive surgery to allow childbearing. In this respect, the importance of counseling is to be emphasized and patients in complete regression should be encouraged to conceive immediately after completion of planned treatment.

The risk of recurrence reported after completion of treatment is relatively high; therefore, women who successfully completed childbearing or who failed in their attempts to conceive should be undergone definitive surgery. The most contemporary meta-analysis showed a pooled recurrence rate of 40.6% after successful fertility-sparing therapy [25]. The safety of fertility-sparing therapy, however, is supported by the findings that almost all recurrences consist of early-stage EC still curable with definitive surgery. In the literature, only 10 patients with stage II or extrauterine recurrent disease after fertility-sparing therapy have been reported [25], four of whom died of disease [22, 26–28]. It is not clear, however, whether these cases were true early, low-grade EC at their initial diagnosis or whether fertility-sparing therapy compromised their survival. It is to be mention the reported occurrence of metachronous OC (early stage, G1) in 2 out of 19 complete responders (10.5%) with intramucous G1 EC, 14 and 44 months after initial negative staging laparoscopy [29]. This data underlines the importance of a careful follow-up and timing of definitive surgery.

EC in younger women is frequently associated with exposure to an excessive unopposed estrogen environment.

As previously mentioned, elimination of such conditions using low-dose cyclic progestin or a progestin-containing IUD may decrease recurrence or de novo development of endometrial cancer. Therefore, if the patients want to delay pregnancy, maintenance therapy using low-dose cyclic progestin or LNG-IUD could be recommended. Furthermore, obesity, which is part of the EC (type 1)-related metabolic syndrome, remains a significant risk factor of endometrial transformation even after primary treatment. This evidence suggests that a program of weight loss intervention in the obese patients should be included into fertility-sparing protocols. It is to mention that a randomized trial is currently running in Australia to detect the additional benefit from a weight loss program associated with LNG-IUD in patients with early-stage type 1 EC not suitable for surgery (feMMe Trial, ANZGOG 1301) [30].

Standard treatment for recurrent disease after fertility-preserving treatment is TAH-BSO. As some women may still wish to maintain their reproductive potential, repeat fertility-sparing treatment may be considered in G1 EC recurrences confined to endometrium. In these circumstances, however, data are even more limited than in the primary setting. Fifty-two to one hundred percent complete response after second-round treatment has been reported, suggesting that conservative retreatment may be feasible and safe, although a temporary approach, for women who decline definitive surgery at the time of uterine-confined recurrence [5, 22, 31].

Some investigators have proposed hysteroscopic surgical excision of the tumor followed by progestin as an alternative conservative management approach in young women with EC. Although limited and based on small series and case reports [32–38], data on this strategy suggest that the addition of hysteroscopic resection (HR) may improve the efficacy of progestin alone, maximizing the likelihood of disease regression. The overall 91% (range 78–100%) complete regression rate, observed in the studies on combined HR and progestin therapy (Table 13.1) [32–38], seems to be higher than that reported in the most recent series including progestin therapy alone (77%; range 43–78%) (Table 13.2) [20, 39–43].

Furthermore, the HR of the tumor before high-dose progestin therapy appears shortening the time between diagnosis and complete response. In particular, the

Table 13.1 Literature review of early, well-differentiated, endometrioid EC conservatively treated by combined hysteroscopic resection and progestin therapy

Author	n	Resectoscopic technique	Adjuvant treatment (mg/day)	Oncologic outcome at 6 months	Relapse	DFI (months)	Pregnancy (n patients)	Live births	Follow-up (months)	Current status
Mazzon et al. [38]	6	Three steps[a]	MA (160)	CR	–	n/a	4	5	21–82	NED
Shan et al. [36]	14	EER	MA (160–200)	11CR; 3PD	3	10–24	2	1	15–66	13NED; 1AWD
Marton et al. [35]	2	EER	MPA (400) or LNG-IUD	CR	2	13–15	2	2	n/r	n/r
Arendas et al. [32]	2	Two steps[a]	MPA (300) or cyclic MPA (20–100)	CR	1	48	1	1	48–57	NED
De Marzi et al. [33]	3	Three steps[a]	MA (160) or LNG-IUD	CR	1	6	1	1	8–37	NED
Wang et al. [34]	6	Three steps[a]	MA (160)	CR	–	n/a	3	3	26–91	NED
Laurelli et al. [29]	20	Three steps[a]	LNG-IUD	19CR; 1PD	2	8–41	11	10	30–114	NED

AWD alive with disease, *CR* complete regression, *DFI* disease-free interval, *EC* endometrial cancer, *EER* extensive endometrial resection, *LNG-IUD* levonorgestrel intrauterine device, *MA* megestrol acetate, *MPA* medroxyprogesterone acetate; n/a: not applicable, *NED* no evidence of disease, n/r not reported, *PD*, persistent disease

[a]Resection of the tumor and of a small layer of the myometrium below the lesion (two steps), and of the endometrium adjacent to the tumor (three steps)

Table 13.2 Most recent series of early, well-differentiated, endometrioid EC conservatively treated by progestin alone

Author	n	Progestin treatment (mg/day)	Oncologic outcome at 6 months	Relapse	DFI (months)	Pregnancy (n patients)	Live births	Follow-up (months)	Current status
Cade et al. [39]	16	MPA (60–400), LNG-IUD, or both	7 CR; 9 PD	2	n/r	3	4	3–134	NED
Koskas et al. [40]	8	MA (160), MPA (10), Ly (15), or NA (5)	5 CR; 1 P; 2 PD	2	12–34	2	3	17–86	NED
Kim et al. [41]	16	Combined MPA (500) / LNG-IUD	9 CR; 7 PD	2	6–7	3	2	16–50	NED
Park et al. [44]	148	MPA (30–1500) or MA (40–240)	115 CR; 33 PD	35	4–61	44	n/r	14–194	NED
Kudesia et al. [42]	10	MA (160–240), LNG-IUD, or both	7 CR; 3 PD	n/r	n/r	n/r	2	3–74	n/r
Ohyagi-Hara et al. [43]	16	MPA (400–600)	11 CR; 1P; 4 PD	9	n/r	1	2	4–154	n/r

CR complete regression, *DFI* disease-free interval, *EC* endometrial cancer, *Ly* Lynestrenol, *LNG-IUD* levonorgestrel intrauterine device, *MA* megestrol acetate, *MPA* medroxyprogesterone acetate, *n/a* not applicable, *NA* nomegestrol acetate, *NED* no evidence of disease, *n/r* not reported, *P* progression, *PD* persistent disease

reduction of tumor load by the initial HR seems to allow an earlier complete regression already achieved after 3 months from the start of adjuvant progestin therapy. Overall, the recurrence rate observed in studies of combined HR and progestins (19%) seems to be lower (Table 13.1) [32–38] than that reported after progestin therapy alone (32%) (Table 13.2) [20, 39–43]. Although such comparisons are not methodologically correct, it may be argued that the hysteroscopic tumor resection gives some additional benefit. Such a potential benefit could be explained by the fact that an earlier complete regression can allow a more precocious attempt to conceive, with the pregnancy itself having a therapeutic effect. In this regard, it has been reported that the addition of HR does not affect reproductive outcomes, if performed with a standardized technique and in selected patients with unifocal EC [29, 37]. In general, data on the pregnancy outcome after fertility-sparing therapy in EC are much less known than those on the oncologic safety. In a meta-analysis including 325 women from 26 studies, a pooled live birth rate of 28% has been reported [25]. This rate, however, would be higher if only women who tried to conceive are considered. Park et al. reported the largest series (141 patients) evaluated in terms of pregnancy outcome after progestin therapy in women with intramucous G1 EC. The overall live birth rate was 26%, but it was 66% when considering only women who tried to conceive [44]. It was reported that use of ART is associated with higher pregnancy and live birth rates compared with spontaneous conception in young women with EC, because of the possible presence of risk factors of infertility (obesity, polycystic ovarian syndrome, chronic anovulation) [25, 44]. To date, only few investigators have assessed the association between the use of fertility drugs and the risk of recurrence after successful conservative EC management, and they did not find any such association. In contrast, it was found that patients who achieved at least one pregnancy had a lower risk of disease recurrence regardless of the use of fertility drugs [44]. The limited data available do not allow to draw definitive conclusions on the safety of ART in these patients. In the light of the considerations above, however, we believe that early referral to reproductive endocrinologist should be mandatory in order to maximize the likelihood of a live birth and minimize the time between diagnosis and definitive EC treatment. In conclusion, although fertility-sparing management is not the current standard of care for young women with EC, it may be considered for those patients with early-stage G1 disease wishing to preserve their reproductive potential. To date, such an approach is still experimental and should be offered only in the framework of scientific protocols conducted in cancer centers. The gynecological oncologist and gynecological pathologist expertise is crucial to ensure the correct decision-making process within a complex algorithm for fertility preservation. Candidates should be carefully selected and counseled about the oncologic risks associated with deviation from the standard of care. Early reproductive and genetic counseling also should be considered as mandatory. Although the ideal fertility-sparing management of EC is yet to be defined, data published so far are very promising. It is to be mentioned that a GCIG (Gynecologic Cancer Inter-Group) project has been recently undertaken with the aim of prospectively register conservatively treated EC cases [45].

References

1. Lee NK, Cheung MK, Shin JY, et al. Prognostic factors for uterine cancer in reproductive-aged women. Obstet Gynecol. 2007;109:655–62.
2. Tomao F, Peccatori F, Pup LD, et al. Special issues in fertility preservation for gynecologic malignancies. Crit Rev Oncol Hematol. 2016;97:206–19.
3. Colombo N, Creutzberg C, Amant F, et al. ESMO-ESGO-ESTRO consensus conference on endometrial cancer: diagnosis, treatment and follow-up. Ann Oncol. 2016;27:16–41.
4. Lajer H, Elnegaard S, Christensen RD, et al. Survival after stage IA endometrial cancer; can follow-up be altered? A prospective nationwide Danish survey. Acta Obstet Gynecol Scand. 2012;91:976–82.
5. Park JY, Nam JH. Progestins in the fertility-sparing treatment and retreatment of patients with primary and recurrent endometrial cancer. Oncologist. 2015;20:270–8.
6. Leitao MM Jr, Kehoe S, Barakat RR, et al. Comparison of D&C and office endometrial biopsy accuracy in patients with FIGO grade 1 endometrial adenocarcinoma. Gynecol Oncol. 2009;113:105–8.
7. Obermair A, Geramou M, Gucer F, et al. Does hysteroscopy facilitate tumor cell dissemination? Incidence of peritoneal cytology from patients with early stage endometrial carcinoma following dilatation and curettage (D&C) versus hysteroscopy and D&C. Cancer. 2000;88:139–43.
8. Chang YN, Zhang Y, Wang YJ, et al. Effect of hysteroscopy on the peritoneal dissemination of endometrial cancer cells: a meta-analysis. Fertil Steril. 2011;96:957–61.
9. Park JY, Kim DY, Kim TJ, et al. Hormonal therapy for women with stage IA endometrial cancer of all grades. Obstet Gynecol. 2013;122:7–14.
10. Koskas M, Yazbeck C, Walker F, et al. Fertility-sparing management of grade 2 and 3 endometrial adenocarcinomas. Anticancer Res. 2011;31:3047–9.
11. Kinkel K, Kaji Y, Yu KK, et al. Radiologic staging in patients with endometrial cancer: a meta-analysis. Radiology. 1999;212:711–8.
12. Eriksson LS, Lindqvist PG, Flöter Rådestad A, et al. Transvaginal ultrasound assessment of myometrial and cervical stromal invasion in women with endometrial cancer: interobserver reproducibility among ultrasound experts and gynecologists. Ultrasound Obstet Gynecol. 2015;45:476–82.
13. NCCN Clinical Practice Guidelines in Oncology. Genetic/familial high-risk assessment: colorectal, version 2. 2015. Available from: http://www.nccn.org/professionals/physician_gls/pdf/genetics_colon.pdf.
14. Lu KH, Schorge JO, Rodabaugh KJ, et al. Prospective determination of prevalence of lynch syndrome in young women with endometrial cancer. J Clin Oncol. 2007;25:5158–64.
15. Evans-Metcalf ER, Brooks SE, Reale FR, et al. Profile of women 45 years of age and younger with endometrial cancer. Obstet Gynecol. 1998;91:349–54.
16. Gitsch G, Hanzal E, Jensen D, et al. Endometrial cancer in premenopausal women 45 years and younger. Obstet Gynecol. 1995;85:504–8.
17. Song T, Seong SJ, Bae DS, et al. Synchronous primary cancers of the endometrium and ovary in young women: a Korean Gynecologic Oncology Group Study. Gynecol Oncol. 2013;131:624–8.
18. Williams MG, Bandera EV, Demissie K, et al. Synchronous primary ovarian and endometrial cancers: a population-based assessment of survival. Obstet Gynecol. 2009;113:783–9.
19. Walsh C, Holschneider C, Hoang Y, et al. Coexisting ovarian malignancy in young women with endometrial cancer. Obstet Gynecol. 2005;106:693–9.
20. Park JY, Kim DY, Kim JH, et al. Long-term oncologic outcomes after fertility-sparing management using oral progestin for young women with endometrial cancer (KGOG 2002). Eur J Cancer. 2013;49:868–74.
21. Chen M, Jin Y, Li Y, et al. Oncologic and reproductive outcomes after fertility-sparing management with oral progestin for women with complex endometrial hyperplasia and endometrial cancer. Int J Gynaecol Obstet. 2016;132:34–8.

22. Ushijima K, Yahata H, Yoshikawa H, et al. Multicenter phase II study of fertility-sparing treatment with medroxyprogesterone acetate for endometrial carcinoma and atypical hyperplasia in young women. J Clin Oncol. 2007;25:2798–803.
23. Baker J, Obermair A, Gebski V, et al. Efficacy of oral or intrauterine device-delivered progestin in patients with complex endometrial hyperplasia with atypia or early endometrial adenocarcinoma: a meta-analysis and systematic review of the literature. Gynecol Oncol. 2012;125:263–70.
24. Koskas M, Uzan J, Luton D, et al. Prognostic factors of oncologic and reproductive outcomes in fertility-sparing management of endometrial atypical hyperplasia and adenocarcinoma: systematic review and meta-analysis. Fertil Steril. 2014;101(3):785–94.
25. Gallos ID, Yap J, Rajkhowa M, et al. Regression, relapse, and live birth rates with fertility-sparing therapy for endometrial cancer and atypical complex endometrial hyperplasia: a systematic review and metaanalysis. Am J Obstet Gynecol. 2012;207:266.e1–12.
26. Cormio G, Martino R, Loizzi V, et al. A rare case of choroidal metastasis presented after conservative management of endometrial cancer. Int J Gynecol Cancer. 2006;16:2044–8.
27. Ferrandina G, Zannoni GF, Gallotta V, et al. Progression of conservatively treated endometrial carcinoma after full term pregnancy: a case report. Gynecol Oncol. 2005;99:215–7.
28. Ota T, Yoshida M, Kimura M, et al. Clinicopathologic study of uterine endometrial carcinoma in young women aged 40 years and younger. Int J Gynecol Cancer. 2005;15:657–62.
29. Laurelli G, Falcone F, Gallo M, et al. Long-term oncologic and reproductive outcomes in young women with early endometrial cancer conservatively treated: a prospective study and literature update. Int J Gynecol Cancer. 2016;26(9):1650–7.
30. Hawkes AL, Quinn M, Gebski V, et al. Improving treatment for obese women with early stage cancer of the uterus: rationale and design of the levonorgestrel intrauterine device ± metformin ± weight loss in endometrial cancer (feMME) trial. Contemp Clin Trials. 2014;39(1):14–21.
31. Park JY, Lee SH, Seong SJ, et al. Progestin re-treatment in patients with recurrent endometrial adenocarcinoma after successful fertility-sparing management using progestin. Gynecol Oncol. 2013;129:7–11.
32. Arendas K, Aldossary M, Cipolla A, et al. Hysteroscopic resection in the management of early-stage endometrial cancer: report of 2 cases and review of the literature. J Minim Invasive Gynecol. 2015;22:34–9.
33. De Marzi P, Bergamini A, Luchini S, et al. Hysteroscopic resection in fertility-sparing surgery for atypical hyperplasia and endometrial cancer: safety and efficacy. J Minim Invasive Gynecol. 2015;22:1178–82.
34. Wang Q, Guo Q, Gao S, et al. Fertility-conservation combined therapy with hysteroscopic resection and oral progesterone for local early stage endometrial carcinoma in young women. Int J Clin Exp Med. 2015;8:13804–10.
35. Marton I, Vranes HS, Sparac V, et al. Two cases of successful pregnancies after hysteroscopic removal of endometrioid adenocarcinoma grade I, stage IA, in young women with Lynch syndrome. J Turk Ger Gynecol Assoc. 2014;15:63–6.
36. Shan BE, Ren YL, Sun JM, et al. A prospective study of fertility-sparing treatment with megestrol acetate following hysteroscopic curettage for well-differentiated endometrioid carcinoma and atypical hyperplasia in young women. Arch Gynecol Obstet. 2013;288:1115–23.
37. Laurelli G, Di Vagno G, Scaffa C, et al. Conservative treatment of early endometrial cancer: preliminary results of a pilot study. Gynecol Oncol. 2011;120:43–6.
38. Mazzon I, Corrado G, Masciullo V, et al. Conservative surgical management of stage IA endometrial carcinoma for fertility preservation. Fertil Steril. 2010;93:1286–9.
39. Cade TJ, Quinn MA, Rome RM, et al. Progestogen treatment options for early endometrial cancer. BJOG. 2010;117(7):879–84.
40. Koskas M, Azria E, Walker F, et al. Progestin treatment of atypical hyperplasia and well-differentiated adenocarcinoma of the endometrium to preserve fertility. Anticancer Res. 2012;32(3):1037–43.

41. Kim MK, Seong SJ, Kim YS, et al. Combined medroxyprogesterone acetate/levonorgestrel-intrauterine system treatment in young women with early-stage endometrial cancer. Am J Obstet Gynecol. 2013;209(4):358.e1–4.
42. Kudesia R, Singer T, Caputo TA, et al. Reproductive and oncologic outcomes after progestin therapy for endometrial complex atypical hyperplasia or carcinoma. Am J Obstet Gynecol. 2014;210(3):255.e1–4.
43. Ohyagi-Hara C, Sawada K, Aki I, et al. Efficacies and pregnant outcomes of fertility-sparing treatment with medroxyprogesterone acetate for endometrioid adenocarcinoma and complex atypical hyperplasia: our experience and a review of the literature. Arch Gynecol Obstet. 2015;291(1):151–7.
44. Park JY, Seong SJ, Kim TJ, et al. Pregnancy outcomes after fertility-sparing management in young women with early endometrial cancer. Obstet Gynecol. 2013;121:136–42.
45. Creutzberg CL, Kitchener HC, Birrer MJ, et al. Gynecologic Cancer InterGroup (GCIG) Endometrial Cancer Clinical Trials Planning Meeting: taking endometrial cancer trials into the translational era. Int J Gynecol Cancer. 2013;23:1528–34.

Part V

Non-surgical Management of Endometrial Cancer

Risk Factors in the Early-Stage Endometrial Cancer

14

Samira Abdel Azim

According to the National Cancer Statistics, endometrial cancer is the most prevalent gynecologic cancer in the western world and the fourth most common malignancy in women worldwide [1]. Endometrial cancer is a surgically staged disease. Fortunately the majority of patients are diagnosed at an early stage. This provides the opportunity to cure a great amount of these women. However, to find the right treatment for every individual patient on one side and to prevent overtreatment on the other requires reliable factors that help us to predict prognosis and course of disease.

14.1 Classic Risk Factors

At present, the following factors are clinically used to assess the individual patient' prognosis and, based upon the risk assessment, further therapeutic decisions and treatment regimens are initiated.

14.1.1 FIGO Stage

The aim of staging cancers by assessing spread and size of disease is to establish prognosis. Surgical stage is the most important prognostic factor for survival in endometrial cancer. Since the revision of the FIGO classification in 2009 parametrial infiltration is also incorporated in the staging. Almost 71% of patients with endometrial cancer are diagnosed in stage I. Patients with early-stage disease show a 5-year-survival rate of at least 85.4% depending on histologic subtype. This declines to 20.1% in stage IV [2].

S. Abdel Azim (✉)
Medizinische Universität Innsbruck, Innsbruck, Austria
e-mail: samira.abdel-azim@i-med.ac.at

© Springer Nature Switzerland AG 2020
M. R. Mirza (ed.), *Management of Endometrial Cancer*,
https://doi.org/10.1007/978-3-319-64513-1_14

Table 14.1 5-year survival rate depending on grade [2]

Grade	Stage I (%)	Stage II (%)	Stage III (%)	Stage IV (%)
1	92.9	86.0	78.6	49.2
2	89.9	80.0	67.3	26.5
3	78.9	66.0	46.4	13.4

14.1.2 Tumor Grade

Poor tumor differentiation is associated with decreased survival. For patients with grade 2 and grade 3 cancers survival is significantly reduced compared to grade 1 tumors (hazard ratio 1.4 and 2.8 respectively) [2], as detailed in Table. 14.1. Tumor grade is also related with deeper myometrial invasion and increased likelihood of lymph node metastasis.

14.1.3 Histologic Subtype

According to histologic differentiation, various subtypes such as endometrioid, mucinous, squamous, serous-papillary, or clear-cell carcinoma can be distinguished.

Depending on the histologic subtype, the 5-year-survival rate differs significantly. It is substantially lower for patients with serous carcinomas with 52.6% compared to those with endometrioid subtypes with a 83.2% 5-year-survival rate [2].

Bokhman further classified endometrial carcinomas on the basis of two distinct pathologic subtypes: Type-I tumors are usually of endometrioid subtype, arise from endometrial hyperplasia as precursor lesions, are estrogen-dependent and are associated with a favorable prognosis. Type-II cancers are of more aggressive behavior caused by higher tumor grade, poor differentiation, deeper myometrial infiltration and therefore prognosis is poor [3].

14.1.4 Myometrial Infiltration

Myometrial invasion of more than 50% of the endometrium reduces survival in stage I cancers significantly (HR 2.0). The extend of myometrial invasion is a significant prognostic factor regarding recurrent disease in early-stage endometrial cancer [4].

14.1.5 Lymphatic Space Involvement (LVSI)

Presence of malignant cells in the lymphatic space crucially influences survival due to increased risk of pelvic and paraaortic lymph node metastasis. Particularly for patients in early stage the detection of LVSI is an important risk factor. It results in a more than twofold increase in risk of recurrent disease [5]. Especially in early-stage endometrial cancer a single institutional study confirmed that lymphatic space involvement is an independent prognostic factor for poor recurrence-free and overall survival (HR, 2.8 for both) [6]. In an intraoperative risk assessment for surgical management of endometrial cancer all patients except for those in the low-risk group underwent lymphonodectomy (LNE). In multivariate analysis LNE did not sustain as a significant factor for survival [7].

14.1.6 Age

Generally, elderly women have an adverse outcome and a reduced disease-specific 5-year survival compared to younger women. Incidence of endometrial cancer increases with age. The mean age of manifestation is 61 years [8]. About 90% of cases occur after the age of 50. Incidence is highest between 75 and 80 years with around 90 cases per 100,000 in western countries [9]. Age at diagnosis remains an independent prognostic factor. According to a SEER database analysis, women older than 40 years of age are more likely to present with more advanced stage of disease, higher tumor grades and histologically more aggressive tumors [10]. Additionally age is associated with recurrent disease in early stage.

14.1.7 Race

The lifetime risk of developing endometrial cancer among all women is lowest for Native Americans. It shows increasing incidence in Asian Pacific Islanders, Hispanics, African-Americans, and is highest in US white population [11]. Nevertheless, the likelihood of dying of endometrial cancer is doubled in the subpopulation of African-American women. Although this subgroup showed a 12% decrease in disease rate, the death rate among these women had an 86% increase. African-American women seem to be more likely to present with type-II tumors, displaying more aggressive subtypes and higher tumor grades [12]. On the basis of molecular analysis it was revealed that African-American women more often show tumors with p53 mutations which are associated with poorer prognosis [13].

14.2 Molecular Risk Factors

In the last decade our knowledge about endometrial cancer has been substantially expanded by the identification of an increasing number of molecules that influence tumor growth and disease spreading. It is desirable to improve the understanding of molecular changes within malignomas to be able to identify patients with a higher risk at an early stage of disease to tailor management after primary surgery.

14.2.1 Hormone Receptors

The identification of estrogen (ER) and progesterone receptors (PR) as independent prognostic factors on recurrence-free survival in early-stage endometrial cancer were among the first molecular markers evaluated more than three decades ago. Presence of both of these steroid molecules improves disease-free survival significantly especially in stages I and II [14]. They further serve as targets for hormonal therapy especially in young women with early-stage disease. Treatment with progestins for instance, presents an option in young women with the desire of fertility preservation.

14.2.2 TP53 Status

Mutation of the p53-tumor-suppressor gene is one of the most common genetic alterations found in type-II carcinomas. Mutation is found in 18.5–46% of endometrial carcinomas [15]. The p53 alterations are more frequently found in non-endometrioid histologic types, are associated with higher-grade tumors and do less likely express progesterone receptors. When p53 is mutated survival is significantly reduced [16]. In three out of four cases of precursor lesions (endometrial intraepithelial carcinoma, EIC) a loss of function heterozygosity for chromosome 17p (region of p53) can be detected indicating that alteration occurs early in carcinogenesis [17].

14.2.3 HER2/neu Status

HER2/neu is a transmembrane glycoprotein, which belongs to the human EGFR tyrosine kinase family. The overexpression that is caused by gene amplification of this molecule increases cell proliferation, differentiation, and cell survival [18]. Highest HER2 gene amplification rates have been identified in serous endometrial carcinomas [19]. In type-II endometrial carcinomas (of non-endometrial histology) HER2 expression was found in up to 40% of cases [18, 20].

14.2.4 PTEN Mutation

This tumor suppressor gene regulates the cell cycle arrest and thereby controls apoptosis. The loss-of-function PTEN mutation is among the most frequent genetic alterations in endometrial carcinomas and can be found in 40–83% of type-I cancers [21, 22]. PTEN mutation is an early event to occur during carcinogenesis and can also be present in precursor lesions like complex atypical endometrial hyperplasia [23, 24].

14.2.5 PI3Kinase Mutation

Phosphatidylinositol 3-kinase pathway is a downstream signal from receptor tyrosine kinases (RTK) that is frequently found activated in endometrial cancer. Mutated

PI3Kinase and PI3K pathway aberrations are found in up to 36% and 80% of ECs, respectively [25, 26]. PTEN loss can be a potential activator of the pathway but also somatic mutations or fibroblast growth factor receptor mutations interfere with the RTK signaling [27]. Apart from diagnostic purpose PI3Kinase can also serve as a therapeutic target, as dual PI3Kinase/mTOR inhibitors are under clinical investigation [28].

14.2.6 Microsatellite Instability (MSI)

Microsatellite instability is caused by a failure of the DNA mismatch repair system leading to formation of novel microsatellite fragments, which are repetitive short DNA segments. Affected DNA mismatch repair genes, for instance, MLH1, MSH2, MSH6, and PMS2, are responsible for Lynch syndrome. This condition increases the risk of multiple malignancies, including endometrial cancer. Women carrying the disease have a 40–60% lifetime risk for developing endometrial cancer [29]. MSI positive tumors are more commonly found in white women and more frequently seen in early stages [30].

14.2.7 Somatic Copy Numbers (SCN)

Data from the Cancer Genome Atlas project on the analysis of endometrial cancers on a molecular level were obtained to further characterize the disease. When analyzing different histologic subtypes it was observed that endometrioid subtypes were similar on a molecular level, frequently displaying PTEN and KRAS mutations, seldom p53 mutations, and low somatic copy number alterations (SCNA). Serous and other subtypes often showed p53 mutations and high SCNA. Tumors that had high CN molecularly resembled serous ovarian carcinomas and the clinical behavior and survival was much akin to that of serous ovarian cancer [31].

14.2.8 POLE Proofreading Mutation

Germline mutation in the exonuclease domain of DNA polymerase POLE predisposes to endometrial cancer. In POLE-mutated cancers polymerase proofreading is impaired leading to an increase of base substitution mutations by a defect in the correction of impaired bases. Sporadic POLE mutations are present in around 7% of EC [32]. POLE-mutant tumors were shown to have a lower risk of recurrent disease although there is a strong correlation with high-grade tumors. POLE proofreading mutation was shown to be of independent prognostic significance predicting favorable prognosis especially in grade 3 endometrial tumors [33].

14.2.9 HE4

Human epididymis protein (HE) 4 is a potential preoperative biomarker for endometrial cancer especially in early stage [34]. It was shown that high levels of HE4 correlated with aggressive biological behavior of endometrial cancer. Hence it was concluded that HE4 may be an independent prognostic predictor for poorly differentiated carcinomas [35]. Furthermore HE4 was preoperatively evaluated in combination with CA125 levels in early-stage endometrial carcinomas. HE4 was an independent prognostic marker for overall survival, (HR 2.4, $p = 0.017$). The combination of HE4 and CA125 even increased the hazard ratio on overall survival (HR 4.0, $p = 0.023$). Especially in the subgroup of endometrioid differentiated ECs HE4 was of significant prognostic value [36].

14.2.10 L1CAM (CD171)

L1CAM is a 200–220 kDA transmembrane glycoprotein that belongs to the Ig superfamily. It is expressed on the cell surface of different human carcinomas but also found in blood and ascites by its shed form, the soluble L1–32 [37, 38]. L1CAM was evaluated in endometrial carcinoma. In all detected cases of cancer, L1CAM was

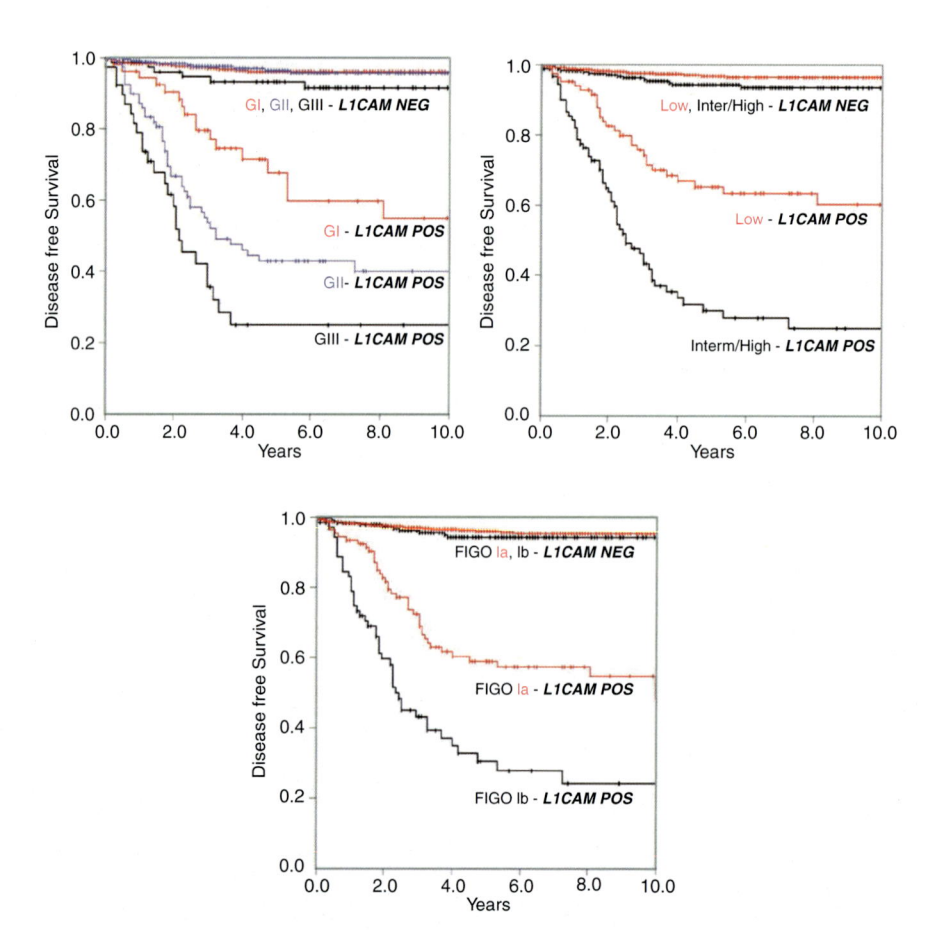

Fig. 14.1 Univariate disease-free survival analyses for FIGO stage, grading and risk assessment according to the L1CAM status [40]

associated with a poor prognosis and adverse outcome [39]. In a large multicenter study L1CAM was evaluated in early-stage endometrioid uterine cancer. Usually this subgroup of patients has a favorable prognosis and very low recurrence rates. About 18% of patients were L1CAM positive and had a significantly reduced disease-free and overall survival with a hazard ratio of 15.8 and 13.6, respectively. L1CAM-negative patients had an excellent prognosis regardless of tumor grade, stage, or risk. However, as soon as L1CAM was present in malignant tissue, disease-free survival decreased significantly with increasing tumor grade, FIGO stage and in high risk patients (see Fig. 14.1) [40]. As a future perspective use of L1CAM as a target itself for antibody therapy seems to be another promising approach. A fully humanized anti-L1CAM antibody has already been successfully synthesized and tested [41].

14.3 Additional Risk Factors

A variety of other prognostic parameters have been investigated but influence on survival remains controversial.

14.3.1 Tumor Size

Chattopadhyay et al. investigated tumor size in endometrioid-type stage-I cancers with a cut-off value of 3.75 cm as a prognostic factor. Tumor size proved to be the only independent significant factor for distant metastasis and disease specific survival in this subset of patients [42]. In a recently published study a 2 cm tumor diameter was used as a cut-off value. Tumors greater than 2 cm were significantly associated with pelvic nodal disease. Additionally the impact of location of uterine mass was assessed. Cases of high-grade endometrial carcinomas located in the lower uterine segment showed a significant correlation with pelvic and paraaortic nodal involvement [43].

14.3.2 DNA Ploidy

Malignant tissue often displays aneuploidy, which predisposes to a more aggressive histologic behavior and a poor prognosis. On evaluation of stage-I endometrioid uterine tumors ploidy proved to be a significantly independent marker for recurrence-free survival, with a hazard ratio of 4.5 (CI 1.3–15.3). In the subgroup analyses of patients regarded as low risk there was still a significant difference in recurrence-free survival in favor for patients with euploid tumors [44].

14.3.3 Positive Peritoneal Cytology

Since the revision of the FIGO classification in 2009, peritoneal cytology is no longer a stage-defining variable as it used to be in the 1988 classification. However, a large retrospective study of 14,704 patients with uterine stage-I cancer showed a significantly reduced disease-specific survival for patients with positive peritoneal cytology (PPC). The hazard ratio was 4.7 for patients with positive cytology compared to negative peritoneal cytology in stage IA over all subtypes. When stratified for histologic subtype, the HR even increased to 5.8 in endometrioid/mucinous subtype and was an independent significant prognostic factor for survival [45].

14.4 Summary

Given all these factors the question of practicability in routine diagnostics remains. The use of molecular factors beyond established classic risk factors can give us a better picture of the individual patient's disease and can help us tailor treatments. This may help to reduce overtreatment in some cases while still permitting to identify high-risk patients at an early stage.

In conclusion, this range of novel molecules used as prognostic markers will provide new therapeutic opportunities for targeted therapies. Anti-HER2 therapies are already state of the art in breast cancer therapy and could potentially be used in EC in selected cases as an additional treatment option. Also anti-L1CAM antibodies are currently under testing. Clinical trials will be needed to evaluate these new approaches. In future, new options will hopefully enable physicians to perform a more "personalized" medicine and get away from the "one size fits all" model.

References

1. Siegel RL, Miller KD, Jemal A. Cancer statistics, 2015. CA Caner J Clin. 2015;65:5–29.
2. Creasman WT, Odicino F, Maisonneuve P, Quinn MA, Beller U, Benedet JL, Heintz APM, Ngan HYS, Pecorelli S. Carcinoma of the corpus uteri. FIGO 26th annual report on the results of treatment in gynecological cancer. Int J Gynecol Obstet. 2006;95(Suppl 1):S105–43.
3. Bokhman JV. Two pathogenetic types of endometrial carcinoma. Gynecol Oncol. 1983;15:10–7.
4. DiSaia PJ, Creasman WT, Boronow RC, Blessing JA. Risk factors and recurrent patterns in stage I endometrial cancer. Am J Obstet Gynecol. 1985;151:1009–15.
5. Morrow CP, Bundy BN, Kurman RJ, Creasman WT, Heller P, Homesley HD, Graham JE. Relationship between surgical-pathological risk factors and outcome in clinical stage I and II carcinoma of the endometrium: a Gynecologic Oncology Group study. Gynecol Oncol. 1991;40:55–65.
6. Weinberg LE, Kunos CA, Zanotti KM. Lymphovascular space invasion (LVSI) is an isolated poor prognostic factor for recurrence and survival among women with intermediate- to high-risk early-stage endometrioid endometrial cancer. Int J Gynecol Cancer. 2013;23:1438–45.
7. Egle D, Grissemann B, Zeimet AG, Müller-Holzner E, Marth C. Validation of intraoperative risk assessment on frozen section for surgical management of endometrial carcinoma. Gynecol Oncol. 2008;110:286–92.
8. Sorosky JI. Endometrial cancer. Obstet Gynecol. 2012;120:383–97.
9. National Cancer Institute. What you need to know about cancer of the uterus. 2007. http://www.cancer.gov/cancertopics/wyntk/uterus.
10. Lee NK, Cheung MK, Shin JY, Husain A, Teng NN, Berek JS, Kapp DS, Osann K, Chan JK. Prognostic factors for uterine cancer in reproductive-aged women. Obstet Gynecol. 2007;109:655–62.
11. Howlader N, Noone AM, Krapcho M, Garshell J, Neyman N, Altekruse SF, Kosary CL, Yu M, Ruhl J, Tatalovich Z, Cho H, Mariotto A, Lewis DR, Chen HS, Feuer EJ, Cronin KE. SEER cancer statistics review, 1975–2010. Bethesda: National Cancer Institute; 2013. Based on

November 2012 SEER data submission—posted to the SEER web site. https://seer.cancer.gov/archive/csr/1975_2014/.
12. Setiawan VW, Pike MC, Kolonel LN, Nomura AM, Goodman MT, Henderson BE. Racial/ethnic differences in endometrial cancer risk: the multiethnic cohort study. Am J Epidemiol. 2007;165:262–70.
13. Clifford SL, Kaminetsky CP, Cirisano FD, Dodge R, Soper JT, Clarke-Pearson DL, Berchuck A. Racial disparity in overexpression of the p53 tumor suppressor gene in stage I endometrial cancer. Am J Obstet Gynecol. 1997;176:S229–32.
14. Creasman WT, Soper JT, McCarty KS, McCarty KS, Hinshaw W, Clarke-Pearson DL. Influence of cytoplasmic steroid receptor content on prognosis of early stage endometrial carcinoma. Am J Obstet Gynecol. 1985;151:922–32.
15. Weigelt B, Banerjee S. Molecular targets and targeted therapeutics in endometrial cancer. Curr Opin Oncol. 2012;24:554–63.
16. Lee E-J, Kim T-J, Kim DS, Choi CH, Lee J-W, Lee J-H, Bae D-S, Kim B-G. p53 alteration independently predicts poor outcomes in patients with endometrial cancer: a clinicopathologic study of 131 cases and literature review. Gynecol Oncol. 2010;116:533–8.
17. Tashiro H, Isacson C, Levine R, Kurman RJ, Cho KR, Hedrick L. p53 gene mutations are common in uterine serous carcinoma and occur early in their pathogenesis. Am J Pathol. 1997;150:177–85.
18. Santin AD, Bellone S, Gokden M, Palmieri M, Dunn D, Agha J, Roman JJ, Hutchins L, Pecorelli S, O'Brien T, Cannon MJ, Parham GP. Overexpression of HER-2/neu in uterine serous papillary cancer. Clin Cancer Res. 2002;8:1271–9.
19. Morrison C, Zanagnolo V, Ramirez N, Cohn DE, Kelbick N, Copeland L, Maxwell GL, Maxwell LG, Fowler JM. HER-2 is an independent prognostic factor in endometrial cancer: association with outcome in a large cohort of surgically staged patients. J Clin Oncol. 2006;24:2376–85.
20. Slomovitz BM, Broaddus RR, Burke TW, Sneige N, Soliman PT, Wu W, Sun CC, Munsell MF, Gershenson DM, Lu KH. Her-2/neu overexpression and amplification in uterine papillary serous carcinoma. J Clin Oncol. 2004;22:3126–32.
21. Mutter GL, Lin MC, Fitzgerald JT, Kum JB, Baak JP, Lees JA, Weng LP, Eng C. Altered PTEN expression as a diagnostic marker for the earliest endometrial precancers. J Natl Cancer Inst. 2000;92:924–30.
22. Tashiro H, Blazes MS, Wu R, Cho KR, Bose S, Wang SI, Li J, Parsons R, Ellenson LH. Mutations in PTEN are frequent in endometrial carcinoma but rare in other common gynecological malignancies. Cancer Res. 1997;57:3935–40.
23. Maxwell GL, Risinger JI, Tong B, Shaw H, Barrett JC, Berchuck A, Futreal PA. Mutation of the PTEN tumor suppressor gene is not a feature of ovarian cancers. Gynecol Oncol. 1998;70:13–6.
24. Levine RL, Cargile CB, Blazes MS, van Rees B, Kurman RJ, Ellenson LH. PTEN mutations and microsatellite instability in complex atypical hyperplasia, a precursor lesion to uterine endometrioid carcinoma. Cancer Res. 1998;58:3254–8.
25. Oda K, Stokoe D, Taketani Y, McCormick F. High frequency of coexistent mutations of PIK3CA and PTEN genes in endometrial carcinoma. Cancer Res. 2005;65:10669–73.
26. Cheung LWT, Hennessy BT, Li J, Yu S, Myers AP, Djordjevic B, Lu Y, Stemke-Hale K, Dyer MD, Zhang F, Ju Z, Cantley LC, Scherer SE, Liang H, Lu KH, Broaddus RR, Mills GB. High frequency of PIK3R1 and PIK3R2 mutations in endometrial cancer elucidates a novel mechanism for regulation of PTEN protein stability. Cancer Discov. 2011;1:170–85.
27. Velasco A, Bussaglia E, Pallares J, Dolcet X, Llobet D, Encinas M, Llecha N, Palacios J, Prat J, Matias-Guiu X. PIK3CA gene mutations in endometrial carcinoma: correlation with PTEN and K-RAS alterations. Hum Pathol. 2006;37:1465–72.
28. Slomovitz BM, Coleman RL. The PI3K/AKT/mTOR pathway as a therapeutic target in endometrial cancer. Clin Cancer Res. 2012;18:5856–64.
29. Lu KH, Dinh M, Kohlmann W, Watson P, Green J, Syngal S, Bandipalliam P, Chen L-M, Allen B, Conrad P, Terdiman J, Sun C, Daniels M, Burke T, Gershenson DM, Lynch H, Lynch P,

Broaddus RR. Gynecologic cancer as a "sentinel cancer" for women with hereditary nonpolyposis colorectal cancer syndrome. Obstet Gynecol. 2005;105:569–74.
30. Basil JB, Goodfellow PJ, Rader JS, Mutch DG, Herzog TJ. Clinical significance of microsatellite instability in endometrial carcinoma. Cancer. 2000;89:1758–64.
31. Kandoth C, Schultz N, Cherniack AD, Akbani R, Liu Y, Shen H, Robertson AG, Pashtan I, Shen R, Benz CC, Yau C, Laird PW, Ding L, Zhang W, Mills GB, Kucherlapati R, Mardis ER, Levine DA, Cancer Genome Atlas Research Network. Integrated genomic characterization of endometrial carcinoma. Nature. 2013;497:67–73.
32. Church DN, Briggs SEW, Palles C, Domingo E, Kearsey SJ, Grimes JM, Gorman M, Martin L, Howarth KM, Hodgson SV, NSECG Collaborators, Kaur K, Taylor J, Tomlinson IPM. DNA polymerase ε and δ exonuclease domain mutations in endometrial cancer. Hum Mol Genet. 2013;22:2820–8.
33. Church DN, Stelloo E, Nout RA, Valtcheva N, Depreeuw J, Haar ter N, Noske A, Amant F, Tomlinson IPM, Wild PJ, Lambrechts D, Jürgenliemk-Schulz IM, Jobsen JJ, Smit VTHBM, Creutzberg CL, Bosse T. Prognostic significance of POLE proofreading mutations in endometrial cancer. J Natl Cancer Inst. 2015;107:402–dju402.
34. Moore RG, Miller CM, Brown AK, Robison K, Steinhoff M, Lambert-Messerlian G. Utility of tumor marker HE4 to predict depth of myometrial invasion in endometrioid adenocarcinoma of the uterus. Int J Gynecol Cancer. 2011;21:1185–90.
35. Bignotti E, Ragnoli M, Zanotti L, Calza S, Falchetti M, Lonardi S, Bergamelli S, Bandiera E, Tassi RA, Romani C, Todeschini P, Odicino FE, Facchetti F, Pecorelli S, Ravaggi A. Diagnostic and prognostic impact of serum HE4 detection in endometrial carcinoma patients. Br J Cancer. 2011;104:1418–25.
36. Mutz-Dehbalaie I, Egle D, Fessler S, Hubalek M, Fiegl H, Marth C, Widschwendter A. Gynecol HE4 is an independent prognostic marker in endometrial cancer patients. Gynecol Oncol. 2012;126(2):186–91. https://doi.org/10.1016/j.ygyno.2012.04.022. Epub 2012 Apr 21.
37. Huszar M, Moldenhauer G, Gschwend V, Ben-Arie A, Altevogt P, Fogel M. Expression profile analysis in multiple human tumors identifies L1 (CD171) as a molecular marker for differential diagnosis and targeted therapy. Hum Pathol. 2006;37:1000–8.
38. Moos M, Tacke R, Scherer H, Teplow D, Früh K, Schachner M. Neural adhesion molecule L1 as a member of the immunoglobulin superfamily with binding domains similar to fibronectin. Nature. 1988;334:701–3.
39. Huszar M, Pfeiffer M, Schirmer U, Kiefel H, Konecny GE, Ben-Arie A, Edler L, Münch M, Müller-Holzner E, Jerabek-Klestil S, Abdel-Azim S, Marth C, Zeimet AG, Altevogt P, Fogel M. Up-regulation of L1CAM is linked to loss of hormone receptors and E-cadherin in aggressive subtypes of endometrial carcinomas. J Pathol. 2010;220:551–61.
40. Zeimet AG, Reimer D, Huszar M, Winterhoff B, Puistola U, Azim SA, Muller-Holzner E, Ben-Arie A, van Kempen LC, Petru E, Jahn S, Geels YP, Massuger LF, Amant F, Polterauer S, Lappi-Blanco E, Bulten J, Meuter A, Tanouye S, Oppelt P, Stroh-Weigert M, Reinthaller A, Mariani A, Hackl W, Netzer M, Schirmer U, Vergote I, Altevogt P, Marth C, Fogel M. L1CAM in early-stage type I endometrial cancer: results of a large multicenter evaluation. J Natl Cancer Inst. 2013;105:1142–50.
41. Doberstein K, Harter PN, Haberkorn U, Bretz NP, Arnold B, Carretero R, Moldenhauer G, Mittelbronn M, Altevogt P. Antibody therapy to human L1CAM in a transgenic mouse model blocks local tumor growth but induces EMT. Int J Cancer. 2015;136:E326–39.
42. Chattopadhyay S, Cross P, Nayar A, Galaal K, Naik R. Tumor size: a better independent predictor of distant failure and death than depth of myometrial invasion in International Federation of Gynecology and Obstetrics stage I endometrioid endometrial cancer. Int J Gynecol Cancer. 2013;23:690–7.
43. Doll KM, Tseng J, Denslow SA, Fader AN, Gehrig PA. High-grade endometrial cancer: revisiting the impact of tumor size and location on outcomes. Gynecol Oncol. 2014;132:44–9.
44. Song T, Lee J-W, Kim H-J, Kim MK, Choi CH, Kim T-J, Bae D-S, Kim B-G. Prognostic significance of DNA ploidy in stage I endometrial cancer. Gynecol Oncol. 2011;122:79–82.
45. Garg G, Gao F, Wright JD, Hagemann AR, Mutch DG, Powell MA. Positive peritoneal cytology is an independent risk-factor in early stage endometrial cancer. Gynecol Oncol. 2013;128:77–82.

Role of Radiation Therapy

15

Mansoor Raza Mirza

Radiation therapy has been historically prescribed as adjuvant therapy in endometrial cancer and is suggested in most of the guidelines. The recently published ESMO-ESGO-ESTRO guidelines [1–3] has recently summarized these indications. These guidelines use the current classification, however the studies reviewed are performed using old FIGO-classification.

15.1 Low-Risk Endometrial Cancer

Low-risk endometrial cancer is stage I endometrioid adenocarcinoma, grade 1 and 2 with <50% myometrial invasion and without lymphovascular invasion (LVSI-negative). Survival in this subgroup is high. There has never been any evidence of benefit of postoperative treatment for these patients.

15.2 Intermediate-Risk Endometrial Cancer

Intermediate-risk endometrial is stage I endometrioid adenocarcinoma, grade 1 and 2 with >50% myometrial invasion and without lymphovascular invasion (LVSI-negative). This group of patients are at risk for local recurrences. Many studies have focused on whether the postoperative irradiation could improve survival, as well as relapse-free survival. The four randomized studies and a meta-analysis are summarized below:

M. R. Mirza (✉)
Department of Oncology, Rigshospitalet, Copenhagen, Denmark

Nordic Society of Gynaecological Oncology (NSGO), Copenhagen, Denmark
e-mail: Mansoor.Raza.Mirza@regionh.dk

© Springer Nature Switzerland AG 2020
M. R. Mirza (ed.), *Management of Endometrial Cancer*,
https://doi.org/10.1007/978-3-319-64513-1_15

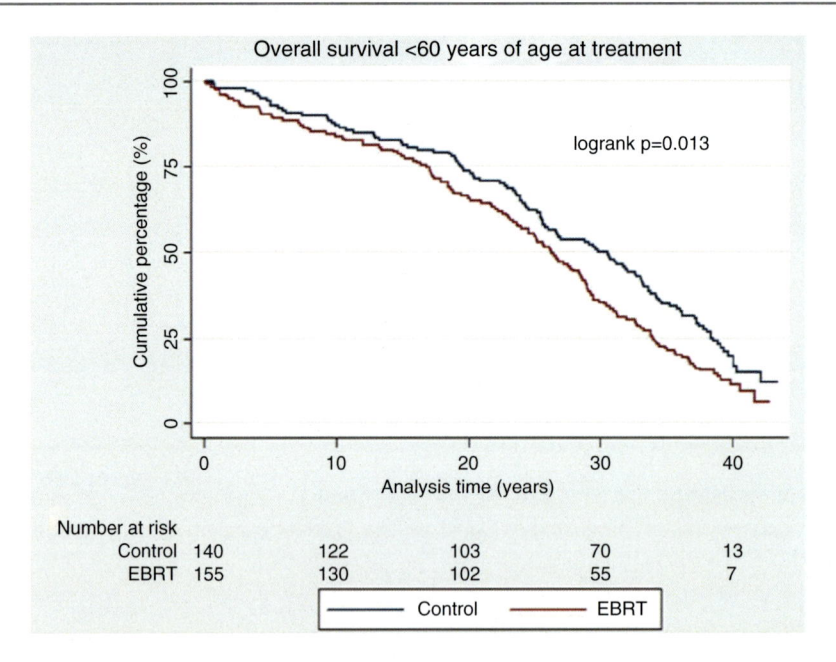

Fig. 15.1 Overall survival in women younger than age 60 years, by treatment arm [5]. *EBR* external beam radiation therapy

15.2.1 The Value of Postoperative External Beam Radiation Therapy (EBRT)

15.2.1.1 The Oslo Trial [4]
540 operated (no lymph node resection) patients with stage I received vaginal brachytherapy. Subsequently, they were randomized to +/− EBRT. There was no survival benefit in the patients receiving EBRT. The 5-year survival rate was 91% vs. 89%; however, significant reduction in pelvic recurrences was achieved by EBRT (6.9% versus 1.9%; $p < 0.01$). A long-term follow-up [5] demonstrated that the women who were <60 years of age at the time of diagnosis had a poorer survival by the addition of EBRT (Fig. 15.1). EBRT group had twice the risk of secondary cancer in the pelvic area and increase in other nonmalignant diseases (Fig. 15.2).

15.2.1.2 PORTEC-1 Study [6]
715 patients with stage I intermediate risk factors were randomized to +/− EBRT. Again surgery in this trial did not mandate lymphadenectomy. Vaginal brachytherapy was allowed. There was no survival benefit on addition of EBRT; the 5-year survival rate was 81% against 85% ($p = 0.31$). This trial also demonstrated a significant reduction in the pelvic recurrence rate from 14 to 4% ($p < 0.001$). The PORTEC group evaluated the results of long-term follow-up of these patients [7]. They included patients from both PORTEC-1 and PORTEC-2 and patients from a study of preoperative irradiation of the rectum. These results did not reveal an increased risk of developing secondary cancers after radiation therapy.

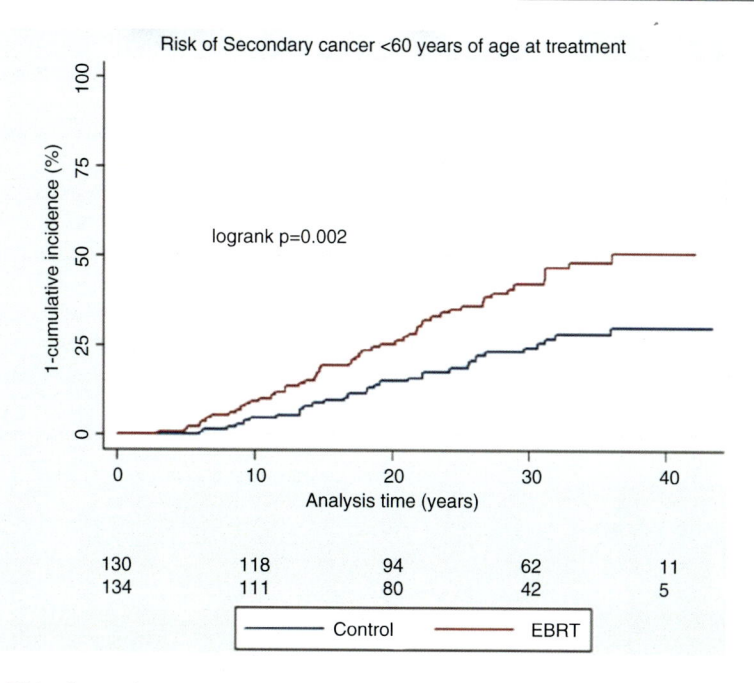

Fig. 15.2 Risk of secondary cancer in women younger than 60 years at treatment [5]. *EBR* external beam radiation therapy

15.2.1.3 GOG-99 Study [8]

90 patients with surgical-stage I and II (surgery including lymphadenectomy) were randomized to +/− EBRT. Vaginal brachytherapy was allowed. The results did not show any survival benefit for patients receiving EBRT. The 3-year survival was, respectively, 96% and 89% ($p = 0.09$). EBRT significantly reduced the pelvic relapse rate from 8.5 to 1.6% ($p < 0.001$).

15.2.1.4 ASTEC Study [9]

905 patients with stage I and II were operated (+/− lymph node resection) and then randomized to +/− EBRT. Vaginal brachytherapy was permitted. The results did not show any survival benefit for patients receiving EBRT. The 5-year survival rate was 84% in both arms ($p = 0.98$). Vaginal-cuff and pelvic relapses were significantly reduced (7–4%; $p < 0.038$) in patients receiving EBRT.

15.2.1.5 Meta-analysis [10]

Cochrane meta-analysis of randomized trials confirmed that the EBRT has no impact on survival, though significantly lowered the risk of local and regional recurrence.

Cochrane analysis of survival with or without EBRT (Fig. 15.3; [10]):

Cochrane analysis of recurrence with or without EBRT (Fig. 15.4; [10]):

Addition of ERBT caused significant increase in toxicity. Acute grade 3–4 toxicity ($n = 1328$) was reported in two studies (HR = 4.68; CI = 1.35–16.16). In six

Study or Subgroup	Log[Hazard Ratio]	SE	EBRT Total	No EBRT Total	Weight	Hazard Ratio IV, Random, 95% CI
EBRT vs no additional treatment						
GOG 99	-0.15	0.25	190	202	15.0%	0.86 [0.53, 1.40]
PORTEC-1	0.2	0.2	354	360	23.5%	1.22 [0.83, 1.81]
Subtotal (95% CI)			544	562	38.5%	1.06 [0.76, 1.48]
Heterogeneity: Tau² = 0.01; Chi² = 1.20, df =1 (P =.27); I² =16%						
Test for overall effect: Z = 0.33 (P = .74)						
EBRT vs no additional treatment (VBT balanced across groups)						
ASTEC/EN.5 (1)	0.05	0.175	452	453	30.7%	1.05 [0.75, 1.48]
Sorbe 2011 (2)	-0.14	0.23	264	263	17.8%	0.87 [0.55, 1.36]
Subtotal(95% CI)			716	716	48.4%	0.98 [0.75, 1.29]
Heterogeneity: Tau² = 0.00; Chi² = 0.43, df =1 (P =.51); I² =0%						
Test for overall effect: Z = 0.14 (P = .89)						
EBRT vs VBT						
PORTEC-2 (3)	-0.16	0.268	214	213	13.1%	0.85 [0.50, 1.44]
Subtotal (95% CI)			214	213	13.1%	0.85 [0.50, 1.44]
Heterogeneity: Not applicable						
Test for overall effect: Z = 0.60 (P = .55)						
Total (95% CI)			1474	1491	100.0%	0.99 [0.82, 1.20]
Heterogeneity: Tau² = 0.00; Chi² = 2.16, df =4 (P =.71); I² =0%						
Test for overall effect: Z = 0.06 (P = .95)						
Test for subgroup differences: Chi² = 0.47, df =2 (P =.79); I² =0%						

(1) 54% in EBRT group and 52% in the No EBRT group received VBT
(2) All women received VBT. This trail expressed HRs in term of VBT; we have expressed the HR in terms of EBRT.
(3) This trail expressed HRs in therm of VBT (VBT vs EBRT); we have expressed the HR in terms of EBRT.

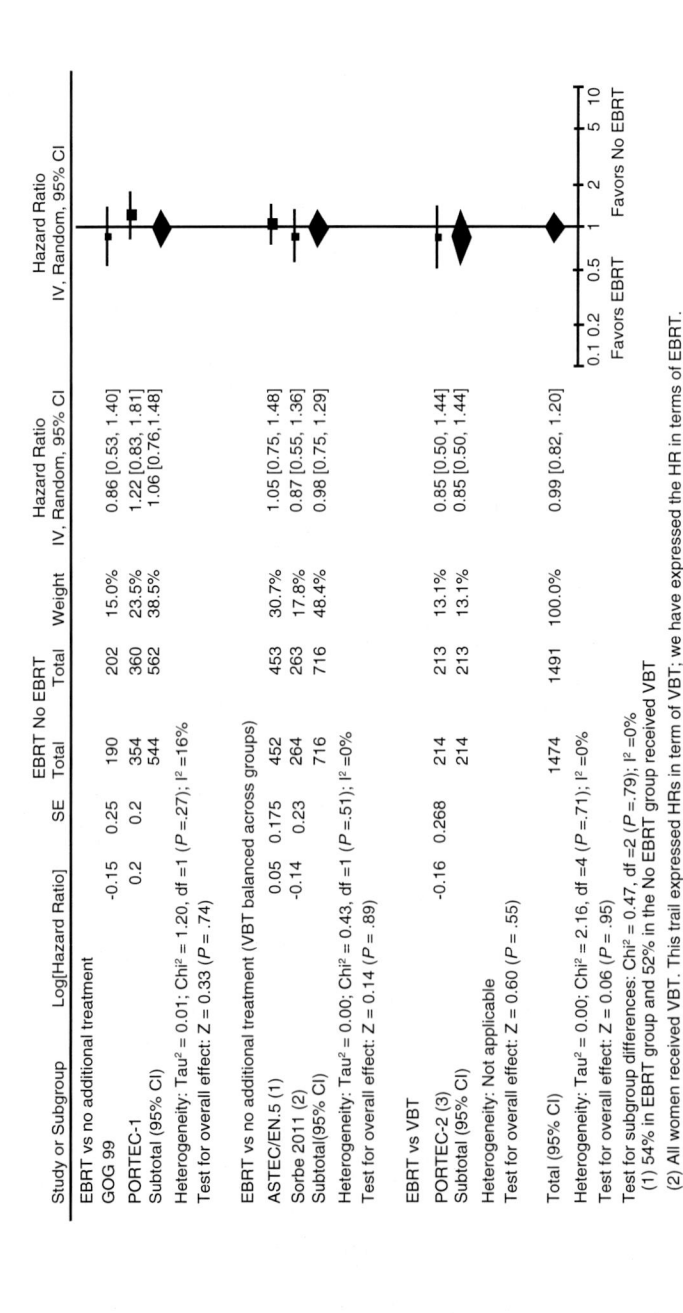

Fig. 15.3 Forest plot of hazard ratios (HRs) comparing overall survival (OS) for stage I endometrial carcinoma patients who received external beam radiotherapy (EBRT) treatment vs. those who received no EBRT treatment. HRs for each trial are represented by the squares, the size of the square represents the weight of the trial in the meta-analysis, and the horizontal line crossing the square represents the 95% confidence interval (CI). The diamonds represent the estimated overall effect based on the meta-analysis random effect of all trials. Inverse variance (IV) and random effects methods were used to calculate HRs, 95% CIs, P values, and the test for overall effect; these calculations were two-sided. The χ^2 test was used to calculate heterogeneity. *Random* random effects method, *SE* standard error, *VBT* vaginal brachytherapy. © The Author 2012. Published by Oxford University Press. All rights reserved

15 Role of Radiation Therapy

Study or Subgroup	Log[Hazard Ratio]	SE	EBRT Total	No EBRT Total	Weight	Hazard Ratio IV, Random, 95% CI	Hazard Ratio IV, Random, 95% CI
EBRT vs no additional treatment							
GOG 99	−1.77	0.63	190	202	9.3%	0.17 [0.05, 0.59]	
PORTEC-1	−1.12	0.34	354	360	31.9%	0.33 [0.17, 0.64]	
Subtotal (95% CI)			544	562	41.2%	0.28 [0.16, 0.51]	
Heterogeneity: Tau² = 0.00; Chi² = 0.82, df = 1 (P = .36); I² = 0%							
Test for overall effect: Z = 4.23 (P < .0001)							
EBRT vs no additional treatment (VBT balanced across groups)							
ASTEC/EN.5 (1)	−0.78	0.34	452	453	31.9%	0.46 [0.05, 0.89]	
Sorbe 2011 (2)	−1.11	0.55	264	263	14.7%	0.33 [0.12, 0.88]	
Subtotal (95% CI)			716	716	46.6%	0.41 [0.24, 0.72]	
Heterogeneity: Tau² = 0.00; Chi² = 0.30, df = 1 (P = .59); I² = 0%							
Test for overall effect: Z = 3.15 (P = .002)							
EBRT vs VBT							
PORTEC-2 (3)	−0.73	0.55	214	213	12.2%	0.48 [0.16, 1.42]	
Subtotal (95% CI)			214	213	12.2%	0.48 [0.16, 1.42]	
Heterogeneity: Not applicable							
Test for overall effect: Z = 1.33 (P = .18)							
Total (95% CI)			1474	1491	100.0%	0.36 [0.25, 0.52]	
Heterogeneity: Tau² = 0.00; Chi² = 2.31, df = 4 (P = .68); I² = 0%							
Test for overall effect: Z = 05.33 (P < .00001)							
Test for subgroup differences: Chi² = 1.19, df = 2 (P = .55); I² = 0%							

(1) 54% in EBRT group and 52% in the No EBRT group received VBT
(2) All women received VBT. This trail expressed HRs in term of VBT; we have expressed the HR in terms of EBRT.
(3) This trail expressed HRs in therm of VBT (VBT vs EBRT); we have expressed the HR in terms of EBRT.

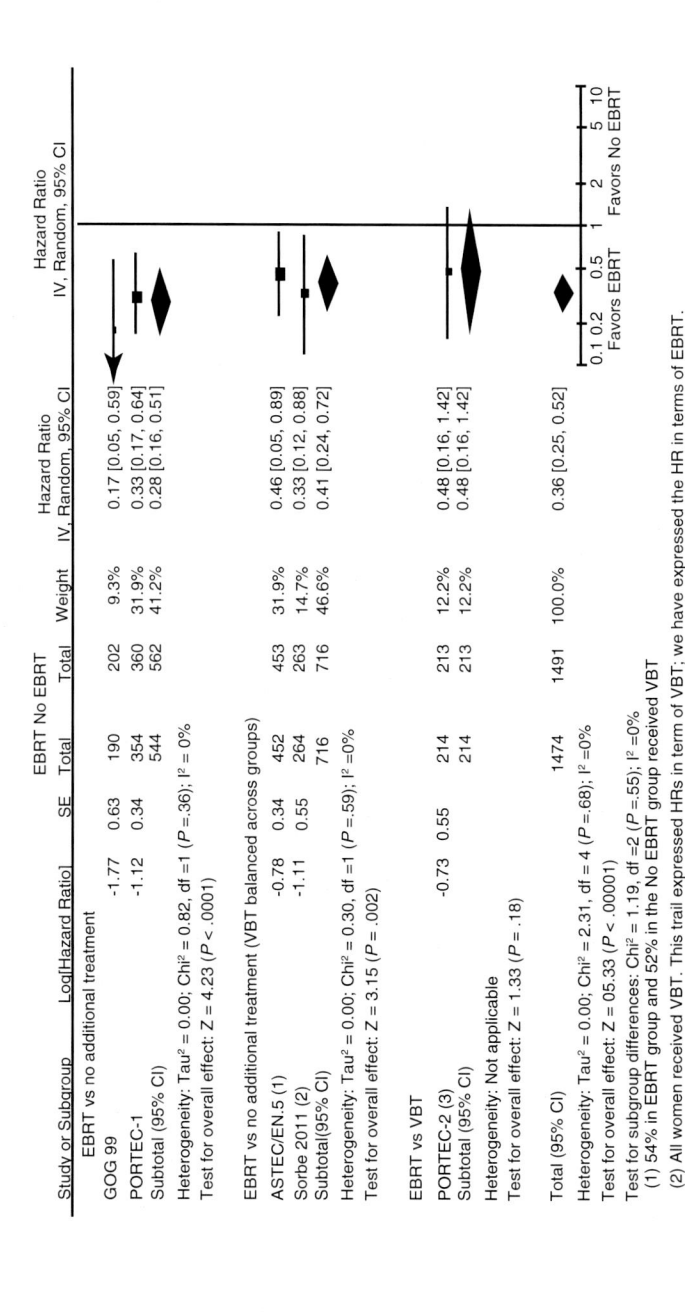

0.1 0.2   0.5   1   2   5 10
Favors EBRT   Favors No EBRT

Fig. 15.4 Forest plot of hazard ratios (HRs) comparing the locoregional recurrence for stage I endometrial carcinoma patients who received external beam radiotherapy (EBRT) treatment vs. those who received no EBRT treatment. HRs for each trial are represented by the squares; the size of the square represents the weight of the trial in the meta-analysis, and the horizontal line crossing the square represents the 95% confidence interval (CI). The diamonds represent the estimated overall effect based on the meta-analysis random effect of all trials. Inverse variance (IV) and random effects methods were used to calculate HRs, 95% CIs, P values, and the test for overall effect; these calculations were two-sided. The χ^2 test and the I^2 statistic were used to calculate heterogeneity. *Random random effects method, SE standard error, VBT vaginal brachytherapy.* © The Author 2012. Published by Oxford University Press. All rights reserved

studies, late side effects of grade 3–4 (n = 3501) were reported (HR = 2.58; CI = 1.61–4.11). Furthermore, EBRT resulted in deterioration in quality of life.

15.2.2 The Value of Postoperative Vaginal Brachytherapy (VBT)

15.2.2.1 PORTEC-2 [11]

427 patients with stage I and II were randomized to EBRT or VBT after surgery. This trial demonstrated that VBT is equally effective in reducing vaginal-cuff relapses with lesser side effects and better quality of life as compared to EBRT. Other studies have shown that VBT reduces quality of life compared to no treatment [8, 12].

15.3 Conclusion and Recommendations

All phase III studies have failed to demonstrate survival benefit of radiation therapy. The significant local control did not translate into survival benefit. One of the reason can be that radiotherapy naïve patients can be effectively salvaged upon local relapse by radiation therapy.

15.4 Medium-High-Risk Endometrial Cancer

There are no prospective independent studies in this subgroup of patients, as the patients were part of the studies reviewed above and thus the evidence is the same as described above.

15.5 High-Risk Endometrial Cancer

This group comprise of the following patients: stage I grade 3 endometrioid adenocarcinoma with more than 50% of myometrial invasion, independent of LVSI status; stage II disease; stage III, radically operated, endometrioid adenocarcinomas, and any stage non-endometrioid carcinomas (serous, clear-cell, undifferentiated carcinomas, carcinosaromas, etc.)

These patients have an increased risk of local relapse as well as of distant metastases. It is a very heterogeneous group of patients with very different survival. The majority of randomized trials have included these patients together with patients of better or worse risk groups. The subgroup analysis of these trials may indicate some benefit of radiation therapy, though more appropriate with the addition of chemotherapy.

References

1. Colombo N, Creutzberg C, Amant F, Bosse T, González-Martín A, Ledermann J, et al. ESMO-ESGO-ESTRO consensus conference on endometrial cancer: diagnosis, treatment and follow-up. Ann Oncol. 2016a;27(1):16–41.
2. Colombo N, Creutzberg C, Amant F, Bosse T, González-Martín A, Ledermann J, et al. ESMO-ESGO-ESTRO consensus conference on endometrial cancer: diagnosis, treatment and follow-up. Int J Gynecol Cancer. 2016b;26(1):2–30.
3. Colombo N, Creutzberg C, Amant F, Bosse T, González-Martín A, Ledermann J, et al. ESMO-ESGO-ESTRO consensus conference on endometrial cancer: diagnosis, treatment and follow-up. Radiother Oncol. 2015;117(3):559–81.
4. Aalders J, Abeler V, Kolstad P, Onsrud M. Postoperative external irradiation and prognostic parameters in stage I endometrial carcinoma: clinical and histopathologic study of 540 patients. Obstet Gynecol. 1980;56(4):419–27.
5. Onsrud M, Cvancarova M, Hellebust TP, Tropé CG, Kristensen GB, Lindemann K. Long-term outcomes after pelvic radiation for early-stage endometrial cancer. J Clin Oncol Off J Am Soc Clin Oncol. 2013;31(31):3951–6.
6. Creutzberg CL, Nout RA, Lybeert ML, Wárlám-Rodenhuis CC, Jobsen JJ, Mens JW, Lutgens LC, Pras E, van de Poll-Franse LV, van Putten WL, PORTEC Study Group. Fifteen-year radiotherapy outcomes of the randomized PORTEC-1 trial for endometrial carcinoma. Int J Radiat Oncol Biol Phys. 2011;81(4):e631–8. https://doi.org/10.1016/j.ijrobp.2011.04.013.
7. Wiltink LM, Nout RA, Fiocco M, Meershoek-Klein Kranenbarg E, Jürgenliemk-Schulz IM, Jobsen JJ, et al. No increased risk of second cancer after radiotherapy in patients treated for rectal or endometrial cancer in the randomized TME, PORTEC-1, and PORTEC-2 trials. J Clin Oncol Off J Am Soc Clin Oncol. 2015;33(15):1640–6.
8. Keys HM, Roberts JA, Brunetto VL, Zaino RJ, Spirtos NM, Bloss JD, et al. A phase III trial of surgery with adjunctive external pelvic radiation therapy in intermediate risk endometrial adenocarcinoma: a Gynecologic Oncology Group study. Gynecol Oncol. 2004;92(3):744–51.
9. Blake P, Swart AM, Orton J, Kitchener H, Whelan T, Lukka H, et al. Adjuvant external beam radiotherapy in the treatment of endometrial cancer (ASTC and NCIC CTG EN.5 randomized trials): pooled trial results, systematic review and meta-analysis. Lancet. 2009;373(9658):137–46.
10. Kong A, Johnson N, Kitchener HC, Lawrie TA. Adjuvant radiotherapy for stage I endometrial cancer: an updated Cochrane systematic review and meta-analysis. J Natl Cancer Inst. 2012;104(21):1625–34.
11. Nout RA, Smit VT, Putter H, Juergenliemk-Schulz IM, Jobsen JJ, Lutgens LC, et al. Vaginal brachytherapy versus pelvic external beam radiotherapy for patients with endometrial cancer or high-intermediate risk (PORTEC-2): an open-label, non-inferiority, randomized trial. Lancet. 2010;375(9717):816–23.
12. Creutzberg CL, van Putten WL, Koper PC, Lybeert ML, Jobsen JJ, Wárlám-Rodenhuis CC, et al. Surgery and postoperative radiotherapy versus surgery alone for patients with stage-1 endometrial carcinoma: multicentre randomized trial. PORTEC Study Group. Post operational radiation therapy in endometrial carcinoma. Lancet. 2000;355(9213):1404–11.

Chemotherapy in Endometrial Cancer

16

Domenica Lorusso and Mansoor Raza Mirza

Management of endometrial cancer has become more complex during the past 10 years for several reasons: changes in histological classification (type 1 vs. type 2) have affected surgical management, adjuvant therapy strategies deeply modified based on data from randomized trials and indications and modalities of lymphadenectomy have changed, even if therapeutic or simply prognostic role of lymphadenectomy remains to be defined.

The estimated cumulative life-time risk to develop endometrial cancer is 0.96%, the corresponding mortality risk is 0.23%, and the mortality to incidence ratio is 0.24 (lower with respect to breast cancer (0.32), ovarian cancer (0.63), and cervical cancer (0.55)) [1, 2].

Survival is dependent on several predictive factors: FIGO stage (5 year overall survival ranges from 74 to 91% for FIGO stage I–II, 57–66% for FIGO stage III, and 20–26% for FIGO stage IV disease) [3, 4]; grade, lymphnodes involvement (5 year disease-free survival is estimated at 90% in patients without lymph node metastasis, 60–70% in those with pelvic-only lymphnode metastasis, and 30–40% in those with para-aortic lymph node metastasis).

Around 55% of patients with endometrial cancer have uterus-confined disease with low-risk factors, and are treated with surgery alone, which is associated with a 95% probability to be relapse-free at 5 years. For patients with uterine limited disease with intermediate- and high-risk factor 4 randomized trials and a Cochrane meta-analysis have evaluated the role of radiation therapy (EBRT) [5–13] concluding that radiation treatment reduces the risk of locoregional recurrence without increasing overall survival.

D. Lorusso (✉)
Fondazione Policlinico Universitario A Gemelli, Rome, Italy

M. R. Mirza
Department of Oncology, Rigshospitalet, Copenhagen University Hospital, Copenhagen, Denmark
e-mail: mansoor@rh.regionh.dk

© Springer Nature Switzerland AG 2020
M. R. Mirza (ed.), *Management of Endometrial Cancer*,
https://doi.org/10.1007/978-3-319-64513-1_16

The lack of benefit of radiation therapy in terms of overall survival is related to the fact that in most of the cases disease relapses as distant metastasis outside the irradiated field: this figure prompts the clinicians to investigate the role of adjuvant chemotherapy as a tool to reduce systemic disease.

16.1 Adjuvant Chemotherapy

The first trial attempting to evaluate the role of chemotherapy in the adjuvant setting was the GOG 34 study, which randomized [14] 224 stage I–III endometrial cancer patients who had undergone surgery with pelvic and para-aortic lymphnodes sampling to receive, after postoperative EBRT, 8 cycles of CT (doxorubicin) vs. observation. The study, which was prematurely closed due to a poor patient's accrual, reported that CT did not provide any additional advantage compared to RT alone in terms of recurrence and survival.

Adjuvant chemotherapy versus pelvic EBRT alone in stage I–IV uterine cancer has been compared in three randomized trials [15–17]. In the Japanese trial [15] 385 patients with IB-IIIC endometrioid uterine cancer, with >50% myometrial invasion were randomized to receive 3 cycles of CAP (cyclophosphamide, doxorubicin, and cisplatin) chemotherapy regimen, vs. EBRT. 55% of the patient population was of stage 1, grade 1 with a significantly high baseline survival with surgery alone. No significant differences were noted in overall survival and progression-free survival between the two treatment arms, nevertheless, in a post-hoc subgroup analysis, the patients with stage IB endometrial cancer and older than 70 years, or with G3 endometrioid tumor, and the patients with stage II endometrial cancer, or with positive cytology, seem to benefit more from chemotherapy than radiation. The Maggi's Italian trial [16] randomized 345 stage IB–II G3 with >50% myometrial invasion and stage III endometrioid uterine tumors to receive 5 cycles of CAP vs. EBRT. 64% of patients received selective nodal sampling and 65% of patients had stage III disease. The median number of chemotherapy cycles was only 3. No significant differences were reported in 5 year overall survival, progression-free survival, or relapse rate. Even if the trial had not the statistical power to detect difference in relapse distribution, it seem to suggest a reduction in locoregional recurrences in patients treated with EBRT and a lower incidence of distant metastasis in patients receiving systemic chemotherapy. According to the actual standard of chemotherapy regimen (Carboplatin-Paclitaxel, CP) both the trials can be considered inadequate for number of cycles and type of chemotherapy; moreover they were designed as superiority trials aiming at demonstrating the advantage of chemotherapy over radiation treatment in survival, so that they are inconclusive in suggesting the equivalence of the two treatments in the adjuvant setting. The third trial [17] was a randomized phase III trial comparing cisplatin-doxorubicyn (CA) chemotherapy vs. EBRT in 422 stage II–IV endometrial cancer patients with <2 cm residual tumor after surgery. The trial reported a significant increase both in progression-free (HR 0.61, $p < 0.01$) and overall survival (HR 0.68 $p < 0.01$) for chemotherapy treated patients.

Recently the results of GOG 249 trial were reported [18]. The trial was a randomized phase II trial comparing in 601 high intermediate and high risk, early stage (I–II, type 1 and 2) endometrial cancer patients EBRT vs. brachytherapy followed by 4 cycles of CP chemotherapy. 89% of patients enrolled in the study had received lymphadenectomy. Unfortunately around half of the patient population was of stage 1, grade 1–2 with a very good baseline survival with surgery alone. The trial reported no significant differences in terms of relapse-free or overall survival at a median follow-up of 24 months but the chemotherapy containing arm revealed more toxic for both haematologic and non haematologic toxicity. The conclusion of the authors suggest that the low risk of systemic recurrences in this population may have reduced the impact of chemotherapy treatment and this strategy should be possibly explored in higher risk patients.

Given the impression that chemotherapy is more prone to reduce distant metastasis while EBRT is able to control locoregional recurrences, the logical evolution of the adjuvant strategy, was to try combine the two treatments.

The NSGO9501/EORTC 55991 trial randomized 382 patients with Stage I, II (occult), IIIa (only for positive peritoneal citology), IIIc (only for pelvic lymphnodes involvement) to receive EBRT vs. the combination of EBRT plus 4 cycles of chemotherapy. Lymphadenectomy was optional and only 26% of patients received it. 90% of patients received a chemotherapy scheme. Progression-free survival was 7% higher in the chemotherapy group ($p = 0.009$), but overall survival did not differ significantly. Similar results were reported in the pooled data analysis with the Italian MaNGO ILIADE-III trial on 534 patients where a significant increase of cancer-related survival was detected (HR 0.55 $p = 0.01$) [19]. Surprisingly no difference in progression-free survival was reported for serous and clear cell carcinomas with whatever treatment.

A Finnish trial randomized 156 FIGO stage IA grade 3 and Stage IB–IIIA grade 1–3 patients to receive RT with or without chemotherapy (PAC for 3 cycles intermittent to radiotherapy). Although a trend toward an increase in PFS by 7 months in the sequential chemoradiotherapy was noted, no OS benefit was observed [20].

A meta-analysis on the role of adjuvant chemotherapy in high risk endometrial cancer including 9 trials and 131,326 patients reported that adjuvant chemotherapy significantly increases overall survival (HR 0.74) and progression-free survival (HR 0.75) and reduce the risk of distant metastasis (HR 0.79) [21]. For additional information on the trials see Tables 16.1 and 16.2.

Recently completed and ongoing trials are focusing on the role of chemotherapy, radiation therapy, or the combination of both in particular setting of high risk endometrial cancer patients.

The recently closed GOG-258 trial evaluated the role of radiation therapy with chemotherapy in high risk disease. 813 patients with stage III–IVA optimally debulked (residual tumor <2 cm) endometrioid tumors and stage I–II serous or clear cell cancer were randomized to receive 6 cycles of adjuvant carboplatin-paclitaxel combination (TC) chemotherapy vs. the combination of concurrent cisplatin-based chemoradiation followed by 4 cycles of systemic TC chemotherapy. The results of this trial revealed that there was no difference in recurrence-free survival or overall

Table 16.1 Summary of randomized phase III trials giving sequential adjuvant CT and radiation as adjuvant treatment for endometrial carcinoma

First author, year (study; years)	Patients	Aggressive histology	LN procedure	Treatment (dosages of CT were per m² unless specified otherwise)	Outcomes	Remarks
1. Morrow et al., 1990 (GOG 34; 1977–1986)	Stage I–II (occult), all grade with any of: ≥50% MI (44%), positive PN or PAN (32%), Cx invasion (24%), adnexal metastases (1%)	33% had tumor grade 3 (3% were clear cell CA)	All had LND	I. EBPRT ± extended field then observation (n = 89) II. EBPRT ± extended field then doxorubicin 45–60 mg × 8 (n = 92) (max cumulated dose of 400–500 mg)	5-year OS: ≅60% both arms 16% (doxorubicin) vs. 23% (no Rx) had distant recurrences	Poor accrual, low statistical power; in chemo arm: higher G3 and positive PN, poor compliance and follow-up. Three deaths in doxorubicin and two deaths in RT
2. Hogberg et al., 2010 (Combined NSGO/EORTC and MaNGO/ILAIDE III)	See 2.1 and 2.2	49% had tumor grade 3 (27% were serous, clear cell or anaplastic CA)	80% had PND, 5% had PAND	See 2.1 and 2.2	HR of CT vs. RT (95% CI) 1. For PFS = 0.63 (0.44–0.89), 2. For OS = 0.69 (0.46–1.03), 3. For CSS = 0.55 (0.35–0.88)	Subgroup analyses showed higher PFS in CT arm in patients with tumor grades 1–2, endometrioide histology or those who had LND
2.1 NSGO-EORTC55991; 1996–2007	1. Stage I, 2. Occult stage II, 3. Stage IIIA from positive peritoneal cytology only, 4. Stage IIIC without para-aortic LN involvement (<2% were stage III)	53% had tumor grade 3 (38% were serous, clear cell or anaplastic CA)	17% had PND, 4% had PAND	I. EBPRT ± ICRT (n = 196) II. EBPRT ± ICRT + either regimen every 3–4 weeks (n = 186) 1. AP (cisplatin ≥50 mg + doxorubicin 50 mg or epirubicin 75 mg) 2. TEP (paclitaxel 175 mg + epirubicin 60 mg + carboplatin AUC 5) 3. TAP (paclitaxel 175 mg + doxorubicin 50 mg + cisplatin ≥50 mg) 4. TP (paclitaxel 175 mg + carboplatin AUC 5–6)	HR of CT vs. RT (95% CI) 1. For PFS = 0.64 (0.41–0.99), 2. For OS = 0.66 (0.40–1.08), 3. For CSS = 0.51 (0.28–0.90)	Only 70% of patients completed chemotherapy; no significant effect of the 2 arms in serous and clear cell CA

2.2 MaNGO-ILAIDE III; 1998–2007	Stage IIB–IIIC (64% were stage III)	39% had tumor grade 3 (3% were serous, clear cell or anaplastic CA)	49% had PND, 5% had PAND	I. EBPRT ± ICRT ± extended field (n = 76) II. EBPRT ± ICRT ± extended field + AP every 3 weeks × 3 (n = 80) (cisplatin 50 mg + doxorubicin 60 mg)	HR of CT vs. RT (95% CI) 1. For PFS = 0.61 (0.33–1.12), 2. For OS = 0.74 (0.36–1.52) 3. For CSS = 0.65 (0.30–1.44)	89% of patients completed chemotherapy
3. Kuoppala et al., 2008 (Finnish trial; 1992–1996)	1. Stage IA–IB (grade 3) 2. Stage IC, II, IIIA (all grades) (12% were stage III)	34% had tumor grade 3 (4% were clear cell CA)	80% had PND, <3% had PAND	I. EBPRT only (n = 72) II. CEP 3 cycles: Before and after EBPRT 1, and after EBPRT 2 (n = 84) (Cyclofosphamide 500 mg + epirubicin 60 mg + cisplatin 50 mg)	Chemoradiation vs. RT: DFS: 25 months vs. 18 months (p = 0.134) OS: 37 months vs. 23 months (0.148)	Higher complications in the combination arm: anemia (22% vs. 78%) and intestinal symptoms (10% vs. 3% needed surgical Rx)

CI confidence interval, *HR* hazard ratio, *MI* myometrial invasion, *PAN* para-aortic node, *PAND* para-aortic node dissection, *PN* pelvic node, *PND* pelvic node dissection, *RFS* recurrence-free survival, *Rx* treatment

Table 16.2 Summary of randomized phase III trials comparing adjuvant CT to radiation therapy for endometrial carcinoma

First author, year (study; years)	Patients	Aggressive histology	LN procedure	Treatment	Outcomes	Remarks
1. Randall et al., 2006 (GOG 122; 1992–2000)	Stage III–IV with the following: no hematogenous to visceral, no inguinal LN, residual ≤2 cm (86% had microscopic diseases, 11% where ≤1 cm)	53% had tumor grade 3 (27% serous, clear cell or undifferentiated CA)	87% had PND, 75% had PAND	I. WAI + EBPRT or extended field (n = 202) (to both sites if positive PN without PAN Bx or no LN Bx at all) II. AP every 3 weeks × 7 cycles then P × 1 more cycle (n = 194) (doxorubicin 60 mg + cisplatin 50 mg) (maximum doxorubicin, 420 mg)	HR of chemo vs. WAI (95% CI): 1. HR of PFS = 0.71 (0.55–0.91) 5-year PFS: 42% vs. 38% 2. HR for OS = 0.68 (0.52–0.89) 5-year OS: 53% vs. 42%	Dose of RT was inadequate; 84% completed RT, 63% with CT; different aspects of toxicity (deaths: 2% in WAI, 4% in CT); peripheral neuropathy lasted in chemo Rx
2. Maggi et al., 2006 (Italian Study; 1990–1997)	Stage IC, G3 or stage II, G3, ≥50% MI or stage III (64%) with no gross residual diseases	56% had tumor grade 3 (aggressive histology not included)	LN sampling (% done not stated)	I. EBPRT ± extended field (n = 166) II. CT every 4 weeks × 5 cycles (n = 174) (Cytoxan 600 mg + doxorubicin 45 mg + cisplatin 50 mg)	5-year PFS: 63% in both arms (p = 0.442) 5-year OS: Chemo 66% vs. RT 69% (p = 0.772)	RT tended to lower locoregional recurrences (12% vs. 16%); CT tended to lower distant recurrences (20% vs. 27%); 84% completed RT, 75% with chemo Rx
3. Susumu et al., 2008 (JGOG 2033; 1994–2000)	Stage IC–IIIC (25% stage III), <75 year old, ≥50% MI, no residual tumor	14% had tumor grade 3 (aggressive histology not included)	96% had PND, 29% had PAND	I. EBPRT ± ICRT (n = 192) II. CT every 4 weeks × ≥3 cycles (n = 193) (cytoxan 333 mg + doxorubicin 40 mg + cisplatin 50 mg)	CT vs. RT: 5-year OS: 87% vs. 85% (p = 0.462) 5-year PFS: 82% vs. 84% (p = 0.726)	95% completed chemoRx; CT does better in HIR[a] 5-year OS: 90% vs. 74% (p = 006) 5-year PFS: 84% vs. 66% (p = 024)

CI confidence interval, *HR* hazard ratio, *MI* myometrial invasion, *PAN* para-aortic node, *PAND* para-aortic node dissection, *PN* pelvic node, *PND* pelvic node dissection, *RFS* recurrence-free survival, *Rx* treatment, *WAI* whole abdominal irradiation

[a]HIR in the Susumu trial included stage IC, >70 years (or G3) or stage II or IIIA with ≥50% myometrial invasion

survival and that external beam radiotherapy is not necessary for the treatment of high-risk early stage or of stage III endometrial cancer [22].

The recently closed Portec 3 trial explores another modality to combine chemotherapy and radiation in the adjuvant treatment of endometrial cancer. 660 patients with high-risk (FIGO Stage IA G3 with LVSI, IB G3, II–III any Grade and any histology) endometrial cancer have been randomly assigned to receive EBRT alone or the combination of concurrent cisplatin-based chemoradiation followed by 4 cycles of carboplatin-paclitaxel (TC) combination chemotherapy. The final overall survival results of the trial [23] revealed no benefit of adding chemotherapy to EBRT. Including 40% of trial population as grade 1–2 early stage disease may have negatively influenced the trial results as these patients have high overall survival after surgery alone and may not require any adjuvant treatment: the experimental arm revealed to be more toxic particularly in terms of gastrointestinal, haematologic and neurologic toxicity with a global decrease of quality of life scores during treatment and until 6 months after the completion of treatment in the experimental arm [24].

The ongoing ENGOT-EN 2 trial [25] is exploring the role of chemotherapy in node-negative stage I–II intermediate or high risk endometrial cancer. 240 endometrioid Stage I G3 and stage II and non endometrioid stage I–II patients will be randomized to receive 6 cycles of CP chemotherapy vs. observation (brachytherapy is optional in both arms according to center policy).

16.2 Metastatic Disease

The overall rate of recurrence for endometrial cancer is about 15%, with more than half occurring within 2 years of primary treatment. Recurrence rates for patients with early stage disease range from 2 to 15%, whereas it is up to 50% in women with advanced stage disease or in patients with aggressive histologies (grade 3 or type 2 tumors) [26, 27].

Women with recurrences can present with an isolated vaginal recurrence, pelvic recurrence, or disseminated metastatic disease. In the first two situations, radiotherapy, if not previously received, and/or surgery may provide excellent tools for treatment. For women with metastatic disease, the predominant modality of treatment is systemic therapy with either endocrine therapy or chemotherapy. However, the prognosis for these patients is poor with median progression-free survival of 12 months and median OS of 32 months.

Cisplatin, carboplatin, paclitaxel, and doxorubicin have all been studied as single-agent in metastatic disease with response rates ranging from 21 to 36% [28]. However, a trend toward an earlier use of chemotherapy in the adjuvant setting has limited the availability of active agents in the context of recurrent disease.

GOG 177 study established the combination of paclitaxel, doxorubicin, and cisplatin (TAP) as the standard of care for women with advanced, metastatic, or recurrent endometrial cancer [29]. The trial randomized 263 advanced/recurrent endometrial cancer patients to receive doxorubicin and cisplatin (CA) vs. TAP: the experimental arm was associated with a higher response rate (57% vs. 34%; $P < 0.01$), an improved PFS (median, 8.3 vs. 5.3 months; $P < 0.01$), and OS (15.3

Table 16.3 Second-line chemotherapy for endometrial carcinoma

First author, year	N	Drug	RR (%)
Homesley et al., 2005	52	Liposomal doxorubicin	11.5
Lincoln et al., 2003	44	Paclitaxel[a]	27.3
Moore et al., 1999	25	Dactinomycin	12
Muggia et al., 2002	42	Liposomal doxorubicin	9.5
Miller et al., 2002	22	Topotecan	9.1
Fracasso et al., 2006	42	Oxaliplatin	13.5
Garcia et al., 2008	26	Docetaxel (weekly)[b]	7.7
Dizon et al., 2009	50	Ixabepilone[b]	12

[a]Patients were taxane-naïve
[b]Patients had received prior taxane

vs. 12.3 months; $P = 0.37$). Unfortunately the triplet was more toxic, particularly in terms in terms of neurological toxicity (12% vs. 1%).

The GOG 209 trial randomized 800 advanced/recurrent endometrial cancer patients to receive TAP regimen vs. the combination of carboplatin and paclitaxel [30]. The two arms appeared equivalent in terms of objective response (about half of the patients in each arm demonstrated objective responses and 30% experienced stable disease) progression-free survival (14 months in both arms) and overall survival (38 versus 32 months for the 3-drug and 2-drug regimens respectively). This study confirmed carboplatin-Paclitaxel as the standard of care for recurrent and advanced disease.

For women who progress after a platinum-based therapy, second line agents have limited activity (see Table 16.3): in general for patients who are anthracycline-naive, doxorubicin is considered the preferred option.; for those who have already received an anthracycline retreatment with paclitaxel, particularly in the weekly schedule, is a commonly administered second-line agent. As a general role in the later line treatment, the patients tend to receive all of these agents in no defined sequence, providing they remain good candidates for treatment.

16.3 Biological Treatments

Targeted therapies, which specifically inhibits molecular abnormalities or pathways of the tumors, have emerged as a novel approach for the medical treatment of several malignancies. Multiple molecular pathways of cellular proliferation have been identified in endometrial cancer, and several targets within these pathways have been explored. In particular the mammalian targets of rapamycin (mTOR) and angiogenesis appear as relevant therapeutic targets in endometrial cancer.

16.4 mTOR Inhibitors

mTOR is an intracellular serine-threonine kinase that acts as an integral part of several signaling pathways, including vascular endothelial growth factor (VEGF), insulinlike growth factor receptor, and phosphoinositol 3-kinase (PI3K)-Akt [31] and has a role in the regulation of cell growth and proliferation, cell metabolism and apoptosis.

A phase II trial of 29 recurrent and metastatic chemo-naive endometrial cancer patients treated with intravenous temsirolimus reported 4 (14%) partial responses, and 20 (69%) stabilizations of disease with a median duration of 5.1 and 9.7 months, respectively [32]. In a phase II study with oral Everolimus in recurrent or metastatic endometrial cancer patients, no partial response was observed; however, 12 out of the 28 (43%) evaluable patients reported prolonged (>8 weeks) stabilization of disease [33]. Dual mTOR inhibitors that target the catalytic domains of mTOR complexes 1 and 2 have recently been developed to maximize mTOR blockade and are now in phase II clinical trials [34].

16.5 Antiangiogenic Agents

Angiogenesis is also a fundamental step in the transition of tumors from a dormant state to a malignant, rapidly proliferative state so that targeting angiogenesis is attractive because it can potentially reduce cancer progression.

Bevacizumab is a humanized monoclonal antibody that binds to circulating VEGF-A. Aghajanian et al. reported 13.5% clinical responses and 40.4% of 6-months progression-free patients with a median PFS and OS of 4.2 and 10.5 months respectively in a population of 52 advanced/recurrent endometrial cancer patients treated with Bevacizumab as single agent [35].

In a phase II single arm trial with CP-Bevacizumab in a population of 38 advanced/recurrent endometrial cancer patients who had undergone primary surgical treatment [36], O'Malley et al. reported a median PFS of 26 months with 55% of patients free of disease at 24 months.

In GOG 86P, presented at ASCO 2015, 349 advanced endometrial cancer patients were randomly assigned to receive CP with either temsirolimus or bevacizumab, or the combination of carboplatin, ixabepilone, plus bevacizumab. With respect to the historical controls the CB- bevacizumab arm reported an increase in PFS (HR 0.805) and OS (22.7 vs. 34 months) [37].

MITO END 2 trial is a multicenter randomized phase II trial comparing CP chemotherapy vs. CP-Bevacizumab in 108 advanced endometrial cancer patients [38] whose results were presented at ASCO 2015. A significant increase in PFS (8.7 vs. 12 months; HR 0.59), response rate (ORR 54.3 vs. 71.7%), 6-months disease control rate (69% vs. 83%) and OS (18 vs. 23.5 months; HR 0.65) were reported in patients treated in the experimental arm. The toxicity profile of the experimental combination, was particularly impacting in terms of cardiovascular events (de novo occurrence of hypertension > grade 2 0 vs. 21%; grade >2 cardiac disorders 0 vs. 3.8%; grade >2 arterial and venous thromboembolic events 0 vs. 11.5% for the standard and experimental arm respectively) and prompt the authors to suggests that a certain caution should be adopted in this population when using antiangiogenic agents.

The ongoing ENGOT-EN1/FANDANGO trial [39] is exploring the role of chemotherapy (CP) with an anti-VEGF tyrosine kinase inhibitor, Nintedanib, or placebo, given both concomitant to chemotherapy as well as maintenance until progression of disease in stage IIIb–IV or at first relapse. The trial shall enroll 146 patients and primary endpoint is PFS.

References

1. Ferlay J, Soerjomataram I, Dikshit R, et al. Cancer incidence and mortality worldwide: sources, methods and major patterns in GLOBOCAN 2012. Int J Cancer. 2015;136:E359–86.
2. Weiderpass E, Antoine J, Bray FI, Oh JK, Arbyn M. Trends in corpus uteri cancer mortality in member states of the European Union. Eur J Cancer. 2014;50:1675–84.
3. Siegel RL, Miller KD, Jemal A. Cancer statistics, 2015. CA Cancer J Clin. 2015;65:5–29.
4. Creasman WT, Odicino F, Maisonneuve P, et al. Carcinoma of the corpus uteri. FIGO 26th annual report on the results of treatment in gynecological cancer. Int J Gynaecol Obstet. 2006;95(suppl 1):S105–43.
5. Creutzberg CL, van Putten WL, Koper PC, et al. Surgery and postoperative radiotherapy versus surgery alone for patients with stage 1 endometrial carcinoma: multicentre randomised trial. PORTEC Study Group. Post operative radiation therapy in endometrial carcinoma. Lancet. 2000;355:1404–11.
6. Keys HM, Roberts JA, Brunetto VL, the Gynecologic Oncology Group, et al. A phase III trial of surgery with or without adjunctive external pelvic radiation therapy in intermediate risk endometrial adenocarcinoma: a Gynecologic Oncology Group study. Gynecol Oncol. 2004;92:744–51.
7. Aalders J, Abeler V, Kolstad P, Onsrud M. Postoperative external irradiation and prognostic parameters in stage I endometrial carcinoma: clinical and histopathologic study of 540 patients. Obstet Gynecol. 1980;56:419–27.
8. Onsrud M, Cvancarova M, Hellebust TP, Tropé CG, Kristensen GB, Lindemann K. Long-term outcomes after pelvic radiation for early-stage endometrial cancer. J Clin Oncol. 2013;31:3951–6.
9. Creutzberg CL, Nout RA, Lybeert ML, the PORTEC Study Group, et al. Fifteen-year radiotherapy outcomes of the randomized PORTEC-1 trial for endometrial carcinoma. Int J Radiat Oncol Biol Phys. 2011;81:e631–8.
10. Blake P, Swart AM, Orton J, the ASTEC/EN.5 Study Group, et al. Adjuvant external beam radiotherapy in the treatment of endometrial cancer (MRC ASTEC and NCIC CTG EN.5 randomised trials): pooled trial results, systematic review, and meta-analysis. Lancet. 2009;373:137–46.
11. Nout RA, Smit VTHB, Putter H, the PORTEC Study Group, et al. Vaginal brachytherapy versus pelvic external beam radiotherapy for patients with endometrial cancer of high-intermediate risk (PORTEC-2): an open-label, non-inferiority, randomised trial. Lancet. 2010;375: 816–23.
12. Sorbe B, Horvath G, Andersson H, Boman K, Lundgren C, Pettersson B. External pelvic and vaginal irradiation versus vaginal irradiation alone as postoperative therapy in medium-risk endometrial carcinoma—a prospective randomized study. Int J Radiat Oncol Biol Phys. 2012;82:1249–55.
13. Kong A, Johnson N, Kitchener HC, Lawrie TA. Adjuvant radiotherapy for stage I endometrial cancer: an updated Cochrane systematic review and meta-analysis. J Natl Cancer Inst. 2012;104:1625–34.
14. Morrow CP, Bundy BN, Homesley HD, et al. Doxorubicin as an adjuvant following surgery and radiation therapy in patients with high-risk endometrial carcinoma, stage I and occult stage II: a Gynecologic Oncology Group study. Gynecol Oncol. 1990;36:166Y171.

15. Susumu N, Sagae S, Udagawa Y, the Japanese Gynecologic Oncology Group, et al. Randomized phase III trial of pelvic radiotherapy versus cisplatin-based combined chemotherapy in patients with intermediate- and high-risk endometrial cancer: a Japanese Gynecologic Oncology Group study. Gynecol Oncol. 2008;108:226–33.
16. Maggi R, Lissoni A, Spina F, et al. Adjuvant chemotherapy vs radiotherapy in high-risk endometrial carcinoma: results of a randomised trial. Br J Cancer. 2006;95:266–71.
17. Randall ME, Filiaci VL, Muss H, the Gynecologic Oncology Group study, et al. Randomized phase III trial of whole-abdominal irradiation versus doxorubicin and cisplatin chemotherapy in advanced endometrial carcinoma: a Gynecologic Oncology Group study. J Clin Oncol. 2006;24:36–44.
18. McMeekin DS, Filiaci VL, Thigpen JT, Gallion HH, Fleming GF, Rodgers WH, the Gynecologic Oncology Group study. The relationship between histology and outcome in advanced and recurrent endometrial cancer patients participating in first-line chemotherapy trials: a Gynecologic Oncology Group study. Gynecol Oncol. 2007;106:16–22.
19. Hogberg T, Signorelli M, de Oliveira CF, et al. Sequential adjuvant chemotherapy and radiotherapy in endometrial cancer—results from two randomised studies. Eur J Cancer. 2010;46:2422–31.
20. Kuoppala T, Mäenpää J, Tomas E, et al. Surgically staged high-risk endometrial cancer: randomized study of adjuvant radiotherapy alone vs. sequential chemo-radiotherapy. Gynecol Oncol. 2008;110:190–5.
21. Johnson N, Bryant A, Miles T, Hogberg T, Cornes P. Adjuvant chemotherapy for endometrial cancer after hysterectomy. Cochrane Database Syst Rev. 2011;(10):CD003175. https://doi.org/10.1002/14651858.CD003175.pub2.
22. Matai D, et al. GOG-258: randomized phase III trial of cisplatin and tumor volume–directed irradiation followed by carboplatin and paclitaxel vs carboplatin and paclitaxel for optimally debulked, advanced EC. J Clin Oncol. 2017;35(suppl):Abstract 5505.
23. De Boer SM, et al. PORTEC-3: adjuvant chemoradiotherapy versus radiotherapy alone for women with high-risk endometrial cancer (PORTEC-3): an open-label, multicentre, randomised, phase 3 trial. J Clin Oncol. 2017;35(suppl):Abstract 5504.
24. de Boer SM, Powell ME, Mileshkin L, the PORTEC Study Group, et al. Toxicity and quality of life after adjuvant chemoradiotherapy versus radiotherapy alone for women with high-risk endometrial cancer (PORTEC-3): an open-label, multicentre, randomised, phase 3 trial. Lancet Oncol. 2016; https://doi.org/10.1016/S1470-2045(16)30120-6.
25. Mirza, et al. ENGOT-EN2/DGCG: chemotherapy or observation in stage I-II intermediate or high risk endometrial cancer. NCT01244789.
26. Creutzberg CL, van Putten WL, Koper PC, PORTEC Study Group, et al. Survival after relapse in patients with endometrial cancer: results from a randomized trial. Gynecol Oncol. 2003;89:201–9.
27. Del Carmen MG, Boruta DM II, Schorge JO. Recurrent endometrial cancer. Clin Obstet Gynecol. 2011;54:266–77.
28. Humber CE, Tierney JF, Symonds RP, et al. Chemotherapy for advanced, recurrent or metastatic endometrial cancer: a systematic review of Cochrane collaboration. Ann Oncol. 2007;18:409–20.
29. Fleming GF, Brunetto VL, Celia D, et al. Phase III trial of doxorubicin plus cisplatin with or without paclitaxel plus filgrastim in advanced endometrial carcinoma: a Gynecologic Oncology Group study. J Clin Oncol. 2004;22:2159–66.
30. Miller D, Filiaci V, Fleming G, et al. Late-breaking abstract 1: randomized phase III noninferiority trial of first line chemotherapy for metastatic or recurrent endometrial carcinoma: a Gynecologic Oncology Group study. Gynecol Oncol. 2012;125:771.
31. Meric-Bernstam F, Gonzalez-Angulo AM. Targeting the mTOR signaling network for cancer therapy. J Clin Oncol. 2009;27:2278–87.
32. Oza AM, Elit L, Tsao MS, et al. Phase II study of temsirolimus in women with recurrent or metastatic endometrial cancer: a trial of the NCIC Clinical Trials Group. J Clin Oncol. 2011;29:3278–85.

33. Slomovitz BM, Lu KH, Johnston T, et al. A phase 2 study of the oral mammalian target of rapamycin inhibitor, everolimus, in patients with recurrent endometrial carcinoma. Cancer. 2010;116:5415–9.
34. Naing A, Aghajanian C, Raymond E, et al. Safety, tolerability, pharmacokinetics and pharmacodynamics of AZD8055 in advanced solid tumours and lymphoma. Br J Cancer. 2012;107:1093–9.
35. Aghajanian C, Sill MW, Darcy KM, et al. Phase II trial of bevacizumab in recurrent or persistent endometrial cancer: a Gynecologic Oncology Group study. J Clin Oncol. 2011;29:2259–65.
36. O'Malley D, McCann G, Fowler J, et al. A phase II evaluation of carboplatin/paclitaxel/bevacizumab in the treatment of advanced stage endometrial carcinoma. Presented at the 42nd annual meeting on women's cancer, Austin; 2013.
37. Aghajanian C, Filiaci VL, Dizon DS, et al. A randomized phase II study of paclitaxel/carboplatin/bevacizumab, paclitaxel/carboplatin/temsirolimus and ixabepilone/carboplatin/bevacizumab as initial therapy for measurable stage III or IVA, stage IVB or recurrent endometrial cancer, GOG-86P. J Clin Oncol. 2015;33(suppl):abstr 5500.
38. Lorusso D, Ferrandina G, Colombo N, et al. Randomized phase II trial of carboplatin-paclitaxel (CP) compared to carboplatin-paclitaxel-bevacizumab (CP-B) in advanced (stage III-IV) or recurrent endometrial cancer: the MITO END-2 trial. J Clin Oncol. 2015;33(suppl):abstr 5502.
39. Mirza, et al. ENGOT-EN1/FANDANGO: a randomized phase II trial of first-line combination chemotherapy with nintedanib/placebo for patients with advanced or recurrent endometrial cancer. NCT02730416.

Role of Hormonal Therapy in Advanced Stage Endometrial Cancer

17

Anouk Gaber-Wagener and Christian Marth

Systemic treatment of advanced disease may be cytotoxic chemotherapy or endocrine therapy. Platinum compounds, taxanes, or anthracyclines are mostly used as single agents or in combination. In patients who have not yet had chemotherapy the response rate is seen up to 20%. The treatment should take account of obesity, irradiation, age, and general condition of the women. Were the objective is palliation or prolongation of survival rather than cure, endocrine therapy is a treatment option, with less toxicity than aggressive chemotherapy. Hormonal therapy is generally better tolerated. These patients typically have some risk factors as obesity, diabetes and hypertension. In postmenopausal women, the principal source of ER is through conversion of androstenedione by aromatase in peripheral adipose tissue. In addition, aromatase is high in endometrial cancer stroma, and locally produced ER may act in a paracrine way to stimulate cancer growth [1, 2].

Endocrine treatment is the treatment used for advanced or recurrent endometroid (Type 1 potentially hormone responsive), estrogen-dependent endometrial cancer. The stage of an endometrial cancer is the most important factor in choosing a treatment plan. The advanced-stage endometrial cancer is a heterogeneous disease that may present as pulmonary metastasis, micro- or macroscopic lymph node metastasis, intra-abdominal metastasis, or inoperable metastasis. Therefore, defining an optimal treatment regimen is difficult. Endometrium cancer is staged during a surgical intervention; it is known as a surgical staging.

Before surgery, often MRI or CT scan are done; to look for signs that the cancer has spread. These imaging tests will show how far the cancer has spread. If we talk about advanced-stage disease then we refer to Stage IV of the FIGO Status.

A. Gaber-Wagener (✉) · C. Marth
Medizinische Universität Innsbruck, Tirol Kliniken, Innsbruck, Austria
e-mail: anouk.gaber-wagener@tirol-kliniken.at

© Springer Nature Switzerland AG 2020
M. R. Mirza (ed.), *Management of Endometrial Cancer*,
https://doi.org/10.1007/978-3-319-64513-1_17

17.1 Stage IV

The cancer has spread to the inner surface of the urinary bladder or the rectum (lower part of the large intestine), to lymph nodes in the groin, and/or to distant organs, such as the bones, omentum, or lungs.

Stage IVA (T4, any N, M0): The cancer has spread to the inner lining of the rectum or urinary bladder (called the mucosa). It may or may not have spread to nearby lymph nodes but has not spread to distant sites. Stage IVB (any T, any N, M1): The cancer has spread to distant lymph nodes, the upper abdomen, the omentum, or to organs away from the uterus, such as the bones, omentum, or lungs. The cancer can be any size and it may or may not have spread to lymph nodes.

Endometrium cancer cells and metastasis show progesterone receptors and/or estrogen receptors. The presence of high levels of progesterone is predictive of a favorable response to hormonal therapy in endometrial cancer. Treatment with progesterone is capable of inhibiting invasion of endometrial cells by downregulating several genes, e.g. integrins or K-cadherin. In well-differentiated endometrial cancer, estrogen and progesterone- receptors are abundant. A significant correlation is found between G-protein coupled with estrogen-receptor and better survival, which are highly expressed in high-grade endometrial cancers [3].

In 1961, Rita Kelley was the first to publish a paper about progestional agents in the treatment of carcinoma of the endometrium. They utilized progesterone dosages in the range of 150–1000 mg. She described for the first time the effects of the female hormone progesterone as an anti-cancer therapy for women with advanced endometrial cancer. The number of trials evaluated oral and parenteral progesterone, mostly in patients with advanced or recurrent disease [4–8].

More recent trials report of a response rate of 20–25% [9–11].

In the GOG 81 trial Thigpen et al. compared MPA Dosage of MPA 1000 mg daily versus MPA 200 mg daily, those 145 patients treated with a lower dose had a better RR of 25% against 15%, a PFS of 3 months and a OS of 11 months. Therefore, a higher dose is not always better.

The GOG 119 (Whitney) trial endorsed 68 patients. They had high RR of 33% and 13 months of OS, while combining or alternating MPA 100 mg bid plus continuous tamoxifen 20 mg daily [12]. The best outcome was obtained GOG trial–Phase II (GOG 153). They tried another regime with a different MA dosage, they enrolled 56 patients and they received 80 mg bid MA (megestrol acetate) × 3 weeks alternating with tamoxifen 20 mg bid × 3 weeks. Here the RR was 27%, PFS of 2.7 months, and a OS of 14 months. This study showed the best survival outcome, the trial in which patients had the highest percentage of grade 1 tumors [13]. Higher dosage of progesterone does not improve the effectiveness of advanced endometrial cancer. There is no superiority in using 1000 mg/day of MPA or 200 mg/day.

Even a hormonal therapy with Tamoxifen (GOG-81F) has shown positive effects on advanced endometrial cancers. There has been a response rate of 10%, these 68 patients only received Tamoxifen 20 mg/day. Low-grade endometrial cancers are more likely to respond to treatments with tamoxifen than compared to high-grade cancers [11]. In advanced or recurrent endometrial cancer hormone therapy is indicated. It is recommended for endometroid type only. For patients with hormone receptor positive tumors—grade 1 or 2 and without rapidly progressive disease, it is the preferred frontline systemic therapy. Grade 3 tumors rarely express hormone receptors and show rather poor response to hormonal treatment. In general, progesterones (medroxyprogesterone acetate 200 mg) are recommended. Higher doses than 200 mg did not show better results. Tamoxifen, fulvestrant, and aromatose inhibitors could also be considered. Before starting a hormonal therapy in advanced resp. recurrent disease, there should be a testing for hormone receptor status. As shown in many studies, patients with positive receptor status for progesterone and estrogen have more effectiveness. The presence of high levels of estrogen (and progesterone) receptors on cancer cells are predictive of a favorable response to hormonal therapy [14].

Best results have been seen in grade 1 or 2 endometroid tumors. The best response is seen in well-differentiated tumors, patients with a long interval before recurrence, respectively those patients with lung and bone metastases. There is an overall response of 25% for progestins. Also, an extended treatment free-interval is predictive for a good response [15].

In the recurrent situation, a biopsy should be done, because there could be a shift/difference between the receptor status in the primary tumor and the recurrent disease. The treatment decision is based on the histologic type of endometroid cancer. A positive ER/PR expression is found in 90% of the tumors. As shown in the recent study data, high response rate of over 60% in ER+/Pr+. G1 and G2 tumors are more likely to respond. Among the studies a response rate of 25%, progression free survival of 3 months and an overall survival of 11 months has been shown. The efficacy is related to hormone receptor status and the grade of the tumor. In progression a loss of receptor (downregulation of progesterone receptor) was detected [16].

17.2 Toxicity Profile of Hormonal Therapy

Hormone therapy has a convenient toxicity profile and provides an excellent benefit/risk ratio. They show minimal toxicity. Hypertension, fluid retention, insomnia, tremor, thrombosis, increased blood sugar, and pulmonary embolic events are described as toxic side effects. Grade 3 or Grade 4 toxicity is described less than 5%. Patients undergoing a therapy with progestational agents complain about weight gain. Progesterone stimulates appetite. High-dose regimens can induce hyperglycemia. It should not be given if patients suffer of liver insufficiency. The objective of treatment is more palliation and prolongation of survival than cure. It is certainly better tolerated than chemotherapy [17, 18].

17.3 Guidelines and Recommendations of the Different Societies

The NCCN (National Comprehensive Cancer Network) recommends in their latest Guideline Version 2.2015 for advanced and recurrent endometrial cancer the following hormonal therapies: progestational agents, tamoxifen, aromatase inhibitors, megestrol/tamoxifen (alternating). This therapy is only for endometroid histology (i.e., not for serous adenocarcinoma, clear-cell adenocarcinoma or sarcoma). These recommendations are level 2A and they believe for patients with disseminated metastatic recurrence respectively advanced stages who have a poor response to hormonal therapy are appropriate for clinical trials or palliative care (BMC).

GOG (Gynecologic Oncology Group) trials established the dosage of progestins and the efficacy for advanced and recurrent endometroid cancer. They demonstrated that there is no difference in the daily dosage of oral medroxyprogesterone. The favorable factors for a good response are well-differentiated cancers and high levels of progesterone receptors (GOG 81, GOG 48, GOG 121). There was shown a high RR in combining or alternating megestrol and tamoxifen (GOG-119, GOG-153).

17.4 Society of Gynecologic Oncology

In April 2015, the SGO implemented the new Practice Bulletin, a new clinical management guideline for endometrial cancer. They reviewed the literature and the trials and created an evidence-based recommendation for treatment. A GOG-119–Phase II Study around Whitney showed a RR of 33% with a median PFS interval of 3 months and a median OS of 13 months. Patients with advanced endometrial carcinoma were treated with alternating weekly cycles of MPA (medroxyprogesterone acetate) and daily doses of tamoxifen. The response rate was 27%, an OS of 14 months. Hormone therapy can be a used for patients with advanced or recurrent endometrial cancer who are unable or unwilling to undergo a chemotherapy, regardless of tumor grade or hormone receptor status [19, 20].

17.5 Mentioned Level A Recommendation

The use of chemotherapy in the treatment of advanced endometrial cancer improves patient outcomes.

17.5.1 ESMO/ESGO/ESTRO Guidelines for Management of Endometrial Cancer

ESGO is collaborating with ESMO and ESTRO to elaborate guidelines for the management of major tumor sites in gynecologic oncology. A consensus conference on endometrial cancer was organized in Milan in December 2014 (submitted for publication in Annals of Oncology). Their recommendations for hormonal therapy:

1. Hormone therapy is indicated in advanced or recurrent endometrioid endometrial cancer, 2A.
2. Hormone therapy is more likely to be effective in grade 1 or 2 endometrioid tumors, 4B.

3. Hormone receptor status should be determined before hormone therapy is initiated, as it is more likely to be effective in patients with positive progesterone and estrogen receptor status, 3B.
4. Biopsy of recurrent disease could be considered, as there may be differences in hormone receptor status in the primary and metastatic tumor, 3C.
5. Hormone therapy is the preferred front-line systemic therapy for patients with hormone receptor positive tumors—grade 1 or 2 and without rapidly progressive disease, 5A.
6. Progestogens (e.g. MPA 200 mg or MA 160 mg) are generally recommended, 3A.
7. Other hormonal agents to consider include tamoxifen, fulvestrant and aromatase inhibitors, 3C.

References

1. Krasner C. Aromatase inhibitors in gynecologic cancers. J Steroid Biochem Mol Biol. 2007;106:76–80.
2. Garret A, Quinn MA. Hormonal therapies and gynaecological cancers. Best Pract Res Clin Obstet Gynaecol. 2008;22:407–21.
3. Murali R, Soslow RA, Weigelt B. Classification of endometrial carcinoma: more than two types. Lancet Oncol. 2014;15(7):e268–78. https://doi.org/10.1016/S1470-2045(13)70591-6.
4. Burke WM, et al. Endometrial cancer: a review and current management strategies: part II SGO Clinical Practice Endometrial Cancer Working Group. Gynecol Oncol. 2014;134:393–402.
5. Kitchener HC, et al. Endometrial cancer state of the science meeting. Int J Gynecol Cancer. 2009;19:134–40.
6. Kelley RM, Baker WH. Progestational agents in the treatment of carcinoma of the endometrium. N Engl J Med. 1961;264:216–8.
7. Kelley RM, Baker WH. The role of progesterone in human endometrial cancer. Cancer Res. 1965;25:1190–2.
8. Taylor RW. Treatment of disseminated, recurrent endometrial cancer with progestational agents. In: Schulz K-D, King RJB, Pollow K, Taylor RW, editors. Endometrial cancer–international symposium Marburg 1986. Munich: W. Zuckschwerdt Verlag; 1986. p. 155–6.
9. Reifenstein EC. The treatment of advanced endometrial cancer with hydroxyprogesterone caproate. Gynecol Oncol. 1974;2:377–414.
10. Thigpen JT, Brady MF, Alvarez RD, et al. Oral medroxyprogesterone acetate in the treatment of advanced or recurrent endometrial carcinoma: a dose response study by the Gynecologic Oncology Group. J Clin Oncol. 1999;17:1736–44.
11. Thigpen T, Brady MF, Homesley HD, Soper JT, Bell J. Tamoxifen in the treatment of advanced or recurrent endometrial carcinoma: a Gynecologic Oncology Group study. J Clin Oncol. 2001;19(2):364–7.
12. Whitney CW, Brunetto VL, Zaino RJ, et al. Phase II study of medroxyprogesterone acetate plus tamoxifen in advanced endometrial carcinoma: Gynecologic Oncology Group study. Gynecol Oncol. 2004;92(1):4–9.
13. Fiorica JV, Brunetto VL, Hanjani P, Lentz SS, Mannel R, Andersen W. Phase II trial of alternating courses of megestrol acetate and tamoxifen in advanced endometrial carcinoma: Gynecologic Oncology Group study. Gynecol Oncol. 2004;92(1):10–4.
14. Decruze, et al. Int J Gynecol. 2007.
15. Markman M. Hormonal therapy of endometrial cancer. Eur J Cancer. 2005;41:673–5.

16. Muggia F, Blank SV. Treatment of advanced and recurrent carcinoma: hormonal therapy, uterine cancer. Curr Clin Oncol. https://doi.org/10.1007/978-1-60327-044-1_11.
17. Sjoquist KM. Hormonal therapy in gynecological cancers. Int J Gynecol Cancer. 2011;21:1328–33.
18. Lentz SS, Brady MF, et al. High-dose megestrol acetate in advanced or recurrent endometrial carcinoma: a GOG study. J Clin Oncol. 1996;14:357–61.
19. Colombo N, Preti E, Landoni F, Carinelli S, Colombo A, Marini C, Sessa C. Ann Oncol. 2013;24(Suppl 6):vi33–8.
20. Burke W, et al. Endometrial cancer: a review and current management strategies: part I SGO Clinical Practice Endometrial Cancer Working Group. Gynecol Oncol. 2014;134:385–92.

Targeted Therapy in Management of Endometrial Cancer

18

Yeh Chen Lee, Stephanie Lheureux, Mansoor Raza Mirza, and Amit M. Oza

18.1 Introduction

18.1.1 Integration of Molecular Classification and Histopathology for Endometrial Cancer

Since 1983, endometrial cancer (EC) has been classified using Bokhman's dualistic model [1] based on clinicopathological characteristics. Type I EC, with endometrioid histology representing up to 80% of the cases, is associated with endometrial hyperplasia secondary to estrogenic stimulation. This estrogen-related pathway in EC is typically low-grade cancers and expresses hormone-receptors, which can be leveraged therapeutically. Type II EC consists of the estrogen-independent non-endometroid carcinomas such as serous, clear cell, carcinosarcoma, mucinous adenocarcinoma, and squamous-cell carcinoma or undifferentiated carcinoma histology.

This estrogen independent pathway in EC arises from an atrophic endometrium and is less common (10–20%) and usually high grade with negative/weak expression of hormone receptors [2, 3]. The most common molecular alterations observed in Type II EC are p53 and p16 mutations, Her-2 overexpression or amplification and loss of E-cadherin. Molecular characterization should now allow perhaps a more accurate classification system. Next-generation sequencing studies and comprehensive analysis performed by the Cancer Genome Atlas consortium (TCGA) has expanded our knowledge of the alterations in signaling pathways in EC. Integrating molecular data to the Bokhman's dualistic model, Type I EC are generally associated with genetic alterations in KRAS, PTEN, PIK3CA, CTNNB1, and MLH1 promoter hypermethylation [4, 5]; whereas Type II EC are mainly characterized by increased levels of mTOR or prototypically TP53 mutations in serous carcinomas [5, 6]. Notably, there is still substantial overlap in genetic alterations between both groups and strong evidence of heterogeneity of EC with respect to their biological, genetic, and pathological features [5]. Therefore, the dualistic model has been adapted into a new molecular classification of four subgroups that more accurately reflect underlying tumor biology and clinical outcome: (1) DNA polymerase epsilon (POLE) ultramutated—a catalytic subunit of DNA polymerase epsilon involved in nuclear DNA replication and repair; (2) microsatellite instability (MSI) hypermutated; (3) copy-number low (endometrioid) and microsatellite stable (MSS); and (4) copy-number high (serous-like) [5]. Figure 18.1 demonstrates the evolution of EC disease characterization over time.

The POLE ultramutated subgroup is the smallest subpopulation characterized by mutations of the exonuclease domain of POLE58, high mutational burden (*PTEN, PIK3R1, PIK3CA, FBXW7 and KRAS*), few copy-number alterations, microsatellite

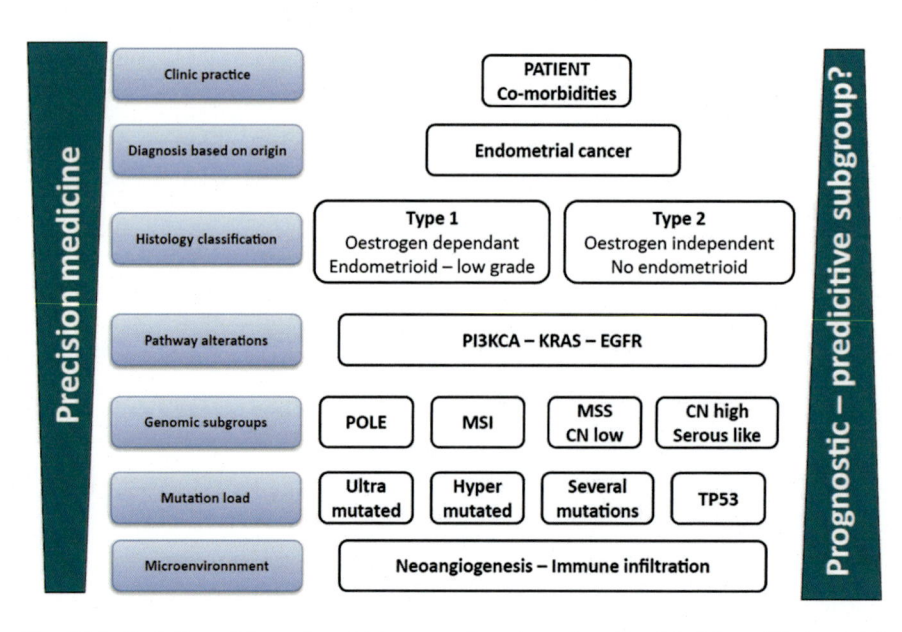

Fig. 18.1 Evolution of the endometrial cancer characterization. Reprinted from "Endometrial cancer-targeted therapies myth or reality? Review of current targeted treatments" by Lheureux et al., 2016, Eur J Cancer, 59: 99–108 [7]. *POLE* polymerase epsilon, *CN* copy number, *MSI* microsatellite instability, *MSS* microsatellite stability

stable and excellent prognosis [8]. In total, 60% of POLE ultramutated EC are high-grade endometrioid lesions and 35% harbor *TP53* mutations. MSI hypermutated subgroup are characterized by a mutation frequency approximately tenfold greater than MSS tumors, few somatic copy-number alterations, frameshift deletions in RPL22, frequent nonsynonymous KRAS mutations and few mutations in FBXW7, CTNNB1, PPP2R1A and TP53 [5]. The copy-number low, MSS, endometrioid subgroup had an unusually high frequency of CTNNB1 mutations (52%) and low mutation rates [5]. The copy-number high group consists of serous tumors and some high-grade endometrioid tumors; characterized by TP53 mutation, high frequencies of somatic copy-number alterations that display genomic instability, few DNA methylation changes and low hormone receptor expression [5].

18.1.1.1 Disease Characterization to Drive Targeted Therapy

Options for treatment of advanced or persistent EC disease remain limited, and survival has not changed in the last decade. Recent years have seen efforts to refine disease characterization to customize therapeutic strategies and thereby improve therapeutic outcomes of EC. Yet, there is an unmet need for effective treatment for EC as the only targeted therapy approved is hormonal therapy [7]. Though hormonal therapy has been a "standard" therapy for four decades, predication of its efficacy with receptor evaluation or understanding mechanisms of resistance remains an important challenge.

Among many targeted agents investigated, antiangiogenic and PI3K/AKT/mTOR pathway inhibitors agents have demonstrated clinical activity and remain under further investigation. Other targeted therapies are explored including metformin, EGFR inhibitors, and nuclear export protein inhibitors. Managing toxicities in this patient population remains challenging and often limits therapeutic options. Targeting the microenvironment, and more recently the immune infiltration, are areas of active interest. The cell cycle and DNA repair pathways and targeted-chemotherapy also constitute potential targets for the development of precision therapies. Patient-derived tumor xenograft models have been developed and will provide opportunities to better understand the molecular and microenvironment characteristics of this cancer [9].

Advances in the understanding of cell biology have allowed EC to be classified into various subtypes that respond differently to targeted therapy. Translational clinical trials that link biology with precision-targeted therapy are key to improving outcome and will require careful analysis of potential biomarkers in early phase studies with subsequent validation in larger randomized trials. This approach requires international collaborative efforts to achieve meaningful improvement in the prognosis of women with EC.

18.2 Targeting Estrogen and Progesterone Receptors

Hormonal therapy is a treatment option in EC, particularly for patients with recurrent low-grade endometrioid histology, and can be considered as the first target-specific therapy in this disease. However, the predictive value of hormone receptor status remains controversial. A significant proportion of EC, in particular Type I tumors, express estrogen receptor (ER) or progesterone receptor (PR). Agents investigated thus far include progestogens, selective estrogen receptor modulators (SERM), aromatase inhibitors (AI), and gonadotropin-releasing hormone (GnRH) inhibitors.

To date, progestogens have demonstrated the most favorable tolerability and efficacy with response rates (RR) ranging from 15 to 30% [10]. Positive receptor status (particularly in PR) and low-grade histology are predictive of response [11–13]. However, it appears that a small number of receptor-negative patients may still derive benefit from this therapy, thus emphasizing the need to explore the mechanisms involved in response and also resistance [12]. In unselected populations, AI (letrozole and anastrozole) or SERM (tamoxifen) had demonstrated low objective RR of approximately 10% [14–16]. The preliminary report from the PARAGON study (ANZGOG 0903) enrolling recurrent gynecological cancers with positive ER/PR receptors demonstrated that patients with EC derived clinical benefit (44% at 3 months) from anastrozole with significant improvement in quality of life [17].

The combination of tamoxifen and megestrol has been proposed to be more efficacious due to upregulation of the PR by tamoxifen but in practice no clear benefit has been seen [18, 19]. The overall RR was 27% with a median progression-free survival (PFS) of 2.7 months and an overall survival (OS) of 14 months [19]. Conversely, a Cochrane review showed no improvement [20] in survival in advanced EC with hormonal therapy. To detect a benefit, large randomized trials would be required but most trials to date have had small sample sizes. Important to note, the ability to demonstrate improvement in quality of life and symptom control was also insufficiently assessed in these studies. As such, continued efforts to clarify the role of hormonal therapy are warranted.

Several novel hormonal agents are currently under investigation. Fulvestrant is a pure estrogen antagonist with a high affinity for ER but in contrast to tamoxifen, has no agonist activity [21]. To date, fulvestrant has been studied in EC in two phase II trials [22, 23]. The first trial detected a RR in PR-positive and ER-positive patients as 20% ($p < 0.02$) and 16% ($p = 0.068$) respectively [22]. The second study including only ER or PR-positive patients demonstrated a partial response of 11.4% in the intent-to-treat population and 15.4% in the per protocol arm [23]. Only 40% of patients had received prior chemotherapy [23].

BN83495 is a first-in-class orally available irreversible steroid sulphatase (STS) inhibitor [24]. The STS pathway has emerged as a novel therapeutic target given its pivotal role in regulating the formation of biologically active steroids from inactive steroid sulfates [25]. A phase II trial was launched in EC comparing the efficacy of BN83495 to megestrol acetate in chemotherapy-naive patients (NCT00910091). However, in this study, patients on megestrol acetate performed much better than BN83495 with a PFS of 40 weeks and 16 weeks respectively.

Onapristone is a type I PR antagonist, which prevents PR-induced DNA transcription. The phase I is completed and currently being assessed in the phase II setting [26].

Given that EC can gradually lose PR or ER expression or develop alternate mechanisms of resistance, several trials have evaluated combinations of hormonal therapies or with other targeting therapies (See Table 18.1).

18 Targeted Therapy in Management of Endometrial Cancer

Table 18.1 Overview of current clinical trials investigating hormonal therapy in endometrial cancer [cut off date Nov 1st, 2016]

Agents	Clinical trial information/study name	Phase	Number of patients	Intervention
Monotherapy				
Anastrozole [17]	ACTRN12610000796088 PARAGON ANZGOG-0903	II	84 Prior 0–3 lines of chemotherapy	Anastrozole
Onapristone [26]	NCT02052128	I–II	60 Stage 1: No limit in line of chemotherapy Stage 2: 0–1 line of chemotherapy	Onapristone
BN83495	NCT00910091	II	73 Prior 0–1 line of chemotherapy	BN83495 vs. Megestrol acetate
Combination hormonal therapy				
Letrozole Palbociclib	NCT02730429	II	80 Any line of chemotherapy	Letrozole +/− Palbociclib
Letrozole Ribociclib (LEE011)	NCT02657928	II	40	Letrozole + Ribociclib
Sodium Cridanimod Megestrol acetate Medroxyprogesterone acetate	NCT02064725	II	58	Sodium cridanimod + megestrol acetate or medroxyprogesterone acetate
Hormonal therapy in combination with other targeted therapy/chemotherapy				
Letrozole [27]	NCT02188550	II	20	Letrozole + Everolimus
Letrozole	NCT02228681	II	74 Prior 0–1 line of chemotherapy	Letrozole + Everolimus vs. Tamoxifen + medroxyprogesterone acetate
Anastrozole	NCT02730923	II	72 0–1 prior line of chemotherapy	Anastrozole +/− AZD2014 (dual mTORC1/2 inhibitor)
Enzalutamide	NCT02684227	II	69 No prior chemotherapy	Enzalutamide + Carboplatin-Paclitaxel

vs. versus

18.3 Targeting the Cyclin-Dependent Kinase (CDK)

Cyclins are a group of proteins that act as activators to cyclin-dependent kinases (CDKs) and are required for normal cell cycle transitions. Cyclin A is involved in the transitions between G1 to S and G2 to M. Its deregulation has been linked to a number of neoplasms, including endometrial cancer. The prognostic significance of cyclin A expression seems to be cancer-specific; however, current knowledge on its impact on survival of endometrial cancer is limited. Preclinical data indicates that high expression of cyclin A is associated with poor prognosis in endometrial endometrioid adenocarcinomas [28].

Palbociclib and other similar molecules are oral and selective inhibitors of the CDKs 4 and 6. Studies in breast cancer have demonstrated superiority of letrozole in combination with palbociclib vs. letrozole monotherapy in ER+ advanced disease. The combination is well tolerated with acceptable toxicity profile [29].

Endometrial endometrioid adenocarcinomas are hormone-dependent, and endocrine therapy with aromatase inhibitors is well established [30].

A double-blind, placebo-controlled randomized trial is enrolling patients to evaluate efficacy of Palbociclib, a CDK4/6 inhibitor, in combination with Letrozole for patients with Estrogen Receptor.

Positive advanced or recurrent Endometrial cancer [31].

18.4 Targeting the Angiogenesis Pathway

Angiogenesis is one of the cardinal processes leading to invasion and metastasis in solid tumors [32]. In EC, elevated vascular endothelial growth factor (VEGF) plasma levels correlate with poor prognosis [33]. Thalidomide was the first anti-angiogenic agent assessed demonstrating a RR of 12.5% with only 8.3% surviving 6 months [34].

Bevacizumab, a recombinant humanized monoclonal antibody against VEGF-A, is the most commonly studied anti-angiogenic agent. From the 52 evaluable patients enrolled in the Gynecology Oncology Group (GOG) 229-E study, a RR of 13.5% and a 6-month PFS rate of 40.4% with single-agent bevacizumab were demonstrated [35] and the median OS was 10.5 months. There were three patients with grade IV toxicities (metabolic and one gastric bleed) but no gastrointestinal fistulae or perforations were seen. While a striking association between elevated VEGR-A and poor outcome was detected this did not correlate with levels in archival tissue [35]. In contrast, higher levels of VEGR-A in the tumor were associated with reduced risk of death [35].

There are a few studies investigating the role of bevacizumab in combination with chemotherapy in EC (See Table 18.2). The GOG-86P (NCT00977574) study compared the combination of paclitaxel/carboplatin/bevacizumab (See arm 1 of Table 18.2), paclitaxel/carboplatin/temsirolimus (See arm 2 of Table 18.2), and ixabepilone/carboplatin/bevacizumab (See arm 3 of Table 18.2) as initial therapy for

Table 18.2 Overview of current clinical trials investigating anti-angiogenic agent in endometrial cancer [cut off date Nov 1st, 2016]

Agents	Targets	Clinical trial information/study name	Phase	Number of patients	Intervention
Monotherapy					
Cabozantinib [36] (XL184)	VEGFR2 RET, MET, AXL, KIT	NCT01935934	II	79 Prior 1 line of chemotherapy	Cabozantinib
Nintedanib (BIBF1120)	VEGFR, FGFR, PDGFR	NCT02866370 NiCCC	II	120 ≥1 line of chemotherapy	Nintedanib vs. Standard chemotherapy
In combination with chemotherapy					
Bevacizumab [37]	VEGF	NCT00977574 GOG-86P	II	349 Chemotherapy-naïve	Carboplatin-Paclitaxel + Bevacizumab vs. Carboplatin-Paclitaxel + Temsirolimus vs. Carboplatin-Ixabepilone + Bevacizumab
Bevacizumab	VEGF	NCT01770171 MITOBEVAEND2	II	108 0–1 prior line of chemotherapy	Carboplatin-Paclitaxel +/− Bevacizumab
Bevacizumab	VEGF	NCT00513786	II	38 Chemotherapy-naïve Postdefinitive surgery	Carboplatin-Paclitaxel +/− Bevacizumab
Nintedanib (BIBF1120)	VEGFR, FGFR, PDGFR	NCT02730416	II	148 Prior 0–1 line of chemotherapy	Carboplatin-Paclitaxel +/− Nintedanib

VEGF vascular endothelial growth factor, *VEGFR* vascular endothelial growth factor receptor, *FGFR* fibroblast growth factor receptor, *PDGFR* platelet derived growth factor receptor, *vs.* versus

measurable stage III or IVA, stage IVB, or recurrent endometrial cancer [37]. The preliminary findings of this trial showed that best activity was seen in arm 1—paclitaxel/carboplatin/bevacizumab, with a high overall RR of 59.5% and a significant improvement in OS compared to historic reference for paclitaxel/carboplatin (OS censoring at 36 months, a secondary end-point, was statistically significantly ($p < 0.039$) [37]). There was no significant improvement in PFS ($p = 0.40$) for this study. A randomized phase II study (NCT01770171), investigated carboplatin/paclitaxel with or without bevacizumab in advanced stage or recurrent disease [38]. The preliminary findings showed that addition of bevacizumab to standard chemotherapy significantly increased PFS from 8.7 months to 13 months (HR 0.57; 95% CI = 0.34–0.96; $p = 0.036$). Given the increase of grade III cardiovascular toxicities in the combination, the patients with preexisting cardiovascular risk factors should be carefully monitored.

The role of bevacizumab in conjunction with either radiation or chemoradiation has also been explored. Women with high-risk EC were treated with pelvic radiation and concurrent cisplatin (day 1 and day 29 of radiation) and bevacizumab (day 1, day 15 and day 29 of radiation, at a dose of 5 mg/kg) followed by adjuvant carboplatin and paclitaxel for 4 cycles [39]. Seven of thirty patients developed grade ≥3 adverse events within the first 90 days, and an additional 6 experienced grade ≥3 adverse events between 90 days and 365 days after treatment. No patient developed a within-field pelvic failure during the follow-up period of 26 months [39]. Another study investigated concurrent bevacizumab and radiation for women with recurrent EC (n = 15) or ovarian cancer (n = 4) with gross disease involving the vaginal cuff and/or pelvic nodes and/or para-aortic nodes [40]. The regimen appears tolerable and the 1-year and 3-year PFS was 80% and 67%, respectively [40]. Studies to further evaluate the role of bevacizumab in this setting are warranted.

Aflibercept, a vascular endothelial growth factor (VEGF) ligand binding fusion protein that serves as a "decoy receptor," is another anti-angiogenic agent that has been studied in EC. It targets VEGF and placental growth factor. In GOG-229F, aflibercept demonstrated a PFS at 6 months of 23% with only a 7% PR rate in 44 patients [41]. Tolerability was an issue with 32% of patients stopping treatment due to toxicity and two cases of posterior reversible leukoencephalopathy were described. Data shows that fibroblast growth factor-1 (FGF-1) expression was associated with the outcome [41].

Sunitinib, an oral tyrosine kinase inhibitor (TKI), has also been investigated with interesting results. In 34 patients, the RR was 15% with a median time to progression of 3 months and a median OS of 19.4 months [42]. However, 60% of patients had a dose reduction with the most common side effects noted being hypertension and fatigue. This drug has currently been compared to temsirolimus in advanced rare tumors (NCT01396408). Preliminary results from 162 patients showed predefined activity seen in medullary thyroid cohort and clear cell carcinomas of the ovary or endometrium [43]. Both drugs appeared to induce response in clear cell carcinomas of the ovary or endometrium [43].

Cediranib, a multi-TKI targeting vascular endothelial growth factor receptor (VEGFR), platelet-derived growth factor receptor (PDGFR), and fibroblast growth factor receptor (FGFR) as a monotherapy treatment for recurrent or persistent endometrial cancer, had median PFS of 3.65 months and median OS of 12.5 months [44]. Microvessel density appears to correlate with longer PFS and may be a useful biomarker for activity [44].

Dovitinib is a potent TKI of VEGFR, PDGFR, and FGFR. While dovitinib did not reach the prespecified efficacy outcome in a second-line setting, single-agent activity was observed in FGFR2 (mutated) and FGFR2 (nonmutated) advanced or metastatic EC [45]. Documented treatment effects seemed independent of FGFR2 mutation status.

Dalantercept, anti-angiogenic with a mechanism distinct from VEGF inhibition, had insufficient single-agent activity in recurrent EC [46]. Dalantercept is a soluble form of the activin receptor-like kinase 1 (ALK1) that binds to the transforming growth factor-b superfamily members BMP9 and BMP10 and prevents these proteins from signaling through ALK1.

A double-blind, placebo-controlled randomized trial is enrolling patients to evaluate efficacy of, a triple-VEGF TKI, Nintedanib in combination with carboplatin-paclitaxel combination chemotherapy for patients with advanced or recurrent endometrial cancer [47].

Newer multitargeted anti-angiogenic agents under investigation include brivanib, lenvatinib and cabozantinib. These agents were investigated in phase II studies and exemplified the importance of integrating correlative studies. Brivanib (BMS-582664) is a potent dual VEGFR/FGFR TKI that showed a PFS rate at 6 months of 30.2% (90% CI 18.9–43.9) and a median OS of 10.7 months in the GOG-2291 study [48]. The study assessed expression of multiple angiogenic proteins and FGFR2 mutation status and found that VEGF and Ang-2 expression may diametrically predict PFS when modeled together [48]. Patients with higher levels of Ang-2 were associated with a lower risk of progression (HR = 0.28) while patients with higher levels of VEGF were associated with a higher risk of progression (HR = 3.1) [48]. It should be noted that patients with high VEGF tended to have high levels of Ang-2, which may have masked these trends when the biomarkers were modeled individually. The interactions between these biomarkers may be explained by the fact that at low levels of VEGF, Ang-2 is anti-angiogenic and can induce endothelial cell death; but at high levels of VEGF, Ang-2 is pro-angiogenic and supports development of blood vessels [48]. Further studies of Ang-2 and VEGF in EC are warranted.

Lenvatanib is an oral receptor TKI targeting VEGFR1–3, FGF1–4, RET, KIT, and PDGFRβ. A RR of 14.3% by independent review with a median PFS of 5.4 months and median OS of 10.6 months was seen in 133 patients [49]. In correlative studies, they identified seven cytokine and angiogenic factors where baseline levels correlate with survival: Ang-2, Il-8, HGR, VEGF-A, PIGF, Tie-2, and TNFa. Only Ang-2 correlated with maximum tumor shrinkage ($P < 0.01$) [50]. Low baseline level of Ang-2 was associated with greater maximal tumor shrinkage with the Overall Response Rate (ORR) 61% versus 18%, median PFS 9.5 months versus 3.7 months, and median OS of 23 months versus 8.9 months [50]. Patients with mutations in PIK3CA showed a trend to worse outcomes ($P = 0.085$) [50].

Cabozantinib, a small molecule inhibitor of the tyrosine kinases c-Met, VEGFR2, RET, and AXL, is being investigated in patients with metastatic EC (NCT01935934, See Table 18.2). The preliminary report showed that cabozantinib is well-tolerated and has achieved the prespecified efficacy; 12-week PFS achieved in 21 out of 29 serous subtype and 23 out of 36 endometrioid subtype [36]. Notable activity was also observed in the exploratory cohort of carcinoma sarcoma subtype in this study [36]. Studies investigating Nintedanib are underway (See Table 18.2).

18.5 Targeting the PI3K/Akt/mTOR Pathway

Among all solid tumors, EC is known to have the highest rate of alteration in the phosphatidylinositide 3-kinases/protein serine-threonine kinase AKT/Mammalian Target of Rapamycin (PI3K/AKT/mTOR) pathway; with alteration described in

92% and 60% of type I and II tumors, respectively [5]. The PI3K/AKT/mTOR signaling pathway regulates central aspects of cancer biology, such as metabolism, cellular growth and survival [33, 51].

Activation of the PI3K/AKT pathway occurs frequently in type I tumors through a variety of mechanisms such as the loss of PTEN that occurs in up to 70% of cases and/or PI3K mutations occurring in upwards of 36% of cases [52, 53]. A large series confirmed that type I tumors are characterized by PTEN loss and showed that type II tumors are characterized by increased levels of mTOR and lower rates of PTEN [6]. This led to the observation that PTEN plays a central role in the pathogenesis of type I ECs while mTOR is primarily involved in etiology of type II EC. Despite these improvements in our understanding of the biology of EC, the contributing role of the microenvironment and pathway alterations to disease remain poorly understood. Table 18.3 lists the agents investigated targeting the PI3K/AKT/mTOR pathway.

18.5.1 mTOR Inhibitors

Based on the central importance of this pathway and biologic rational in EC, several mTOR inhibitors have been investigated, including temsirolimus [54, 61], everolimus [55, 56, 63] and more recently ridaforolimus [57–59]. mTOR inhibitors show anti-tumor activity across histologic subtypes, predominantly stable disease with an objective RR from 0 to 25%, higher in chemotherapy-naïve patients [54–59, 61, 63]. A phase II study investigating temsirolimus in a heavily pretreated population of patients with ovarian cancer and EC did not demonstrate clinical benefit [61]; while another study investigating ridaforolimus (compared to progestin or physicians' choice chemotherapy) demonstrated a significantly better PFS improvement (3.6 months vs. 1.9 months, $p = 0.008$) but with a considerable toxicity profile [57]. Toxicity included pneumonitis, mucositis, fatigue, diarrhea, rash, thrombocytopenia, anemia, and metabolic abnormalities, such as hyperglycemia and hyperlipidemia. To date, the correlative analysis of specimens on these trials have suggested that tumor histology subtypes or molecular factors (such as PTEN or PI3KCA alterations) are not reliable biomarkers for predicting response to mTOR inhibitors [64, 65]. However, EC patients with K-RAS mutations do not seem to derive benefit from treatment with rapalogs [63].

18.5.2 PI3K Inhibitors

Pilaralisib (XL147), a selective and reversible PI3K inhibitor, was investigated in a single-arm phase II study and showed modest anti-tumor activity with an overall RR of 6.0% [66]. Similarly, BKM120, a pan-PI3K inhibitor, has demonstrated minimal anti-tumor activity in recurrent EC with unfavorable toxicities including cutaneous rash (54%), depressive events (47%) and anxiety (40%) [67].

18 Targeted Therapy in Management of Endometrial Cancer

Table 18.3 Overview of the therapeutic agents investigated targeting the PI3K/AKT/mTOR pathway in endometrial cancer

Agents	Targets	Phase	Number of patients	Intervention	Study outcome	Correlative studies
Studies that have met prespecified efficacy in phase II setting						
Temsirolimus [54]	mTOR	II	33 in chemotherapy naïve (CN) 27 in chemotherapy-treated (CT)	Temsirolimus	CN: ORR 14% mPFS 7.33 months (meet prespecified efficacy) CT: ORR 4% mPFS 3.25 months	PTEN loss and molecular markers of PI3K/Akt/mTOR pathway did not correlate with clinical outcome
Everolimus [55]	mTOR	II	35 Prior 1–2 lines of chemotherapy	Everolimus	ORR 0% SD 43% CBR at 20 weeks 22%	N/A
Everolimus [56]	mTOR	II	44 Prior 1–2 lines of chemotherapy	Everolimus	ORR 5% SD 32% mPFS 2.8 months	PTEN loss did not correlate with study outcome Patient with K-Ras do not seem to benefit from everolimus
Ridaforolimus [57]	mTOR	II	130 Prior 1–2 lines of chemotherapy	Ridaforolimus vs. Control arm (progestin or investigator's choice chemo)	ORR 0% mPFS 3.6 vs. 1.9 months ($p = 0.008$)	N/A
Ridaforolimus [58]	mTOR	II	45 Prior 1–3 lines of chemotherapy	Ridaforolimus	ORR 11% SD 18% 6 months PFS 18%	N/A
Ridaforolimus [59]	mTOR	II	34 No prior chemotherapy	Ridaforolimus	ORR 8% SD 52.9%	N/A
GDC0980 [60]	PI3K/ mTOR	II	56 Prior 1–2 lines of chemotherapy	GDC0980	ORR 9% mPFS 3.5 months Limited by toxicity	Patients with PI3K pathway mutation may derived enhanced benefit from GDC0980

(continued)

Table 18.3 (continued)

Agents	Targets	Phase	Number of patients	Intervention	Study outcome	Correlative studies
Studies that failed to meet prespecified efficacy in phase II setting (insufficient activity)						
Temsirolimus [61]	mTOR	II	44 (22 with EC) Prior 1–2 lines of chemotherapy	Temsirolimus	Insufficient activity	N/A
Pilaralisib (SAR245408; XL147)	PI3K	II	67 Prior 1–2 lines of chemotherapy	Pilaralisib	ORR 6% CBR 13.4% 6-month PFS 11.9%	PTEN loss and PIK3R1 mutation did not correlate with study outcome
MK2206 [62]	AKT	II	11 PIK3CA mutation stratified Prior 1–2 lines of chemotherapy	MK2206	ORR 5.4%	Stratification of PIK3CA mutation did not predict drug response

CN chemotherapy naïve, *CT* chemotherapy-treated, *EC* endometrial cancer, *vs.* versus, *ORR* objective response rate, *mPFS* median progression-free survival, *SD* stable disease, *CBR* clinical benefit rate, *N/A* not applicable

18.5.3 AKT Inhibitor

Newer classes of PI3K/AKT pathway inhibitors are being investigated. This is in part due to an increase in our understanding that the mTOR complex is composed of mTORC1 (Raptor complex primary coordinator of translational control via 4EBP1 and p70S6K) and mTORC2 (Rictor complex likely regulating cell proliferation and survival in part by AKT activation) [68, 69]. Indeed, mTORC1 is sensitive to inhibition by rapamycin and its analogs, while mTORC2 is not. In the presence of selective mTORC1 inhibition, mTORC2 can exert a positive feedback on AKT [70]. Results from a phase II study of MK-2206, an allosteric AKT inhibitor, showed that 4 in 36 patients enrolled onto study were on treatment for more than 6 months [62]. Interestingly, these patients had tumors of serous histology, a subtype associated with worse OS. This study found stratification by PI3KCA mutations did not predict drug response.

Another study investigating AZD5363 (AKT inhibitor) in selected patients with gynecological cancers and PIK3CA or AKT mutation showed some clinical benefit (NCT01226316). There were 9 out of 11 patients with AKT1 E17K mutation who demonstrated target lesion shrinkage, including three confirmed partial response [71].

18.5.4 Dual PI3K/mTOR Inhibitor

A phase II trial assessing a dual PI3K/mTOR inhibitor (GDC-0980) in 56 patients with advanced EC, showed a median PFS at 3.5 months. The 3 patients with confirmed response had at least one alteration in a PI3K pathway gene [60]. The evaluation of the anti-tumor activity of GDC-0980 was limited by tolerability, especially in diabetic patients. There was significant frequency of grade 3/4 adverse events reported including hyperglycemia (46%), rash (30%), colitis (5%) and pneumonitis (4%).

18.6 Targeting the Glucose Metabolism

Metformin, an oral biguanide, is classically known for its role in the management of diabetes and insulin resistance, known to be a risk factor of EC [72]. Epidemiologic data suggests that use of metformin reduces the risk of EC death [73, 74] but may not decrease the risk of EC [75]. The anti-cancer effects of metformin are associated with direct and indirect insulin-dependent actions of the drug [76, 77]. Metformin has demonstrated inhibition of proliferation and induction of apoptosis of EC cell lines [78, 79]. The insulin-lowering effects of metformin may contribute to its anti-cancer efficacy given insulin has mitogenic and pro-survival effects. In addition to its effect on glucose uptake and glycolysis, metformin activates AMP-activated protein kinase (AMPK) leading to phosphorylation of acetyl CoA carboxylase resulting in increased fatty acid oxidation [76, 77]. It affects cell growth by inducing p53-dependent autophagy and inhibiting mTOR and protein synthesis [76, 77].

Metformin was shown to reduce proliferation in preoperative studies in women with EC with a mean reduction in Ki67 of 11–17% [80, 81]. A total of 65% of patients responded to metformin as defined by a decrease in Ki67 staining in their endometrial tumors post-treatment [80]. Although Ki67 is not an established surrogate marker in EC, high Ki67 is linked to high-grade tumor in EC. Metformin decreased expression of phosphorylated (p)-AMPK, p-Akt, p-S6, p-4EBP1, and ER but not PR expression [80]. Currently, Burnett et al. are investigating the role of metformin in a randomized neoadjuvant trial in 40 grade I/II EC patients. The aim is to evaluate immunohistochemistry-based (IHC) tissue markers of proliferation: Ki67, phosphorylated histone H3, ER, PrR, and telomerase (hTERT). To be eligible, patients must be obese (body mass index ≥ 30 kg/m^2) with no history of diabetes (NCT01877564).

The clinical safety, known pharmacodynamic properties and preclinical and retrospective data make metformin a promising therapeutic option. Currently, the therapeutic role of metformin in EC is being explored in different disease settings (See Table 18.4): (1) neoadjuvant setting (NCT01877564), (2) in combination with standard chemotherapy for first-line setting in a phase II/III study conducted by the GOG (NCT02065687), and (3) in the recurrent setting in combination with other targeted therapies (NCT01797523, NCT02755844). Retrospective analysis of patients diagnosed with EC and on metformin for diabetes have suggested statistically longer survival (45.6 months vs. 12.5 months, $p = 0.006$) compared to those on

Table 18.4 Overview of current clinical trials investigating metformin in endometrial cancer [cut off date Nov 1st, 2016]

Clinical trial information/ study name	Phase	Number of patients	Intervention
Neoadjuvant setting			
NCT01877564	II	40 Obese but no history of diabetes	Metformin vs. no treatment
First line therapy setting			
NCT02065687	II/III	540 Chemotherapy naïve	Carboplatin-paclitaxel +/− metformin
NCT02874430	II	74 Chemotherapy naïve	Metformin + doxycycline
NCT01686126	II	165 Grade 1 endometrioid EC	Levonorgestral +/− metformin Levonorgestral + weight loss intervention
NCT02035787	II	30 Nonsurgical grade 1 EC	Levonosgestral-releasing intrauterine device + metformin
Recurrent disease setting			
NCT01797523	II	62 Prior 1–2 lines of chemotherapy	Metformin + letrozole + everolimus
NCT02755844 ENDOLA	II	36 Any line of chemotherapy	Metformin + metronomic cyclophosphamide + olaparib

EC endometrial cancer

other treatment for diabetes [82]; however, these findings have important limitations and should be interpreted cautiously. In light of this, findings do support a linkage between EC and the metabolism pathway that warrant further investigation to identify a potential target for treatment and prevention.

18.7 Targeting the Epidermal Growth Factor Receptor

The epidermal growth factor receptor (EGFR) is a family of four tyrosine kinase receptors which is important in growth and metastases [83]. EGFR are commonly overexpressed in EC, ranging between 36–87%, with conflicting reports on the impact of its expression on prognosis [84]. To date, results with agents targeting this pathway in EC have been relatively disappointing [84–89].

Gefitinib and erlotinib are orally active inhibitors of EGFR tyrosine kinase activity. While Gefitinib was found to be tolerable it did not demonstrate sufficient results to pursue further with an ORR of only 3.8% and a PFS at 6 months of 15.3% [87]. Erlotinib demonstrated a higher ORR of 12.5% lasting 2–36 months in 32 patients [84]. Molecular analysis did not identify EGFR mutations in responders or correlation of response with gene amplification [84]. A phase II study investigating the activity of cetuximab, a monoclonal antibody targeted against EGFR failed to show significant activity of cetuximab (5% partial response) [89].

The HER2 gene is amplified and overexpressed in approximately 30% and 40–80% of serous EC, respectively [90, 91]. Trastuzumab is a humanized monoclonal antibody that targets the HER2/neu receptor. In a small single-agent study no activity was detected [92]. HER2 positivity was defined by either immunohistochemistry or Fluorescence In Situ Hybridization (FISH) amplification but 45.5% had no gene amplification questioning the efficacy relevance of the results in this small population [93]. A randomized phase II trial is ongoing assessing the interest to add trastuzumab to carboplatin/paclitaxel chemotherapy in patients with advanced HER-positive EC (NCT01367002). Lapatinib is the first dual inhibitor in clinical use acting as a TKI of EGFR and HER2. In a small unselected population, lapatinib demonstrated a PFS at 6 months of only 10% with an objective RR of 3.3% [88]. HER2 expression was only seen in 8% of patients. The patient with a partial response was found to have a specific EGFR mutation (exon 18, E690K). As a single agent in an unselected population, lapatinib has insufficient activity. A patient diagnosed with recurrent serous EC with lung metastasis has been reported to have durable response to afatinib, a HER2 tyrosine kinase inhibitor. Her tumor was positive for HER2 gene amplification [94]. A phase II assessing the activity of afatinib in patients with recurrent serous EC overexpressing HER2 is ongoing (NCT02491099).

18.8 Combination of Targeted Therapies

Rational approach for combination therapy may be necessary to improve treatment effect particularly in EC given the tumor heterogeneity and cross-regulation of molecular pathways (See Table 18.5). Combination therapy with mTOR and an AI

Table 18.5 Overview of the combination targeted therapy agents investigated in endometrial cancer

Agents	Targets	Phase	Number of patients	Intervention	Study outcome (or clinical trial information)	Correlative studies
Studies that have met prespecified efficacy in phase II setting						
Letrozole Everolimus [27]	ER, PR mTOR	II	38 Prior 0–2 lines of chemotherapy	Letrozole + everolimus	CBR 40% ORR 32%	Endometroid histology and *CTNNB1* mutation respond well to this combination Serous histology appear to derive no benefit
Letrozole Everolimus Metformin [95]	ER, PR mTOR AMPK, mTOR	II	62 Prior 1–2 lines of chemotherapy	Letrozole + everolimus + metformin	Data from 49 pts., CBR 60% ORR 29%	
Temsirolimus Megestrol acetate Tamoxifen [96]	mTOR ER, PR	II	71 Prior 1 line of chemotherapy	Temsirolimus +/− Alternating megestrol acetate and tamoxifen	ORR 14% (closed early due to excess toxicity)	AKT1 mutation was associated with increased PFS and RR; CTNNB1 mutation was associated with increased PFS but not RR
Temsirolimus Bevacizumab [97]	mTOR VEGF	II	53 Prior 1–2 lines of chemotherapy	Temsirolimus + bevacizumab	ORR 24.5% 6 month PFS 46.9% mPFS 5.6 months mOS 16.9 months	
Studies that failed to meet prespecified efficacy in phase II setting (insufficient activity)						
Temsirolimus Bevacizumab [98]	mTOR VEGF	II	26 Prior 1 line of chemotherapy	Temsirolimus + bevacizumab	ORR 20% SD 20%	

Ongoing studies

MLN0128 MLN1117	Dual mTORC1/2 inhibitor PI3Kα inhibitor	II	260 Prior 1–2 lines of chemotherapy	MLN0128 and paclitaxel +/− MLN1117	NCT02725268
AZD2014 AZD5363 Olaparib	Dual mTORC1/2 inhibitor AKT inhibitor PARP	I/II	150 Any lines of chemotherapy	AZD2014 + Olaparib vs. AZD5363 + olaparib	NCT02208375
AZD 2014 Anastrozole	Dual mTORC1/2 inhibitor ER, PR	II	72 Prior 1 line of chemotherapy	Anastrozole +/− AZD2014	NCT02730923

ER estrogen receptor, *PR* progesterone receptor, *mTOR* mechanistic target of rapamycin, *AM*, *PK* AMP-activated protein kinase, *VEGF* vascular endothelial growth factor, *CBR* clinical benefit rate, *ORR* objective response rate, *mPFS* median progression-free survival, *mOS* median overall survival, *SD* stable disease

has been evaluated based on preclinical evidence showing that mTOR inhibition overcomes hormonal resistance [99]. The combination of everolimus 10 mg and letrozole 2.5 mg demonstrated a clinical benefit rate (CBR) of 40% at 4 months in the 35 evaluable patients among 38 patients enrolled in the trial and a RR of 32% [27]. Women with endometrioid histology and CTNNB1 mutations responded well to this combination; in contrast to the 11 serous cases who had no clinical benefit. The most common drug-related toxicities were fatigue, nausea, stomatitis, hypertriglyceridemia, and hyperglycemia [27]. Another study investigating combination of everolimus, letrozole, and metformin showed a higher clinical benefit of 60% at 4 months and manageable toxicity [95]. The combination of temsirolimus with megestrol acetate/tamoxifen was investigated but closed prematurely due to an unacceptable rate of venous thrombosis and insufficient activity to offset this risk [96]. Activating mutations in AKT1 are rare in EC, but may predict clinical benefit from temsirolimus. CTNNB1 mutations were associated with longer PFS on temsirolimus [100]. Currently, a phase I/II study investigating combination of a dual mTORC1/mTORC2 inhibitor and anastrazole is underway (NCT02730923).

The combination of an mTOR inhibitor and anti-angiogenic agent has also been investigated. Temsirolimus (25 mg weekly) with bevacizumab (10 mg/kg every 2 weeks) demonstrated a promising objective RR of 24.5% and PFS at 6 months of 46.9% [97]. Median OS determined was 16.9 months. This combination had significant associated toxicity resulting in 38.8% (19 in 49) of patients discontinuing treatment. Adverse events were consistent with those expected with bevacizumab and temsirolimus treatment and independent of the number of previous treatment lines or history of radiation. Two gastrointestinal–vaginal fistulas, two intestinal perforations, and one grade IV thrombosis were reported. Three patient deaths were possibly treatment-related [97]. A similar study investigating the same combination in 26 women showed a partial RR of 20% and PFS at 6 months of 48% [98]; however, this did not meet the prespecified efficacy criteria as the assumption criteria set was different from the former study. One duodenal perforation was reported for this study [98].

More recently, preclinical data exploring combination therapy such as dual PI3K/mTOR inhibitor (SAR245409) and MEK inhibitor (pimasertib) showed evidence of synergistic anti-tumor effect in EC cell lines, particularly in cells with high sensitivity to MEK inhibitor [101]. This combination is currently been investigated in low-grade serous ovarian cancer (NCT01936363), but yet been tested in EC. Other combination of interest currently being investigated in EC include combination of dual mTORC1/2 inhibitor and PI3Ka inhibitor (NCT02725268), and combination of dual mTORC1/2 inhibitor, AKT inhibitor, and PARP inhibitor (NCT02208375).

18.9 Treatment Concepts Under Investigation

18.9.1 MSI, POLE Ultramutated EC, and Immunotherapy

Recent data seems to show a significant association between microsatellite mismatch repair (MMR) status and outcome in EC, contrary to a previous meta-analysis

[102]. Correlation between MMR-related protein expression and clinicopathologic features in EC using IHC found a significant improvement in 5-year OS, 94% versus 78% ($p = 0.009$), in MMR-deficient (i.e. MSI) patients compared to MMR-proficient (i.e. MSS) patients [103]. Although, inter-study heterogeneity in histology subtypes and adjuvant treatment received in the meta-analysis [102] may have influenced the study outcome. The significantly improved OS reported [103] may be attributable to the majority of patients with intermediate-to-high-risk disease receiving postoperative chemotherapy as adjuvant treatment.

There is heightened interest to explore the therapeutic potential for immunotherapy in EC. The presence of tumor-infiltrating lymphocytes (TILs) was associated with favorable outcome in EC [104]. It is known that patients with POLE ultramutated EC exhibit a striking mutational burden and an enhanced anti-tumor T-cell response [105]. In addition, the immune microenvironment in EC tumor with MSI exhibits elevated CD8 and granzyme B-cells [106]. POLE ultramutated and MSI are associated with high neo-antigen loads and number of TILs, which is counterbalanced by overexpression of PD-1 and PD-L1. These subgroups of EC tumors may be excellent candidates for PD-1 targeted immunotherapies [107]. Supportive of this statement, there is a case report detailing the genomic profiling result of a patient with EC who had an exceptional response to anti-PD-1 antibody (pembrolizumab) [108]. The tumor sample from this individual was found to carry mutation in POLE [108]. The preliminary results from KEYNOTE-028 study (NCT02054806) investigating pembrolizumab in patient with advanced solid tumors showed clinical benefit in the EC cohort who had failed prior systemic chemotherapy [109]. These patients with EC had an ORR of 13% with 6-month PFS at 19% [109]. The clinical benefit of pembrolizumab in EC is being further investigated in phase II study KEYNOTE-158 (NCT02628067). There are multiple studies underway (See Table 18.6) which will hopefully provide insight to the complex immune landscapes of these tumors.

Two phase 3 randomized trials (ENGOT-EN6/TSR-042 and ENGOT-EN7) are planned to evaluate the role of immune checkpoint inhibitors both concomitant to

Table 18.6 Overview of current clinical trials investigating immunotherapy in endometrial cancer [cut off date Nov 1st, 2016]

Clinical trial information/study name	Phase	Number of patients	Intervention
NCT02549209	II	46 Chemotherapy naïve	Pembrolizumab + carboplatin/paclitaxel in endometrial cancer
NCT02899793	II	25 At least 1 line of chemotherapy	Pembrolizumab in POLE ultramutated and/or MSI endometrial cancer
NCT02628067	II	1100 Any prior lines of chemotherapy	Pembrolizumab in solid tumors including endometrial cancer
NCT02912572	II	70 Any prior lines of chemotherapy	Avelumab in POLE ultramutated vs. MSS endometrial cancer

chemotherapy (CP) as well as maintenance therapy until progression of disease in locally advanced and relapsed endometrial cancer. Both MSI-H as well as MSS population will be enrolled [110, 111].

18.9.2 Homologous Recombination DNA Repair Pathway in EC

Based on the recent advances in EC characterization, the genes implicated in DNA repair, cell proliferation, and cell cycle pathways are of interest in EC [112].

Olaparib is a potent Polyadenosine 5′diphosphoribose [poly (ADPribose)] polymerize (PARP) inhibitor and its mechanism of action exploit synthetic lethality to target DNA repair defects [113]. At the nexus of DNA repair and DNA replication, homologous recombination constitutes a key pathway to maintain genomic stability [114]. In a retrospective analysis, high homologous recombination deficiency (HRD) score appears to correlate with adverse outcome in EC [115]. In endometrial cell lines and an orthotopic mouse model with high HRD score, olaparib treatment decreased tumor growth and may be a potential therapeutic target [115, 116]. While similar hallmarks of DNA repair deficiencies are seen in serous EC as in serous ovarian cancer, there is also evidence that loss of PTEN function as seen in endometrioid histology predicts sensitivity to PARP inhibition, via the RAD51-mediated DNA repair pathway, particularly in a low estrogenic hormonal setting [117, 118]. Therefore, it is proposed that a PI3K inhibitor could be paired with a PARP inhibitor recapitulating the synthetic lethality observed upon PARP inhibition for BRCA1- or BRCA2-associated tumors (NCT01623349). The frequency of PI3K pathway activation and the high prevalence of PTEN loss in EC represents a promising strategy toward improving clinical outcomes and also suggests a "new use" of PI3K pathway inhibitors as sensitizers to alternate therapies, such as PARP inhibition [119].

18.9.3 Targeting the Nuclear Export Protein: Exportin 1 (XPO1)

Multiple tumor suppressor proteins and growth regulatory proteins are altered in EC, some of which are attributable to the overexpression or increased activity of XPO1 [120]. Selinexor, is an oral first-in-class, selective inhibitor of nuclear export (SINE) drug that binds to and inhibits XPO1 function. The initial phase II data demonstrate meaningful single agent anti-tumor activity of selinexor (NCT02025985) in patients with heavily pretreated gynecological malignancies, including EC which showed a 62% disease control rate [121]. The side effects of selinexor were reasonably tolerated and were predominantly nausea, anorexia, fatigue, and thrombocytopenia.

A phase 3 randomized placebo-controlled trial, ENGOT-EN5/ SIENDO [122], is evaluating the role of Selinexor as maintenance therapy followed by chemotherapy in locally advanced or relapsed endometrial cancer.

18.9.4 Targeted Chemotherapy

The expression of luteinizing hormone-releasing hormone (LHRH) and its receptors has been demonstrated in 80% of EC [123]. Recently, LHRH receptors have been used for the development of targeted chemotherapy. AEZS-108 (formerly known as AN-152) is a targeted cytotoxic LHRH-analog in which doxorubicin is linked to the LHRH agonist [D-Lys6]LHRH. AEZS-108 binds with high-affinity to LHRH-specific receptors on EC cell lines and upon internalization, induces apoptosis in EC cell lines [124]. In a phase II study involving 44 patients with advanced or recurrent EC, 23% patients had objective response to treatment and the median PFS was 7 months [125]. The most frequently reported grade 3/4 adverse events were neutropenia (12%) and leucopenia (9%) [125].

18.10 Conclusion

The overall survival in advanced stage or recurrent EC has not changed over the last several decades. Whilet different targeted therapies have been investigated in EC, none have resulted in a change in clinical practice to date. Investigations are ongoing for combinations of therapies that are effective with tolerable toxicity. The recent advances in molecular characterization of EC may help better identify the subset of patients that will most likely respond to these treatment approaches (See Fig. 18.1).

Currently, no phase III trial of a targeted agent has been initiated following the preliminary results from the multiple phase II trials performed. As such, future trials should leverage growing recognition of disease biology and designed to impact clinical practice. Additional efforts are needed to incorporate current knowledge of tumor molecular classification and a robust biomarker-associated translational testing to refine patient selection and treatment combination.

References

1. Bokhman JV. Two pathogenetic types of endometrial carcinoma. Gynecol Oncol. 1983;15(1):10–7.
2. Colombo N, Creutzberg C, Amant F, Bosse T, Gonzalez-Martin A, Ledermann J, et al. ESMO-ESGO-ESTRO consensus conference on endometrial cancer: diagnosis, treatment and follow-up. Ann Oncol. 2016;27(1):16–41.
3. Silva JL, Paulino E, Dias MF, Melo AC. Endometrial cancer: redefining the molecular-targeted approach. Cancer Chemother Pharmacol. 2015;76(1):1–11.
4. Minaguchi T, Yoshikawa H, Oda K, Ishino T, Yasugi T, Onda T, et al. PTEN mutation located only outside exons 5, 6, and 7 is an independent predictor of favorable survival in endometrial carcinomas. Clin Cancer Res. 2001;7(9):2636–42.
5. Cancer Genome Atlas Research N, Kandoth C, Schultz N, Cherniack AD, Akbani R, Liu Y, et al. Integrated genomic characterization of endometrial carcinoma. Nature. 2013;497(7447):67–73.

6. Peiro G, Peiro FM, Ortiz-Martinez F, Planelles M, Sanchez-Tejada L, Alenda C, et al. Association of mammalian target of rapamycin with aggressive type II endometrial carcinomas and poor outcome: a potential target treatment. Hum Pathol. 2013;44(2):218–25.
7. Lheureux S, Oza AM. Endometrial cancer-targeted therapies myth or reality? Review of current targeted treatments. Eur J Cancer. 2016;59:99–108.
8. Hussein YR, Weigelt B, Levine DA, Schoolmeester JK, Dao LN, Balzer BL, et al. Clinicopathological analysis of endometrial carcinomas harboring somatic POLE exonuclease domain mutations. Mod Pathol. 2015;28(4):505–14.
9. Depreeuw J, Hermans E, Schrauwen S, Annibali D, Coenegrachts L, Thomas D, et al. Characterization of patient-derived tumor xenograft models of endometrial cancer for preclinical evaluation of targeted therapies. Gynecol Oncol. 2015;139(1):118–26.
10. Podratz KC, O'Brien PC, Malkasian GD Jr, Decker DG, Jefferies JA, Edmonson JH. Effects of progestational agents in treatment of endometrial carcinoma. Obstet Gynecol. 1985;66(1):106–10.
11. Thigpen JT, Brady MF, Alvarez RD, Adelson MD, Homesley HD, Manetta A, et al. Oral medroxyprogesterone acetate in the treatment of advanced or recurrent endometrial carcinoma: a dose-response study by the Gynecologic Oncology Group. J Clin Oncol. 1999;17(6):1736–44.
12. Decruze SB, Green JA. Hormone therapy in advanced and recurrent endometrial cancer: a systematic review. Int J Gynecol Cancer. 2007;17(5):964–78.
13. Temkin SM, Fleming G. Current treatment of metastatic endometrial cancer. Cancer Control. 2009;16(1):38–45.
14. Rose PG, Brunetto VL, VanLe L, Bell J, Walker JL, Lee RB. A phase II trial of anastrozole in advanced recurrent or persistent endometrial carcinoma: a Gynecologic Oncology Group study. Gynecol Oncol. 2000;78(2):212–6.
15. Ma BB, Oza A, Eisenhauer E, Stanimir G, Carey M, Chapman W, et al. The activity of letrozole in patients with advanced or recurrent endometrial cancer and correlation with biological markers—a study of the National Cancer Institute of Canada Clinical Trials Group. Int J Gynecol Cancer. 2004;14(4):650–8.
16. Thigpen T, Brady MF, Homesley HD, Soper JT, Bell J. Tamoxifen in the treatment of advanced or recurrent endometrial carcinoma: a Gynecologic Oncology Group study. J Clin Oncol. 2001;19(2):364–7.
17. Mileshkin LR, Edmondson RJ, O'Connell R, Sjoquist KM, Cannan D, Jyothirmayi R, et al., editors. Phase II study of anastrozole in recurrent estrogen (ER)/progesterone (PR) positive endometrial cancer: the PARAGON trial—ANZGOG 0903. In: ASCO annual meeting proceedings; 2016.
18. Whitney CW, Brunetto VL, Zaino RJ, Lentz SS, Sorosky J, Armstrong DK, et al. Phase II study of medroxyprogesterone acetate plus tamoxifen in advanced endometrial carcinoma: a Gynecologic Oncology Group study. Gynecol Oncol. 2004;92(1):4–9.
19. Fiorica JV, Brunetto VL, Hanjani P, Lentz SS, Mannel R, Andersen W, et al. Phase II trial of alternating courses of megestrol acetate and tamoxifen in advanced endometrial carcinoma: a Gynecologic Oncology Group study. Gynecol Oncol. 2004;92(1):10–4.
20. Kokka F, Brockbank E, Oram D, Gallagher C, Bryant A. Hormonal therapy in advanced or recurrent endometrial cancer. Cochrane Database Syst Rev. 2010;12:CD007926.
21. Wakeling AE, Dukes M, Bowler J. A potent specific pure antiestrogen with clinical potential. Cancer Res. 1991;51(15):3867–73.
22. Covens AL, Filiaci V, Gersell D, Lutman CV, Bonebrake A, Lee YC. Phase II study of fulvestrant in recurrent/metastatic endometrial carcinoma: a Gynecologic Oncology Group study. Gynecol Oncol. 2011;120(2):185–8.
23. Emons G, Gunthert A, Thiel FC, Camara O, Strauss HG, Breitbach GP, et al. Phase II study of fulvestrant 250 mg/month in patients with recurrent or metastatic endometrial cancer: a study of the Arbeitsgemeinschaft Gynakologische Onkologie. Gynecol Oncol. 2013;129(3): 495–9.

24. Woo LW, Ganeshapillai D, Thomas MP, Sutcliffe OB, Malini B, Mahon MF, et al. Structure-activity relationship for the first-in-class clinical steroid sulfatase inhibitor Irosustat (STX64, BN83495). ChemMedChem. 2011;6(11):2019–34.
25. Purohit A, Woo LW, Potter BV. Steroid sulfatase: a pivotal player in estrogen synthesis and metabolism. Mol Cell Endocrinol. 2011;340(2):154–60.
26. Cottu PH, Italiano A, Varga A, Campone M, Leary A, Floquet A, et al., editors. Onapristone (ONA) in progesterone receptor (PR)-expressing tumors: efficacy and biomarker results of a dose-escalation phase 1 study. In: ASCO annual meeting proceedings; 2015.
27. Slomovitz BM, Jiang Y, Yates MS, Soliman PT, Johnston T, Nowakowski M, et al. Phase II study of everolimus and letrozole in patients with recurrent endometrial carcinoma. J Clin Oncol. 2015;33(8):930–6.
28. Santala S, et al. High expression of cyclin a is associated with poor prognosis in endometrial endometrioid adenocarcinoma. Tumour Biol. 2014;35(6):5395–9.
29. Beaver JA, et al. FDA approval: palbociclib for the treatment of postmenopausal patients with estrogen receptor-positive, HER2-negative metastatic breast cancer. Clin Cancer Res. 2015;21(21):4760–6.
30. Bogliolo S, et al. Effectiveness of aromatase inhibitors in the treatment of advanced endometrial adenocarcinoma. Arch Gynecol Obstet. 2016;293(4):701–8.
31. Mirza MR, et al. ENGOT-EN3/PALEO: a randomized phase II placebo-controlled trial of palbociclib in combination with letrozole for patients with estrogen receptor positive advanced or recurrent endometrial cancer. NCT02730429.
32. Hanahan D, Weinberg RA. Hallmarks of cancer: the next generation. Cell. 2011;144(5):646–74.
33. Engelman JA, Luo J, Cantley LC. The evolution of phosphatidylinositol 3-kinases as regulators of growth and metabolism. Nat Rev Genet. 2006;7(8):606–19.
34. McMeekin DS, Sill MW, Benbrook D, Darcy KM, Stearns-Kurosawa DJ, Eaton L, et al. A phase II trial of thalidomide in patients with refractory endometrial cancer and correlation with angiogenesis biomarkers: a Gynecologic Oncology Group study. Gynecol Oncol. 2007;105(2):508–16.
35. Aghajanian C, Sill MW, Darcy KM, Greer B, McMeekin DS, Rose PG, et al. Phase II trial of bevacizumab in recurrent or persistent endometrial cancer: a Gynecologic Oncology Group study. J Clin Oncol. 2011;29(16):2259–65.
36. Dhani N, Hirte H, Butler M, Lheureux S, editors. Phase II study of cabozantinib in recurrent/metastatic endometrial cancer (EC): a study of the Princess Margaret, Chicago and California Phase II Consortia. ASCO annual meeting proceedings. J Clin Oncol. 2016;34:5586.
37. Aghajanian C, Filiaci VL, Dizon DS, Carlson J, Powell MA, Secord AA, et al., editors. A randomized phase II study of paclitaxel/carboplatin/bevacizumab, paclitaxel/carboplatin/temsirolimus and ixabepilone/carboplatin/bevacizumab as initial therapy for measurable stage III or IVA, stage IVB or recurrent endometrial cancer, GOG-86P. In: ASCO annual meeting proceedings; 2015.
38. Lorusso D, Ferrandina G, Colombo N, Pignata S, Salutari V, Maltese G, et al., editors. Randomized phase II trial of carboplatin-paclitaxel (CP) compared to carboplatin-paclitaxel-bevacizumab (CP-B) in advanced (stage III-IV) or recurrent endometrial cancer: the MITO END-2 trial. In: ASCO annual meeting proceedings; 2015.
39. Viswanathan AN, Moughan J, Miller BE, Xiao Y, Jhingran A, Portelance L, et al. NRG oncology/RTOG 0921: a phase 2 study of postoperative intensity-modulated radiotherapy with concurrent cisplatin and bevacizumab followed by carboplatin and paclitaxel for patients with endometrial cancer. Cancer. 2015;121(13):2156–63.
40. Viswanathan AN, Lee H, Berkowitz R, Berlin S, Campos S, Feltmate C, et al. A prospective feasibility study of radiation and concurrent bevacizumab for recurrent endometrial cancer. Gynecol Oncol. 2014;132(1):55–60.
41. Coleman RL, Sill MW, Lankes HA, Fader AN, Finkler NJ, Hoffman JS, et al. A phase II evaluation of aflibercept in the treatment of recurrent or persistent endometrial cancer: a Gynecologic Oncology Group study. Gynecol Oncol. 2012;127(3):538–43.

42. Castonguay V, Lheureux S, Welch S, Mackay HJ, Hirte H, Fleming G, et al. A phase II trial of sunitinib in women with metastatic or recurrent endometrial carcinoma: a study of the Princess Margaret, Chicago and California Consortia. Gynecol Oncol. 2014;134(2):274–80.
43. Dancey J, Krzyzanowska MK, Provencher DM, Cheung WY, Macfarlane RJ, Alcindor T, et al., editors. NCIC CTG IND. 206: a phase II umbrella trial of sunitinib (S) or temsirolimus (T) in advanced rare cancers. In: ASCO annual meeting proceedings; 2015.
44. Bender D, Sill MW, Lankes HA, Reyes HD, Darus CJ, Delmore JE, et al. A phase II evaluation of cediranib in the treatment of recurrent or persistent endometrial cancer: an NRG Oncology/Gynecologic Oncology Group study. Gynecol Oncol. 2015;138(3):507–12.
45. Konecny GE, Finkler N, Garcia AA, Lorusso D, Lee PS, Rocconi RP, et al. Second-line dovitinib (TKI258) in patients with FGFR2-mutated or FGFR2-non-mutated advanced or metastatic endometrial cancer: a non-randomised, open-label, two-group, two-stage, phase 2 study. Lancet Oncol. 2015;16(6):686–94.
46. Makker V, Filiaci VL, Chen LM, Darus CJ, Kendrick JE, Sutton G, et al. Phase II evaluation of dalantercept, a soluble recombinant activin receptor-like kinase 1 (ALK1) receptor fusion protein, for the treatment of recurrent or persistent endometrial cancer: an NRG Oncology/Gynecologic Oncology Group study 0229N. Gynecol Oncol. 2015;138(1):24–9.
47. Mirza MR. ENGOT-EN1/FANDANGO: a randomized phase II trial of first-line combination chemotherapy with nintedanib/placebo for patients with advanced or recurrent endometrial cancer. NCT02730416.
48. Powell MA, Sill MW, Goodfellow PJ, Benbrook DM, Lankes HA, Leslie KK, et al. A phase II trial of brivanib in recurrent or persistent endometrial cancer: an NRG Oncology/Gynecologic Oncology Group study. Gynecol Oncol. 2014;135(1):38–43.
49. Vergote I, Teneriello M, Powell MA, Miller DS, Garcia AA, Mikheeva ON, et al., editors. A phase II trial of lenvatinib in patients with advanced or recurrent endometrial cancer: angiopoietin-2 as a predictive marker for clinical outcomes. In: ASCO annual meeting proceedings; 2013.
50. Funahashi Y, Penson RT, Powell MA, Miller DS, Fan J, Ren M, et al., editors. Analysis of plasma biomarker and tumor genetic alterations from a phase II trial of lenvatinib in patients with advanced endometrial cancer. In: ASCO annual meeting proceedings; 2013.
51. Slomovitz BM, Coleman RL. The PI3K/AKT/mTOR pathway as a therapeutic target in endometrial cancer. Clin Cancer Res. 2012;18(21):5856–64.
52. Dancey J. mTOR signaling and drug development in cancer. Nat Rev Clin Oncol. 2010;7(4):209–19.
53. Kong D, Suzuki A, Zou TT, Sakurada A, Kemp LW, Wakatsuki S, et al. PTEN1 is frequently mutated in primary endometrial carcinomas. Nat Genet. 1997;17(2):143–4.
54. Oza AM, Elit L, Tsao MS, Kamel-Reid S, Biagi J, Provencher DM, et al. Phase II study of temsirolimus in women with recurrent or metastatic endometrial cancer: a trial of the NCIC Clinical Trials Group. J Clin Oncol. 2011;29(24):3278–85.
55. Slomovitz BM, Lu KH, Johnston T, Coleman RL, Munsell M, Broaddus RR, et al. A phase 2 study of the oral mammalian target of rapamycin inhibitor, everolimus, in patients with recurrent endometrial carcinoma. Cancer. 2010;116(23):5415–9.
56. Ray-Coquard I, Favier L, Weber B, Roemer-Becuwe C, Bougnoux P, Fabbro M, et al. Everolimus as second-or third-line treatment of advanced endometrial cancer: ENDORAD, a phase II trial of GINECO. Br J Cancer. 2013;108(9):1771–7.
57. Oza AM, Pignata S, Poveda A, McCormack M, Clamp A, Schwartz B, et al. Randomized phase II trial of Ridaforolimus in advanced endometrial carcinoma. J Clin Oncol. 2015;33(31):3576–82.
58. Colombo N, McMeekin DS, Schwartz P, Sessa C, Gehrig PA, Holloway R, et al. Ridaforolimus as a single agent in advanced endometrial cancer: results of a single-arm, phase 2 trial. Br J Cancer. 2013;108(5):1021–6.
59. Tsoref D, Welch S, Lau S, Biagi J, Tonkin K, Martin LA, et al. Phase II study of oral ridaforolimus in women with recurrent or metastatic endometrial cancer. Gynecol Oncol. 2014;135(2):184–9.

60. Makker V, Recio FO, Ma L, Matulonis U, Lauchle JOH, Parmar H, et al., editors. Phase II trial of GDC-0980 (dual PI3K/mTOR inhibitor) in patients with advanced endometrial carcinoma: final study results. In: ASCO annual meeting proceedings; 2014.
61. Emons G, Kurzeder C, Schmalfeldt B, Neuser P, de Gregorio N, Pfisterer J, et al. Temsirolimus in women with platinum-refractory/resistant ovarian cancer or advanced/recurrent endometrial carcinoma. A phase II study of the AGO-study group (AGO-GYN8). Gynecol Oncol. 2016;140(3):450–6.
62. Myers AP, Broaddus R, Makker V, Konstantinopoulos PA, Drapkin R, Horowitz NS, et al., editors. Phase II, two-stage, two-arm, PIK3CA mutation stratified trial of MK-2206 in recurrent endometrial cancer (EC). In: ASCO annual meeting proceedings; 2013.
63. Tredan O, Treilleux I, Wang Q, Gane N, Pissaloux D, Bonnin N, et al. Predicting everolimus treatment efficacy in patients with advanced endometrial carcinoma: a GINECO group study. Target Oncol. 2013;8(4):243–51.
64. Mackay HJ, Eisenhauer EA, Kamel-Reid S, Tsao M, Clarke B, Karakasis K, et al. Molecular determinants of outcome with mammalian target of rapamycin inhibition in endometrial cancer. Cancer. 2014;120(4):603–10.
65. Myers AP. New strategies in endometrial cancer: targeting the PI3K/mTOR pathway—the devil is in the details. Clin Cancer Res. 2013;19(19):5264–74.
66. Matulonis U, Vergote I, Backes F, Martin LP, McMeekin S, Birrer M, et al. Phase II study of the PI3K inhibitor pilaralisib (SAR245408; XL147) in patients with advanced or recurrent endometrial carcinoma. Gynecol Oncol. 2015;136(2):246–53.
67. Heudel P-E, Fabbro M, Roemer-Becuwe C, Treilleux I, Kaminsky M-C, Arnaud A, et al., editors. Phase II study of the PI3K inhibitor BKM120 monotherapy in patients with advanced or recurrent endometrial carcinoma: ENDOPIK, GINECO Study. In: ASCO annual meeting proceedings; 2015.
68. Montero JC, Chen X, Ocana A, Pandiella A. Predominance of mTORC1 over mTORC2 in the regulation of proliferation of ovarian cancer cells: therapeutic implications. Mol Cancer Ther. 2012;11(6):1342–52.
69. Sarbassov DD, Guertin DA, Ali SM, Sabatini DM. Phosphorylation and regulation of Akt/PKB by the rictor-mTOR complex. Science. 2005;307(5712):1098–101.
70. Sun SY, Rosenberg LM, Wang X, Zhou Z, Yue P, Fu H, et al. Activation of Akt and eIF4E survival pathways by rapamycin-mediated mammalian target of rapamycin inhibition. Cancer Res. 2005;65(16):7052–8.
71. Hyman DM, Smyth L, Bedard PL, Oza A, Dean E, Armstrong A, et al. AZD5363, a catalytic pan-AKT inhibitor, in AKT1 E17K mutation positive advanced solid tumors. Mol Cancer Ther. 2015;14:Abstract nr B109.
72. Nead KT, Sharp SJ, Thompson DJ, Painter JN, Savage DB, Semple RK, et al. Evidence of a causal association between insulinemia and endometrial cancer: a Mendelian randomization analysis. J Natl Cancer Inst. 2015;107(9):djv178.
73. Ko EM, Walter P, Jackson A, Clark L, Franasiak J, Bolac C, et al. Metformin is associated with improved survival in endometrial cancer. Gynecol Oncol. 2014;132(2):438–42.
74. Nevadunsky NS, Van Arsdale A, Strickler HD, Moadel A, Kaur G, Frimer M, et al. Metformin use and endometrial cancer survival. Gynecol Oncol. 2014;132(1):236–40.
75. Ko EM, Sturmer T, Hong JL, Castillo WC, Bae-Jump V, Funk MJ. Metformin and the risk of endometrial cancer: a population-based cohort study. Gynecol Oncol. 2015;136(2):341–7.
76. Dowling RJ, Goodwin PJ, Stambolic V. Understanding the benefit of metformin use in cancer treatment. BMC Med. 2011;9:33.
77. Ben Sahra I, Le Marchand-Brustel Y, Tanti JF, Bost F. Metformin in cancer therapy: a new perspective for an old antidiabetic drug? Mol Cancer Ther. 2010;9(5):1092–9.
78. Cantrell LA, Zhou C, Mendivil A, Malloy KM, Gehrig PA, Bae-Jump VL. Metformin is a potent inhibitor of endometrial cancer cell proliferation—implications for a novel treatment strategy. Gynecol Oncol. 2010;116(1):92–8.
79. Sarfstein R, Friedman Y, Attias-Geva Z, Fishman A, Bruchim I, Werner H. Metformin down-regulates the insulin/IGF-I signaling pathway and inhibits different uterine serous carcinoma

(USC) cells proliferation and migration in p53-dependent or -independent manners. PLoS One. 2013;8(4):e61537.
80. Schuler KM, Rambally BS, DiFurio MJ, Sampey BP, Gehrig PA, Makowski L, et al. Antiproliferative and metabolic effects of metformin in a preoperative window clinical trial for endometrial cancer. Cancer Med. 2015;4(2):161–73.
81. Sivalingam VN, Kitson S, McVey R, Roberts C, Pemberton P, Gilmour K, et al. Measuring the biological effect of presurgical metformin treatment in endometrial cancer. Br J Cancer. 2016;114(3):281–9.
82. Ezewuiro O, Grushko TA, Kocherginsky M, Habis M, Hurteau JA, Mills KA, et al. Association of metformin use with outcomes in advanced endometrial cancer treated with chemotherapy. PLoS One. 2016;11(1):e0147145.
83. Lindsey S, Langhans SA. Epidermal growth factor signaling in transformed cells. Int Rev Cell Mol Biol. 2015;314:1–41.
84. Oza AM, Eisenhauer EA, Elit L, Cutz JC, Sakurada A, Tsao MS, et al. Phase II study of erlotinib in recurrent or metastatic endometrial cancer: NCIC IND-148. J Clin Oncol. 2008;26(26):4319–25.
85. Tsoref D, Oza AM. Recent advances in systemic therapy for advanced endometrial cancer. Curr Opin Oncol. 2011;23(5):494–500.
86. Lheureux S, Wilson M, Mackay HJ. Recent and current phase II clinical trials in endometrial cancer: review of the state of art. Expert Opin Investig Drugs. 2014;23(6):773–92.
87. Leslie KK, Sill MW, Fischer E, Darcy KM, Mannel RS, Tewari KS, et al. A phase II evaluation of gefitinib in the treatment of persistent or recurrent endometrial cancer: a Gynecologic Oncology Group study. Gynecol Oncol. 2013;129(3):486–94.
88. Leslie KK, Sill MW, Lankes HA, Fischer EG, Godwin AK, Gray H, et al. Lapatinib and potential prognostic value of EGFR mutations in a Gynecologic Oncology Group phase II trial of persistent or recurrent endometrial cancer. Gynecol Oncol. 2012;127(2):345–50.
89. Slomovitz B, Schmeler K, Miller D, Lu K, Ramirez P, Caputo T, et al., editors. Phase II study of cetuximab (Erbitux) in patients with progressive or recurrent endometrial cancer. Gynecol Oncol. 2010;116:S8–8.
90. Diver EJ, Foster R, Rueda BR, Growdon WB. The therapeutic challenge of targeting HER2 in endometrial cancer. Oncologist. 2015;20(9):1058–68.
91. Growdon WB, Groeneweg J, Byron V, DiGloria C, Borger DR, Tambouret R, et al. HER2 over-expressing high grade endometrial cancer expresses high levels of p95HER2 variant. Gynecol Oncol. 2015;137(1):160–6.
92. Fleming GF, Sill MW, Darcy KM, McMeekin DS, Thigpen JT, Adler LM, et al. Phase II trial of trastuzumab in women with advanced or recurrent, HER2-positive endometrial carcinoma: a Gynecologic Oncology Group study. Gynecol Oncol. 2010;116(1):15–20.
93. Santin AD. Letter to the editor referring to the manuscript entitled: "phase II trial of trastuzumab in women with advanced or recurrent HER-positive endometrial carcinoma: a Gynecologic Oncology Group study" recently reported by Fleming et al., (Gynecol Oncol., 116;15-20;2010). Gynecol Oncol. 2010;118(1):95–6. Author reply 6–7.
94. Talwar S, Cohen S. Her-2 targeting in uterine papillary serous carcinoma. Gynecol Oncol Case Rep. 2012;2(3):94–6.
95. Soliman PT, Westin SN, Iglesias DA, Munsell MF, Slomovitz BM, Lu KH, et al., editors. Phase II study of everolimus, letrozole, and metformin in women with advanced/recurrent endometrial cancer. In: ASCO annual meeting proceedings; 2016.
96. Fleming GF, Filiaci VL, Marzullo B, Zaino RJ, Davidson SA, Pearl M, et al. Temsirolimus with or without megestrol acetate and tamoxifen for endometrial cancer: a Gynecologic Oncology Group study. Gynecol Oncol. 2014;132(3):585–92.
97. Alvarez EA, Brady WE, Walker JL, Rotmensch J, Zhou XC, Kendrick JE, et al. Phase II trial of combination bevacizumab and temsirolimus in the treatment of recurrent or persistent endometrial carcinoma: a Gynecologic Oncology Group study. Gynecol Oncol. 2013;129(1):22–7.

98. Einstein MH, Wenham RM, Morgan R, Cristea MC, Strevel EL, Oza AM, et al., editors. Phase II trial of temsirolimus and bevacizumab for initial recurrence of endometrial cancer. In: ASCO annual meeting proceedings; 2012.
99. Boulay A, Rudloff J, Ye J, Zumstein-Mecker S, O'Reilly T, Evans DB, et al. Dual inhibition of mTOR and estrogen receptor signaling in vitro induces cell death in models of breast cancer. Clin Cancer Res. 2005;11(14):5319–28.
100. Myers AP, Filiaci VL, Zhang Y, Pearl M, Behbakht K, Makker V, et al. Tumor mutational analysis of GOG248, a phase II study of temsirolimus or temsirolimus and alternating megestrol acetate and tamoxifen for advanced endometrial cancer (EC): an NRG Oncology/Gynecologic Oncology Group study. Gynecol Oncol. 2016;141(1):43–8.
101. Inaba K, Oda K, Ikeda Y, Sone K, Miyasaka A, Kashiyama T, et al. Antitumor activity of a combination of dual PI3K/mTOR inhibitor SAR245409 and selective MEK1/2 inhibitor pimasertib in endometrial carcinomas. Gynecol Oncol. 2015;138(2):323–31.
102. Diaz-Padilla I, Romero N, Amir E, Matias-Guiu X, Vilar E, Muggia F, et al. Mismatch repair status and clinical outcome in endometrial cancer: a systematic review and meta-analysis. Crit Rev Oncol Hematol. 2013;88(1):154–67.
103. Kato M, Takano M, Miyamoto M, Sasaki N, Goto T, Tsuda H, et al. DNA mismatch repair-related protein loss as a prognostic factor in endometrial cancers. J Gynecol Oncol. 2015;26(1):40–5.
104. de Jong RA, Leffers N, Boezen HM, ten Hoor KA, van der Zee AG, Hollema H, et al. Presence of tumor-infiltrating lymphocytes is an independent prognostic factor in type I and II endometrial cancer. Gynecol Oncol. 2009;114(1):105–10.
105. van Gool IC, Bosse T, Church DN. POLE proofreading mutation, immune response and prognosis in endometrial cancer. Oncoimmunology. 2016;5(3):e1072675.
106. Pakish JB, Chisholm GB, Zhang Q, Celestino J, Mok SC, Yates MS, et al., editors. Altered immune environment in Lynch syndrome-related endometrial cancer: implications for immunotherapy? In: ASCO annual meeting proceedings; 2016.
107. Howitt BE, Shukla SA, Sholl LM, Ritterhouse LL, Watkins JC, Rodig S, et al. Association of polymerase e-mutated and microsatellite-instable endometrial cancers with neoantigen load, number of tumor-infiltrating lymphocytes, and expression of PD-1 and PD-L1. JAMA Oncol. 2015;1(9):1319–23.
108. Mehnert JM, Panda A, Zhong H, Hirshfield K, Damare S, Lane K, et al. Immune activation and response to pembrolizumab in POLE-mutant endometrial cancer. J Clin Invest. 2016;126(6):2334–40.
109. Ott PA, Bang Y, Berton-Rigaud D, Elez E, MPishvaian MJ, Rugo HS, et al., editors. Pembrolizumab in advanced endometrial cancer: preliminary results from the phase Ib KEYNOTE-028 study. 2016 ASCO annual meeting. J Clin Oncol. 2016;34:5581.
110. Mirza MR. A study of dostarlimab (TSR-042) plus carboplatin-paclitaxel versus placebo plus carboplatin-paclitaxel in patients with recurrent or primary advanced endometrial cancer (RUBY). NCT03981796.
111. Colombo N. Atezolizumab trial in endometrial cancer: AtTEnd (AtTEnd). NCT03603184.
112. Jones NL, Xiu J, Reddy SK, Burke WM, Tergas AI, Wright JD, et al. Identification of potential therapeutic targets by molecular profiling of 628 cases of uterine serous carcinoma. Gynecol Oncol. 2015;138(3):620–6.
113. Lheureux S, Oza AM. Olaparib for the treatment of ovarian cancer. Expert Opin Orphan Drugs. 2014;2(5):497–508.
114. Li X, Heyer WD. Homologous recombination in DNA repair and DNA damage tolerance. Cell Res. 2008;18(1):99–113.
115. Hansen JM, Ring KL, Baggerly KA, Wu S, Timms K, Neff C, et al., editors. Clinical significance of homologous recombination deficiency (HRD) score testing in endometrial cancer patients. In: ASCO annual meeting proceedings; 2016.
116. Miyasaka A, Oda K, Ikeda Y, Wada-Hiraike O, Kashiyama T, Enomoto A, et al. Anti-tumor activity of olaparib, a poly (ADP-ribose) polymerase (PARP) inhibitor, in cultured endometrial carcinoma cells. BMC Cancer. 2014;14(1):1.

117. Dedes KJ, Wetterskog D, Mendes-Pereira AM, Natrajan R, Lambros MB, Geyer FC, et al. PTEN deficiency in endometrioid endometrial adenocarcinomas predicts sensitivity to PARP inhibitors. Sci Transl Med. 2010;2(53):53ra75.
118. Janzen DM, Paik DY, Rosales MA, Yep B, Cheng D, Witte ON, et al. Low levels of circulating estrogen sensitize PTEN-null endometrial tumors to PARP inhibition in vivo. Mol Cancer Ther. 2013;12(12):2917–28.
119. Rodriguez-Freixinos V, Karakasis K, Oza AM. New targeted agents in endometrial cancer: are we really making progress? Curr Oncol Rep. 2016;18(4):23.
120. Crochiere ML, Baloglu E, Klebanov B, Donovan S, Del Alamo D, Lee M, et al. A method for quantification of exportin-1 (XPO1) occupancy by selective inhibitor of nuclear export (SINE) compounds. Oncotarget. 2016;7(2):1863–77.
121. Vergote I, Lund B, Havsteen H, Ujmajuridze Z, Leunen K, Aaquist Haslund C, et al., editors. Preliminary phase II results of selinexor, an oral selective inhibitor of nuclear export in patients with heavily pretreated gynecological cancers. In: ASCO annual meeting proceedings; 2015.
122. Vergote I, et al. ENGOT-EN5/SIENDO: an investigator sponsored randomized phase 3 trial of maintenance with selinexor/placebo after combination chemotherapy for patients with advanced or recurrent endometrial cancer. EudraCT: 2017-000607-2.
123. Emons G, Ortmann O, Schulz KD, Schally AV. Growth-inhibitory actions of analogues of luteinizing hormone releasing hormone on tumor cells. Trends Endocrinol Metab. 1997;8(9):355–62.
124. Westphalen S, Kotulla G, Kaiser F, Krauss W, Werning G, Elsasser HP, et al. Receptor mediated antiproliferative effects of the cytotoxic LHRH agonist AN-152 in human ovarian and endometrial cancer cell lines. Int J Oncol. 2000;17(5):1063–9.
125. Emons G, Gorchev G, Harter P, Wimberger P, Stähle A, Hanker L, et al. Efficacy and safety of AEZS-108 (LHRH agonist linked to doxorubicin) in women with advanced or recurrent endometrial cancer expressing LHRH receptors: a multicenter phase 2 trial (AGO-GYN5). Int J Gynecol Cancer. 2014;24(2):260–5.

Management of Rare Uterine Malignant Tumors

19

Frederic Amant, Martee Hensley, Patricia Pautier, Michael Friedlander, Satoru Sagae, Keiichi Fujiwara, Dominique Berton Rigaud, Domenica Lorusso, and Isabelle Ray-Coquard

F. Amant (✉)
Department of Oncology, University Hospitals Leuven, Leuven, Belgium

Center for Gynecologic Oncology, Netherlands Cancer Institute and Amsterdam University Medical Centers, Amsterdam, The Netherlands
e-mail: frederic.amant@uzleuven.be

M. Hensley
Department of Medicine, Memorial Sloan-Kettering Cancer Center, Weill Cornell Medical College, New York, NY, USA
e-mail: hensleym@MSKCC.ORG

P. Pautier
Department of Medical Oncology, Gustave Roussy, Villejuif, France
e-mail: patricia.pautier@gustaveroussy.fr

M. Friedlander
Department of Medical Oncology, Royal Hospital for Women, Sydney, NSW, Australia
e-mail: m.friedlander@unsw.edu.au

S. Sagae
Department of Gynecologic Oncology, Hokkaido Ohno Memorial Hospital, Nishi-ku, Sapporo, Japan
e-mail: s_sagae@kojinkai.or.jp

K. Fujiwara
Department of Gynecologic Oncology, Saitama Medical University International Medical Center, Hidaka, Saitama, Japan
e-mail: fujiwara@saitama-med.ac.jp

D. Berton Rigaud
ICO Centre René Gauducheau Bd Jacques Monod, Saint-Herblain, France
e-mail: berton-rigaud@ico.unicancer.fr

D. Lorusso
Gynecologic Oncology Unit, Fondazione IRCCS National Cancer Institute of Milan, Milan, Italy
e-mail: domenica.lorusso@istitutotumori.mi.it

I. Ray-Coquard
Centre Léon Bérard and University Claude Bernard Lyon 1, Lyon, France
e-mail: isabelle.ray-coquard@lyon.unicancer.fr

© Springer Nature Switzerland AG 2020
M. R. Mirza (ed.), *Management of Endometrial Cancer*,
https://doi.org/10.1007/978-3-319-64513-1_19

19.1 Introduction

With 16.1/100,000 new cases diagnosed annually in the EU, rare gynecologic tumors (RGT), including ovarian, fallopian, uterine, cervix, vaginal, and vulvar, represent more than 50% of all gynecologic cancers [1]. These cancers are commonly associated with a poor prognosis, and represent 25% of all gynecologic cancer deaths [2, 3]. It is often difficult to clearly define the natural history, the prognostic factors, and definitive histological diagnosis, as these tumors are so rare. Amongst these rare tumors, there are often considerable variability in patients' age, the histological subtype, anatomical localization, and stage, making it difficult to determine optimal treatment strategies from the literature.

Patient management is largely based on expert opinion and by extrapolating from therapeutic advances made in treating other similar tumors as it has not been feasible to conduct large-scale randomized trials in women with rare gynecologic cancers. The lack of solid evidence to guide treatment decisions remain a significant limitation to making recommendations regarding patient management. There are several reasons to explain the relatively poor prognosis of patients with rare gynecological malignancies including: delayed or incorrect diagnosis due to clinical inexperience; the need for a second opinion which delays the time to initiate treatment; or the absence of good data regarding the best therapeutic options leading to suboptimal treatment.

The histological diagnosis of rare tumors is often complex and in the absence of clearly delineated prognostic or predictive factors to help guide the selection of therapies, it is vital that patients with rare tumors are discussed within a multidisciplinary team comprising experts in the field of pathology, surgery and therapeutics [4]. This poses a huge burden to the health care system, especially in developing countries. Molecular studies have also shown that these rare cancers may actually be quite heterogeneous, and that our perceived clinical understanding of these entities may be incorrect and biased, further compounding the problem [5].

Moreover, inconsistencies in practice may also lead to poorer outcomes [2]. Lack of level 1 evidence from randomized-phase III trials (RCT) to support recommendations leads to variations in treatment practice which may negatively impact on outcomes. Accrual to RCT in rare tumors is difficult, and unfortunately the rarity of these tumors also provides little incentive for the pharmaceutical industry to invest in clinical trials due to the low return. Harmonization of research activities, medical practice and education of all professionals are therefore essential to improve knowledge of these diseases and their management. A global approach is needed to share information and collect research data if we are to make any progress.

In spite of the fact that oncologists and gynecologists managing RGT are usually well-organized at a national level, there are no specific structured collaborations that exist internationally to study rare tumors. The continuous efforts of GCIG have facilitated significant progress in numerous international intergroup clinical trials; development of internationally accepted position papers (such as CA125 response and progression criteria); performance of meta-analyses, and the conduct of Consensus Conferences (in Ovarian and Endometrial Cancers). Consequently, the

GCIG decided in 2012 to promote research and clinical trials for patients with uncommon and rare cancers at the international level under the auspices of the GCIG. All the 20 national groups received the draft version for final comments and validation. At the end of 2013, all the documents were approved by all the national groups as GCIG recommendations for management of rare gynecologic cancers. A final review was organized by the editorial team for harmonization and editing before publishing in 2015 and this provides information on the prognosis and management of rare uterine tumors [6–12]. These include the mesenchymal tumors, high-grade serous carcinoma, carcinosarcoma, and gestational trophoblastic disease which are reviewed below.

19.2 Mesenchymal Tumors

19.2.1 Leiomyosarcoma (LMS)

19.2.1.1 Introduction

Leiomyosarcomas are the most common subtype of uterine sarcomas. Uterine sarcomas of any histologic subtype are rare diseases representing about 8% of uterine cancers, with an incidence of about 0.4 per 100,000 women [13]. Most leiomyosarcomas are high-grade malignancies with a high risk for recurrence and progression. Overall survival is dependent on stage at diagnosis with 5-year survival estimates of 76% for stage I, 60% for stage II, 45% for stage III, and 29% for stage IV. Uterine leiomyosarcomas are staged using the FIGO 2009 uterine sarcoma staging system, although it is recognized that anatomic staging systems perform poorly in terms of survival prognostication. Other factors that have been evaluated for their potential prognostic impact include tumor morcellation [14], mitotic index, and tumor grade [15]. A nomogram that includes additional nonanatomic prognostic factors such as patient age, tumor grade, and mitotic rate provides better estimates of overall survival [15, 16].

19.2.1.2 Initial Treatment

Surgery

Hysterectomy is recommended for patients whose disease appears limited to the uterus. Intact removal of the uterus is preferred, particularly if there is suspicion of malignancy prior to surgery. Morcellation procedures have been associated with intraoperative spread of malignant tissue [17] and poorer survival outcomes. Routine lymph node dissection is not generally required because the risk of occult metastatic disease to lymph nodes is very low. However, it is recommended that lymph nodes that appear enlarged or suspicious for malignant involvement be resected [18]. Bilateral salpingo-oophorectomy (BSO) is reasonable in peri-menopausal and postmenopausal women, although it is recognized that there is no data to show that oophorectomy improves survival outcomes [19]. Estrogen receptors and/or progesterone receptors have been reported to be positive in 40–70% of uterine leiomyosarcoma, and may have prognostic significance [20]. Although oophorectomy may be reasonable to consider in pre-menopausal women, it is acknowledged that retrospective data have not shown survival differences among women under age 50 with uterus-limited disease who did or did not undergo BSO [21].

For disease that appears locally advanced but potentially completely resectable, an attempt to resect all visible disease is reasonable. Retrospective data, albeit representing patient selection bias, have shown longer overall survival among women whose disease is completely resected compared to those with residual disease at the end of the resection attempt [22]. For women who present with multisite metastatic, unresectable disease, there generally is no role for hysterectomy.

Post-resection Management of Uterus-Limited Disease
Although it is recognized that the risk for recurrence after resection of uterus-limited high-grade LMS exceeds 50% [23], no adjuvant intervention has been shown to alter progression-free or overall survival outcomes. Standard management after complete resection of uterus-limited disease is observation. Nearly one-third of patients who are found at time of hysterectomy to have uterine LMS will have evidence of metastatic disease on post-resection imaging. Therefore CT and/or PET/CT and/or MRI is recommended to rule out distant metastases once the diagnosis of uterine LMS has been made. PET imaging has not been shown to be superior to conventional imaging (CT or MRI) for detection of recurrent disease in patients undergoing surveillance or being imaged for suspected recurrence [6]. PET imaging may not detect small volume lung metastases. Adjuvant pelvic radiation was evaluated in a prospective randomized trial for women with uterine carcinosarcoma, leiomyosarcoma, or endometrial stromal sarcoma. Survival outcomes were not improved by adjuvant radiation, and among the patients with uterine LMS, there was no difference in local recurrence rates between patients assigned to adjuvant pelvic RT and those assigned to observation [24].

A prospective phase II study of adjuvant gemcitabine-docetaxel for four cycles, followed by doxorubicin for four cycles, demonstrated a 2-year progression-free survival (PFS) rate of 78% and 3-year PFS rate of 58%. It is not known whether this 3-year PFS rate is superior to what would be expected with observation [25]. A small randomized phase III including 81 patients with a variety of uterine sarcoma histologies and FIGO stages (only 52 stage I, 16 stage II, 13 stage III; 53 leiomyosarcoma, 9 undifferentiated sarcomas, 19 carcinosarcoma), undergoing chemotherapy with doxorubicin plus ifosfamide plus cisplatin followed by radiation, was superior to radiation alone at 3 years for disease-free survival (55% vs. 41%) but not for overall survival [26]. This data cannot be used to support a recommendation for adjuvant chemotherapy as standard treatment given the heterogeneity of the tumor types and stages, the very small sample size and no overall survival benefit. An international, randomized, phase III trial of observation versus adjuvant chemotherapy (gemcitabine-docetaxel for four cycles followed by doxorubicin for four cycles) is ongoing with primary endpoint of overall survival (GOG 0277/IRCI study 001).

For patients with locally advanced, completely resected uterine LMS, there are no prospective data upon which to base management recommendations. Choices would include observation (with treatment at time of recurrence), adjuvant radiation, adjuvant hormone blockade, or adjuvant chemotherapy. The location of the disease, the grade of the tumor, the estrogen receptor and progesterone receptor status, patient preferences, organ function, and comorbidities would be incorporated into the decision.

19.2.1.3 Metastatic Disease

Patients found to have metastatic disease should be evaluated to determine whether resection of metastases may be appropriate. In general, resection should be considered for patients with a relatively long disease-free interval, an isolated site of disease that is amenable to complete resection, with an acceptably low risk of morbidity.

Potentially Resectable Metastatic Disease

Retrospective data show that survival may be prolonged among patients who undergo resection of metastatic disease. These data have inherent patient selection bias, but nevertheless support consideration of metastatectomy for selected patients. Outcomes are more favorable for those patients who have had a long disease-free interval, have a paucity of metastatic sites, and for whom the resection is likely to render them measurably disease-free [27].

Recent advances have been made in nonsurgical treatment of isolated metastatic disease. Radiofrequency ablation and other interventional radiology techniques may be appropriate for certain patients. There are no prospective studies of these interventions, or randomized trials comparing outcomes with surgical outcomes. Unless a separate pre-ablation biopsy is performed, ablation will not provide tissue confirmation of metastatic disease, cannot ensure negative margins, and will leave residual radiographic changes that require follow-up to confirm the site of metastasis was completely ablated. There is no data evaluating adjuvant systemic treatment after metastatectomy. The standard approach is surveillance.

Systemic Treatment for Unresectable Metastatic Disease

Objective response rates can be achieved with systemic treatment for metastatic uterine LMS. In patients with symptomatic disease, chemotherapy provides a reasonable probability for palliation of symptoms. There is no established best first-line chemotherapy regimen. Treatment recommendations for an individual patient should take into consideration the patient's preferences for the treatment schedule, drug side effects, venous access, comorbidities, disease burden, and organ function. Reasonable regimens to consider for first-line therapy include doxorubicin, doxorubicin plus ifosfamide, gemcitabine, gemcitabine plus docetaxel. Other treatment options, which may be used as second-line therapy or after, include pazopanib, trabectedin, dacarbazine or gemcitabine, and eribulin. Enrollment in clinical trials is highly recommended for eligible patients.

Doxorubicin 60 mg/m^2 every 3 weeks achieved objective response in 19% of patients with uterine sarcoma whether given as a single agent or combined with cyclophosphamide. Median overall survival was 12 months [28].

Doxorubicin plus ifosfamide achieved objective response in 30% of patients with uterine LMS [29]. The choice between single-agent doxorubicin and doxorubicin plus ifosfamide should incorporate the disease burden and the patient's risk for toxicity from dual-agent treatment.

Gemcitabine 1000 mg/m^2 IV over 30 min on a 3-week on or 1-week off schedule achieved objective response in 20% of patients with uterine LMS in a phase II trial [30].

Fixed dose-rate gemcitabine plus docetaxel achieved objective response in 27% of patients with uterine LMS when given as second-line therapy (90% of patients had progressed on or after doxorubicin) in a phase II trial [31]. The objective response rate was 36% in the phase II trial as first-line therapy [32]. Gemcitabine was given at 10 mg/m^2/min in these studies. A randomized trial in patients with metastatic soft tissue sarcoma showed superior objective response rates, progression-free, and overall survival among patients treated with gemcitabine plus docetaxel compared to those assigned to gemcitabine alone [33]. Another randomized trial in second-line therapy after doxorubicin in leiomyosarcoma did not find a difference between gemcitabine vs. gemcitabine-docetaxel but the very small sample size, and the imbalance in the treatment arms for important variables such as the percentage of patients who had had prior adjuvant chemotherapy make these data difficult to interpret [34] (all patients were second line after either adjuvant (less than 1 year) or one line for metastatic disease). The toxicity of gemcitabine plus docetaxel is greater than that of single-agent gemcitabine.

Ifosfamide 1.5 g/m^2 IV for 5 days with Mesna, every 3 weeks achieved objective response in 17% of patients with uterine LMS [29].

Pazopanib 800 mg oral daily achieved objective response in about 8% of patients with metastatic soft tissue sarcoma in a phase III trial comparing pazopanib to placebo. The PFS was 20 weeks among patients assigned to pazopanib and 7 weeks among those assigned to placebo. There was no differences in overall survival [35]. Pazopanib is approved by the EMEA and FDA for treatment of soft tissue sarcoma.

Trabectedin 1.5 mg/m^2 IV over 24 h every 3 weeks achieved objective response in 10% of patients with uterine LMS as first-line therapy [36]. The study closed after first stage of accrual for failure to meet the objective response rate goal. The study was not designed to evaluate progression-free survival, however among the 20 patients enrolled in the study, the median PFS was 5.8 months. By contrast, in a retrospective study among patients with uterine LMS who had had prior treatment, trabectedin was associated with a 16% response rate but only a 3 month PFS [37]. Trabectedin by 3 h infusion plus doxorubicin in first-line therapy yielded an objective response in 57% of patients with leiomyosarcoma of either uterine or soft tissue origin as first-line treatment [38]. However in a randomized trial, this combination was not superior to single-agent doxorubicin. Trabectedin was compared to dacarbazine in a phase III trial for patient with LMS or liposarcoma and achieved longer

PFS (4.2 months vs. 1.5 months) but no difference in overall survival (12.4 months vs. 12.9 months) [39]. The data led to FDA approval of trabectedin for patients with metastatic leiomyosarcoma or liposarcoma who have received prior anthracycline treatment.

Dacarbazine and Temozolomide have modest activity in soft tissue sarcomas and in uterine LMS, although prospective data are limited for these agents in the uterine LMS population [40].

Eribulin was compared to dacarbazine in a phase III trial for LMS or liposarcoma patients. Eribulin treatment was associated with longer overall survival (13.5 months vs. 11.5 months), but no difference in PFS. A planned subset analysis showed that the benefit was seen in the liposarcoma group. Eribulin was approved by the FDA for patients with liposarcoma but not for patients with leiomyosarcoma [41].

Hormonal blockade may also be considered for patients with uterine LMS who have a low disease burden that appears to have an indolent disease pace, particularly if their tumors are ER and/or PR positive. In a retrospective study, aromatase inhibition treatment was associated with objective response in fewer than 10% of patients. The time to progression was longer among patients that were hormone receptor positive than among those who were receptor negative. The relatively prolonged PFS that was observed could be attributed to the inherent biology of the uterine LMS in these cases rather than to the hormonal intervention. A small prospective study of letrozole in ER and/or PR positive uterine LMS patients showed a 12-week progression-free survival rate of 50% with median duration of treatment being 2.2 months [42].

19.2.2 Endometrial Stromal Sarcoma (ESS)

19.2.2.1 Introduction
Endometrial stromal sarcoma (ESS) arises from the endometrial epithelial lining and typically has an indolent and hormone-sensitive nature. A separate staging system was proposed by the Fédération Internationale de Gynécologie et d'Obstétrique (FIGO) [43] (See Table 19.1). Abnormal uterine bleeding and infertility are common symptoms of ESS. Women in their reproductive ages and also teenagers can suffer from ESS.

19.2.2.2 Initial Treatment
Figure 19.1 summarizes the treatment strategy for early stage and recurrent ESS [44]. Surgery with hysterectomy, either open or by a minimal invasive technique, is the cornerstone of treatment for localized ESS [44]. Since imaging studies cannot reliably diagnose ESS preoperatively, surgical resection for a presumed fibroid is a reality. This can result in inadvertent tumor morcellation of ESS, a technique used for presumed benign disease which has an adverse impact on the patient outcomes, should be avoided [14]. The benefit of lymphadenectomy for ESS is controversial. The lymphatic system is commonly involved in ESS as the invasion of lymphatic

Table 19.1 FIGO staging for endometrial stromal sarcoma

Stage		Definition
I		Tumor limited to uterus
	IA	≤5 cm
	IB	>5 cm
II		Tumor extends to the pelvis
	IIA	Adnexal involvement
	IIB	Tumor extends to extrauterine pelvic tissue
III		Tumor invades abdominal tissues (not just protruding into the abdomen)
	IIIA	One site
	IIIB	>One site
	IIIC	Metastasis to pelvic and/or para-aortic lymph nodes
IV	IVA	Tumor invades bladder and/or rectum
	IVB	Distant metastasis

Fig. 19.1 The treatment strategy for early-stage and recurrent endometrial stromal sarcoma (ESS) [1]. *Retention of the ovaries can be considered in young women with small ESS. °Adjuvant hormonal treatment can be considered

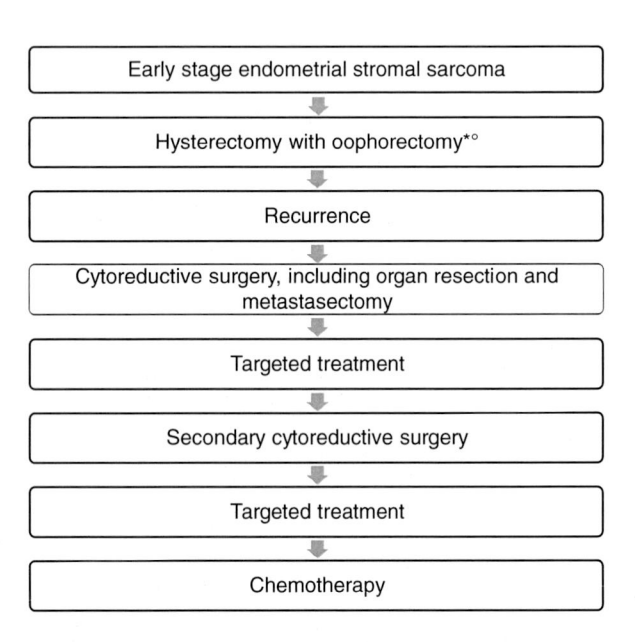

Early stage endometrial stromal sarcoma
↓
Hysterectomy with oophorectomy*°
↓
Recurrence
↓
Cytoreductive surgery, including organ resection and metastasectomy
↓
Targeted treatment
↓
Secondary cytoreductive surgery
↓
Targeted treatment
↓
Chemotherapy

vessels is a pathognomonic microscopic characteristic, as exemplified by the prior pathologic designation of endolymphatic stromal myosis. Nodal involvement designates a higher stage of disease, and results in a worse outcome. The incidence of lymph node metastases in ESS is generally low, with rates of 9.9% (28/282) [45] and 7% (7/100) [46] in recent series. Systematic lymphadenectomy in ESS does not appear to confer a therapeutic benefit [45, 46]. Although prospective studies are lacking, it seems that routine lymphadenectomy is not indicated unless lymph nodes are pathologically enlarged on preoperative imaging studies and as part of a cytoreductive procedure in patients with metastases.

Traditionally, the ovaries were removed at initial surgery as ESS typically express estrogen and progesterone receptors as there were concerns of higher relapse rates if the ovaries were retained. Although this issue has less importance in peri- and postmenopausal women, the question regarding bilateral oophorectomy deserves particular consideration in young pre-menopausal women. In contrast to previous belief, it appears from both small and large series that leaving the ovaries in situ does not worsen survival [46]. Oncological outcome aside, maintenance of quality of life is important especially with the challenges involved in the management of menopausal symptoms in young women undergoing oophorectomy. This is particularly the case as hormone replacement therapy has been associated with higher relapse rates in one series with five patients and it is generally contraindicated in ESS patients [7, 47].

19.2.2.3 Role of Radiotherapy

Adjuvant pelvic radiotherapy does not influence overall survival since ESS typically recurs distantly. Although a modest benefit in locoregional control can be achieved by postoperative radiotherapy, overall survival is not improved [48]. Palliative radiotherapy can be used for recurrent or metastatic ESS when symptoms of local disease reduce quality of life. When systemic treatment and/or surgical resection insufficiently reduce symptoms, radiotherapy is a valuable option. Overall, however, the role for radiotherapy is limited.

19.2.2.4 Role of Adjuvant Hormonal Therapy

There is a very high rate of hormone receptor positivity in ESS, up to 100% in some series [1], which has led to interest in using hormonal therapies for both advanced disease and as adjuvant therapy in patients with early stage disease [48]. The use of adjuvant hormonal therapy has been reported in several studies. A small study reported on 22 patients with ESS, of whom 31% (4/13) of patients receiving adjuvant progestins recurred, compared with 67% (6/9) recurrence in patients who did not receive hormonal therapy [7]. Another study that included 30 ESS patients who received adjuvant hormonal therapy, reported a nonsignificant trend to improved overall survival of 97 months for patients receiving hormonal therapy as compared with 72 months for those who did not ($p = 0.07$) [49]. A recent report summarizing data on the use of aromatase inhibitors found an overall response rate of 67% in a total of 28 ESS patients [48]. The data support the current practice in some centers to recommend adjuvant hormonal treatment to selected patients. This seems reasonable, given that hormonal therapies (tamoxifen is contraindicated) are generally well tolerated. However, several questions remain, such as optimal dose of progestins, which hormonal therapy (progestins or aromatase inhibitors) and duration of therapy. Most clinicians consider progestins as the standard of care in ESS. ESS is not an approved indication for aromatase inhibitors. While some consider 2 year duration of hormonal treatment sufficient in the absence of solid data, others believe the treatment should be lifelong. Uterine sparing surgery in young women is experimental.

19.2.2.5 Metastatic Disease and Relapse

The benefit of cytoreductive surgery in locally advanced ESS is controversial, with little published evidence to support the practice. However, knowledge of tumor biology and natural history (indolent disease with primarily trans peritoneal spread) suggests that cytoreductive surgery might be beneficial because of the "low grade" nature of the disease and the efficacy of additional hormonal therapy [49]. If the ovaries were previously left in situ, they need to be removed when recurrence is diagnosed. Extensive surgery with organ resection (for example, splenectomy, and bowel resection) can be considered in selected patients, particularly if this contributes to achieving complete resection with no residual tumor. However, the impact of resection of locally advanced disease on prolongation of survival is not proven, and so the decision to undertake extensive resection should be taken on an individual patient basis, depending on the relative morbidity of such surgery.

A series studying the benefit of adjuvant hormonal treatment in 31 ESS patients, also included information according to stage [46]. The authors showed benefit for patients with stage III/IV disease who received adjuvant hormonal treatment after surgical resection.

Recurrences of ESS are common even in early-stage disease, with a predilection for lungs and abdomen. Relapse can occur in 36–56% of patients with early stage disease, with a median time to recurrence of 65 and 9 months for stages I and III–IV, respectively [44]. Although supportive data are lacking, repeat surgery for a disease that is indolent and hormone sensitive appears to be an acceptable approach. Secondary and tertiary cytoreductive procedures, including resection of distant metastases should be considered in selected patients. Intervals between surgeries can be extended by the addition of hormonal therapies [7].

There are a number of case reports showing responses to progestins, gonadotrophin-releasing hormone agonists, and aromatase inhibitors [7]. The median time to progression is typically 24 months. The data suggests that hormonal therapies are effective for metastatic disease and can be administered for long periods as they are typically well tolerated in most patients.

The data on the response of ESS to chemotherapy are scarce since the literature dates back to the era where high- and low-grade ESS were pooled and analyzed as a single disease entity. Piver et al. reported on patients with recurrent ESS, including two patients who had durable responses to doxorubicin, methotrexate and megesterol acetate, and doxorubicin and chlorambucil, respectively. However, another ten patients did not respond to chemotherapy [50]. More recently, Cheng et al. reported on ten patients with recurrent ESS who received a range of chemotherapy regimens including doxorubicin, gemcitabine and docetaxel, actinomycin D, and paclitaxel and liposomal doxorubicin. Four patients achieved stable disease, but six patients showed disease progression, with a median time to progression of 6.5 months. Thus, response rates to chemotherapy are low and chemotherapy should only be considered and prescribed when the hormonal therapies have become ineffective and there is clear evidence of resistance to hormonal treatment.

19.2.3 High-Grade Undifferentiated Sarcoma (HGUS)

As specific molecular abnormalities were described, modifications have been made to the classification. Since 2003, endometrial stromal tumors have been divided into three subtypes: stromal nodule, endometrial stromal sarcoma, and undifferentiated endometrial sarcoma [49, 51, 52].

In contrast to ESS, which demonstrates a good prognosis and an indolent clinical course, HGUS are characterized by aggressive behavior and poor prognosis [51, 52]. These differences might be related to a distinct genetic background favoring the development of two clinical pathologic entities.

19.2.3.1 Early Stage and Adjuvant Treatment

Standard management for HGUS consists of total hysterectomy and bilateral-salpingoophorectomy. The role of surgical regional lymphadenectomy remains unknown [53]. Most relapses in patients with complete resection are visceral. Thus, systematic lymphadenectomy is not recommended unless there is a clinical or radiological suspicion of nodal involvement. In the case of extensive disease, abdominal debulking is recommended if feasible. Residual disease has a negative prognostic impact [52] and resection of distant metastasis should be considered as for other sarcomas. However, controversy exists regarding the role of radical surgery in the setting of disseminated disease for endometrial cancer in general, and in uterine sarcoma more specifically [54].

In this particular poor prognosis disease with a high rate of local and metastatic relapse, adjuvant therapy in patients with localized tumors may have a role. In one of the published retrospective studies, postoperative pelvic radiotherapy with or without brachytherapy was the only prognostic factor associated with improved PFS and OS among HGUS patients after surgical resection. To date, external pelvic irradiation has been widely used as adjuvant treatment for high-grade sarcoma, an approach reported to decrease local recurrence but no benefit proved for OS. In the randomized study conducted by the EORTC, adjuvant external pelvic irradiation did not improve PFS and OS among women with high-grade uterine sarcoma. However, this treatment reduced local recurrence rates among patients with carcinosarcoma, but not those with leiomyosarcoma [54]. No data on HGUS were available. Thus, adjuvant radiotherapy may be speculated to decrease locoregional recurrence, but impact on survival is unknown.

The benefit of adjuvant chemotherapy in this particularly aggressive disease has been investigated in a recent phase-III trial. In a study of 81 patients with FIGO stage I–III uterine sarcoma (9 HGUS) randomly allocated to adjuvant chemotherapy (doxorubicin, ifosfamide and cisplatin) followed by pelvic radiotherapy or pelvic radiotherapy alone, the addition of chemotherapy to radiotherapy increased the 3-year DFS rate (55% vs. 41%; $P = 0.048$); there was a trend towards an improvement in OS (3 year OS: 81% vs. 69%, p = NS) [55]. The data suggests that the use of adjuvant chemotherapy followed by pelvic radiotherapy could be recommended for treatment of HGUS. However, given the limited data available to date, the benefit of adjuvant treatment in uterine sarcomas (pelvic radiotherapy and/or chemotherapy) remains poorly defined and deserves further investigation.

19.2.3.2 Metastatic Phase

Despite the absence of specific studies and although responses are short-lived, HGUS are reported to be sensitive to doxorubicin-ifosfamide-based regimens and, more recently, to the combination of gemcitabine and docetaxel with partial and complete responses to therapy [52]. Specific response to second-line agents used in sarcomas such as trabectedin or pazopanib is not well known; however, these patients could be included in PALETTE trial [35]. A prospective randomized trial is ongoing (IRCI project) evaluating cabozantinib in maintenance phase for patients with response or stabilization in first-line chemotherapy including doxorubicine (EORTC 62113-55115).

19.2.4 Adenosarcoma

Mullerian adenosarcomas of the female genital tract are rare malignancies. In 1974 Clement and Scully described the adenosarcoma to be most common in the uterus, but may also arise in extrauterine locations including the cervix, ovary, vagina, fallopian tube, and intestinal serosa [56]. Uterine adenosarcoma make up 5% of uterine sarcomas and tend to occur in post-menopausal women; however, may also be diagnosed in adolescents and young women [57]. They are usually low-grade tumors and are characterized by a benign epithelial component with a malignant mesenchymal component, which is typically a low-grade endometrial stromal sarcoma, but can also occasionally be a high-grade sarcoma [58, 59]. Tumors that exhibit a high-grade sarcomatous overgrowth have a worse outcome.

19.2.4.1 Initial Treatment

The treatment for uterine adenosarcomas is a hysterectomy and bilateral salpingo-oophorectomy. Ovarian metastases appear to be very uncommon and a good case can be made for not removing the ovaries in a pre-menopausal women. There have been individual case reports of more conservative surgery with a hysterectomy alone with ovarian preservation in pre-menopausal women [60] and the treatment decisions need to be individualized based on age and clinicopathological parameters. The incidence of lymph node involvement is reported to be low in Stage 1 uterine adenosarcomas and in the SEER study was only 3%, indicating that lymphadenectomy is not required for the vast majority of patients. The role of adjuvant irradiation, chemotherapy or hormonal therapy is unclear and unlikely will ever be addressed in a clinical trial as they are so uncommon. Given that most uterine adenosarcomas have a low-grade ESS component, the principles of management of these tumors should follow the guidelines for ESS as described by Amant [7]. Arguably, these tumors should be included in studies of ESS but stratified as adenosarcoma or ESS, while the alternative is that they be included with the carcinosarcomas. In a historical series of 100 patients, recurrent tumor occurred in 23 patients at a mean interval after diagnosis of 3.4 years (range 0.5–9.5 years) with most recurrences being local recurrences [59] The only factor associated with local recurrence was the presence of myometrial invasion which raises the question regarding the role of adjuvant pelvic radiation or brachytherapy in these patients. It is even more difficult to make recommendations on the management of extrauterine adenosarcomas as they are so rare and management should be based on surgical principles.

It is unlikely that the diagnosis would be known prior to surgery in most of these patients and would only be made on the final histopathology [10].

19.2.4.2 Metastatic Disease

The management of patients with metastatic adenosarcoma is essentially based on first principles and depends on multiple factors including: age and comorbidities of the patient, the site/s of recurrence, time to recurrence, the number of metastases as well as the sarcomatous subtype. Given that ESS is the most common subtype, the treatment would be similar to the management of patients with metastatic ESS with hormonal therapy including progestogens and/or aromatase inhibitors. The management of patients with high-grade metastatic sarcomas is similar to the management of patients with metastatic high-grade sarcomas. These are all so rare and the literature contains only a number of individual case reports of responses to trabectedin, liposomal doxorubicin as well as anthracyclines and ifosfamide [61, 62]. It is likely that there may be reporting bias as the few reports of chemotherapy in metastatic high-grade adenosarcoma suggest high response rates and very durable remissions and even apparent cures. In contrast, one of the larger case series describing the treatment of 13 patients with recurrent adenosarcomas has been recently reported [63]. Six patients had disease confined to the abdomen or pelvis and had surgical resection at the time of recurrence and had a time to second recurrence of 29.7 months versus 12.7 months for patients treated with nonsurgical therapy alone. This suggests that secondary cytoreduction may be beneficial in selected patients. 11 of 13 patients with measureable disease received chemotherapy, hormonal therapy, or radiation. Only one of five patients had a durable response to hormonal therapy. There were partial responses of short duration observed with ifosfamide and doxorubicin in two patients with a high-grade sarcomatous component and a brief response to gemcitabine and docetaxel in one patient [63]. It seems unlikely that there is anything intrinsically different between high-grade sarcomas arising in adenosarcomas and their histological counterparts that arise de novo and a similar approach to management as in other sarcomas is reasonable.

19.3 Rare Epithelial Tumors

19.3.1 High-Grade Uterine Serous Carcinoma (USC)

USC represents an aggressive histologic subtype of endometrial cancer. A total genome analysis has indicated that it most closely resembles high-grade endometrioid adenocarcinoma [64]. Although USC (previously named as uterine papillary serous carcinoma, and now called uterine serous carcinoma, as not only papillary lesions exist) represents less than 10% of all endometrial cancers, it accounts for more than 50% of relapses and deaths attributed to endometrial carcinoma [65]. The estimated 5-year overall survival rate for patients with USC is 18–27%. Likely due to the clinical observation that approximately 60–70% of women with USC present with disease outside the uterus. Even in cases where disease is apparently confined to the corpus, the rate of recurrence is high and is estimated to be 31–80% [66].

19.3.1.1 Initial Treatment

As USC is relatively rare, USC has been included in prospective trials of endometrial cancer. However no randomized trials limited to only USC have been performed. Most of the currently available data are in the form of small, retrospective single- and multi-institutional studies. In some large randomized studies, this histologic subtype is grouped with other subtypes of endometrial cancer. The percentage of patients with USC accrued to these trials is only about 10–20%, making it difficult to have sufficient power to analyze this subgroup separately and be able to draw specific conclusions regarding therapy and outcome. However because of its aggressive behavior and pattern of recurrence, multimodality treatment, including surgery, chemotherapy, and radiotherapy, has been employed in the management of USC.

Surgery

The initial management for the majority of women with USC is surgical exploration and comprehensive staging for early-stage disease or debulking for advanced cases (including omentectomy). A small number of reports describe neoadjuvant chemotherapy for patients who were supposed to be poor surgical candidates for upfront debulking. Though treatment of lymph nodes in the pelvis does not confer a survival benefit, diagnosis of positive nodes changes management and is therefore advised for high-risk patients. In USC cases, prognostic factors such as myometrial invasion or lymphovascular-space invasion are important determinants of the risk of nodal disease. However, distant metastatic disease may be encountered even in the absence of these risk factors. In a series of 52 surgically staged women with USC, similar rates of lymph node and intraperitoneal metastases were reported in cases with either no myometrial invasion or deep invasion (36% vs. 40% and 43% vs. 35%, respectively) [67]. A study of 84 patients with clinical Stage I USC reported an overall survival advantage benefiting women undergoing comprehensive surgical staging compared to those treated only with hysterectomy and bilateral salpingo-oophorectomy (16.4 years vs. 2.76 years) [68]. Another study of 206 women with surgically staged I–II USC demonstrated that recurrence and progression-free survival were not associated with an increasing percentage of USC in the histologic specimen, lymphovascular-space invasion, or tumor size. Similar to epithelial ovarian cancer, USC often shows metastatic disease outside the pelvis. In one of the largest series of patients with advanced-stage USC, optimal cytoreduction was associated with a median survival of 39 months compared to 12 months in patients who underwent suboptimal surgery ($p = 0.0001$) [69]. Maximal cytoreduction efforts should be made at the time of primary surgery for advanced-stage disease.

Adjuvant Therapy

USC presents a high risk of recurrence outside the pelvis, often in multiple sites, whereas recurrence in most women with early-stage endometrioid endometrial carcinoma (EEC) is in the vagina or pelvis. In this view, adjuvant therapy for USC should be more widely applied with chemotherapy and/or radiation therapy.

The role of adjuvant chemotherapy in the management of early-stage (I/II) USC lacks data from randomized studies. In the largest retrospective series of USC patients to date, significant survival benefits were reported with the use of chemotherapy and radiation [9]. Other retrospective series with Stage I USC only, have reported improved relapse-free survival with platinum/taxane chemotherapy [69]. Among women with surgical Stage I USC, significantly improved rates of both recurrence and overall survival were associated with the addition of platinum/taxane chemotherapy with or without radiation [69]. Both PFS and cause-specific survival rates were better for women treated with chemotherapy. The impact chemotherapy had on recurrence rate, PFS and cause-specific survival was most pronounced in patients with Stages IB/IC USC. A recurrence rate of 43% was reported in patients with Stage IA USC with residual cancer in the uterine specimen not offered adjuvant therapy. Using FIGO 1988 staging, the authors proposed that platinum-based chemotherapy and brachytherapy should be considered in all women with Stage IA USC, except for those with no residual cancer in the uterus at time of hysterectomy [70]. It may be appropriate to offer chemotherapy and radiation to women with Stage IA USC platinum-taxane-based, with the possible exception of those USC with no residual disease in the uterine specimen. However, rigorous data in this small subgroup is lacking. Several studies have reported high recurrence rates for patients with Stages IB/IC USC, as staged according to the FIGO 1988 criteria. Reported 5-year survival rates for Stages IA, IB and IC are 81.5%, 58.6%, and 34.3%, respectively. The fact that 10–20% of women with Stage I USC treated without systemic adjuvant therapy will recur, suggests that USC may be offered platinum-based chemotherapy or brachytherapy. However, we do not have prospective studies to demonstrate such proposals and these studies are needed.

Retrospective studies show that adjuvant treatment for women with stage IB USC could be treated with platinum-taxane-based systemic therapy with consideration of brachytherapy if patients have had a lymph node dissection. In the absence of nodal dissection, pelvic radiation is recommended in the U.S. (NCCN Guidelines). Adjuvant chemotherapy and radiation are used in the management of Stage II USC. In a retrospective study, with a median follow-up time of 33 months, 20 of 55 women (36%) with Stage II USC had recurrent disease [71]. Most of the recurrences were detected within 2 years (85%) and were observed outside the pelvis (70%). In women treated with chemotherapy +/− radiation therapy, the reported recurrence rate was 11%, in contrast to 50% in those treated with radiation therapy only or by observation ($p = 0.013$). None of the women treated with multimodality therapy experienced a recurrence.

The GOG has completed a series of five phase III randomized prospective trials of chemotherapy for advanced-stage or recurrent endometrial carcinoma, of which 18–20% were USC [67]. Studies of paclitaxel plus either carboplatin or cisplatin have shown response rates of 50% or higher, an improved PFS rate, and possibly prolonged survival compared to historical experience with other non-paclitaxel-containing regimens. Paclitaxel-based regimens may be more active in non-endometrioid adenocarcinoma histologies which tend to have a lower response to doxorubicin and/or cisplatin-based regimens. Paclitaxel-containing regimens have been reported to have response rates as high as 80% in recurrent or advanced USC

[67]. In a study of 19 women with locally advanced or recurrent USC treated with carboplatin and paclitaxel, with or without radiation therapy, response rates were 60% and 50% for women with primarily advanced and recurrent USC respectively [67]. In a prospective phase III GOG study with 13% USC cases in each arm, the addition of paclitaxel to cisplatin and doxorubicin (TAP) following cytoreductive surgery and tumor-volume-directed radiation therapy was not associated with improvement in recurrence-free survival but resulted in greater toxicity as compared to carboplatin/paclitaxel (GOG184). Relative to grade 1 EEC, the rate of recurrence for USC was 4.43 times higher. Subgroup analysis revealed that TAP was associated with a 50% reduction in the risk of recurrence or death among patients with gross residual disease. There was a trend towards improved outcomes in women with USC, though this did not reach statistical significance (HR 0.73). Another phase III randomized trial (GOG 177) compared TAP to cisplatin and doxorubicin in women with advanced/metastatic or recurrent endometrial carcinoma. The 3-drug regimen was associated with an improved response rate (57% vs. 34%), longer PFS (8.3 months vs. 5.3 months) and a slight improvement in survival (15.3 months vs. 12.3 months), but with significantly increased toxicity. In the recent Phase III trial, TAP was compared to carboplatin and paclitaxel (TC) in women with advanced-stage or recurrent endometrial cancer. A higher percentage of patients on TC were able to complete all seven planned courses of treatment (69% vs. 62% for TAP). The less-toxic two-drug (TC) regimen is not less effective, and may offer greater clinical benefit in terms of side effects than the three-drug (TAP) regimen. However, each of the phase III GOG trials has included different histologies. Approximately 12–18% of the study populations in each of these trials were patients with USC. Although in one of these trials, recurrence-free survival varied with histology and grade. With USC having the poorest outcome, analysis of the combined data from four earlier GOG phase III trials failed to show an association between histology and response rate. These conflicting results and the continued controversy as to the best management strategy in USC, indicate the need for prospective trials inclusive only of this histology.

Radiation therapy is commonly used as adjuvant treatment in the management of endometrial cancer. Retrospective series show a survival benefit to the combination of radiation with chemotherapy in USC [72]. Because of the tendency for USC to recur within the peritoneal cavity, historical studies of radiation therapy in the management of this disease has explored the role of whole-abdominal radiotherapy with a pelvic boost (WAPI). In the EORTC study of early-stage, high-risk uterine cancer including USC, the combination of radiation therapy and chemotherapy was superior to radiation therapy alone. The hazard ratio for PFS was 0.58 favoring combination radiation and chemotherapy ($p = 0.046$). This translated to an estimated 7% absolute difference in 5-year PFS from 75 to 82%. In the only prospective study of adjuvant radiation in women with early-stage USC, 21 patients were treated with WAPI [73]. Out of 19 patients with evaluable disease, 9 died of recurrent USC, 5 patients developed recurrent disease within the irradiated field and 10 patients remained disease free. Several studies have investigated the role of radiation therapy, ranging from tumor-directed radiation to WAPI, in the treatment of advanced-stage USC. In a prospective study carried out by the GOG, 8 of 20 women with optimally cytoreduced Stages III/IV USC treated with adjuvant WAPI died of disease between 9.6 months and 35.2 months following diagnosis. Forty-seven percent of the recurrences were within the irradiated field. The authors concluded that WAPI, as delivered in the study, was curative only in a minority of patients highlighting the need for randomized studies to explore multimodality treatment options. The GOG conducted a randomized phase III trial (GOG 122) comparing whole abdominal pelvis irradiation (WAPI) to doxorubicin and cisplatin in women with Stages III/IV endometrial cancer (residual disease <2 cm in greatest diameter) with 20% having USC [74]. A statistically meaningful subset analysis of patients with USC could not be carried out, given the small number of patients with USC. The currently accruing GOG 258 phase III study compares adjuvant chemotherapy plus radiation to chemotherapy alone. Both the appropriate timing of initiating chemotherapy and the most appropriate agents to use remain controversial. The potential benefit of multimodality treatment and the optimal sequence remain unclear. Further investigation via additional prospective trials are needed.

19.3.1.2 Management of Metastatic Disease

USC often exhibits HER-2/neu overexpression, which has led some investigators to propose the use of the anti-HER2 monoclonal antibody, trastuzumab, in the management of USC. In the largest reported series of USC patients, HER-2/neu was overexpressed in 47% but rates of 26–62% positivity have been observed depending on disease stage [75]. A clinical study failed to show single-agent activity of trastuzumab in patients with advanced-stage or recurrent endometrial carcinoma whose tumors over-expressed HER2/neu. However, of all endometrial cancer subtypes, HER-2/neu appears to be most commonly expressed in USC. Therefore, there is a scientific rationale for studying platinum/taxane-based regimens with trastuzumab in this patient population. In a phase II trial of bevacizumab in recurrent or persistent endometrial cancer, seven patients (13.5%) experienced clinical responses, which were seen across histologic type. Although interestingly, the one patient with a complete response and three of six patients with a partial response, had serous histology. Additionally, the percentage of patients alive and progression-free at 6 months was similar for serous and endometrioid histologies [76]. Patient numbers were too small to formally evaluate the role of histologic subtype and response to bevacizumab in that trial, but it is worthy of further study. Recent whole-exome sequencing studies [77] have demonstrated gain of function of the HER2/NEU gene, as well as driver mutations in the PIK3CA/AKT/mTOR and cyclin E /FBXW7 oncogenic pathways in a large number of USCs. These results emphasize the relevance of these novel therapeutic targets for biologic therapy of chemotherapy-resistant recurrent USC.

19.3.2 Clear Cell Carcinoma

Clear cell carcinoma (CCC) of the uterine corpus and cervix, is a rare gynecologic cancer. The incidence of uterine CCC is reported to be 1–6% of all endometrial cancer and the incidence of cervical CCC has been reported to be approximately 4% of all cervical cancer [11]. The pathogenesis has not been fully elucidated. In early stage disease, surgical resection is the standard treatment. However, there is no standard approach for advanced or recurrent disease [11].

19.3.2.1 Initial Surgical Treatment

Approximately 75% of patients are diagnosed with stage I/II disease and are treated surgically. A laparoscopic radical trachelectomy has been reported in properly selected young patients with early stage CCC of the cervix.

In general, clinical staging of women with endometrial cancer carries a large margin of error with regard to the true extent of disease, therefore surgical staging is recommended. It has been reported that 52% of patients presenting with UCCC clinically confined to the uterus were found to have extrauterine disease during comprehensive surgical staging, and patients with clinically stage I and II upstaged to III or IV in 39% of UCCC compared to 12% for those with endometrioid subtype [78].

The importance of comprehensive surgical staging and maximal cytoreductive surgery in UCCC was emphasized in a recent review by Thomas et al., but not confirmed by prospective studies. They recommended total hysterectomy and bilateral salpingo-oophorectomy with comprehensive surgical staging, including pelvic and para-aortic lymph node dissection and omentectomy, if patients were medically fit.

Although, no evidence for survival benefit with staging surgery was shown and worse prognosis was often seen with omental metastasis and lymph node metastasis. If extrauterine disease is present, cytoreductive surgery is also recommended. Women with advanced stage disease who were completely cytoreduced had a superior progression-free and overall survival compared with patients with residual disease at the end of surgery [78].

Patients without lymphatic dissemination have excellent prognosis irrespective of the use of adjuvant chemotherapy (3-year overall survival was reported to be about 90%). Lymphatic involvement appears to portend a worse survival, which indicates that lymphadenectomy may be a useful prognostic indicator but it is not known whether lymphadenectomy has a therapeutic effect.

Since UCCC is more likely to present with extrauterine spread compared to lower grade endometrial histology, management with aggressive adjuvant therapy may be recommended after complete surgical staging. Most of the evidence for surgery comes from studies on women with less-aggressive endometrioid carcinoma.

19.3.2.2 Adjuvant Treatment

There is limited evidence for the adjuvant treatment of UCCC. Most reports have assessed clear cell together with serous histologic subtypes. Only a few studies were published solely on UCCC. In general, management with aggressive adjuvant therapy may be recommended. Some UCCC may benefit from adjuvant chemotherapy and radiotherapy (RT). Observation, chemotherapy, or tumor-directed RT is recommended for stage IA UCCC without myometrial invasion [11]. Chemotherapy ± tumor-directed RT are recommended for stage IA, IB, II, III, and IV UCCC. Two retrospective studies have evaluated radiotherapy for UCCC. Those data suggest that adjuvant radiotherapy may provide local disease control. GOG122 favored chemotherapy compared with radiation [74]. The NSGO/EORTC trial compared pelvic radiation with or without chemotherapy [79]. Improved survivals were generally seen in patients treated with adjuvant chemotherapy. Combination of radiation plus chemotherapy approaches may provide patients with the best chance of improved survival; however, there are no randomized controlled trials in this specific subtype to guide therapy.

Thus far, it is unclear if radiotherapy should be added to adjuvant chemotherapy. Adjuvant radiotherapy alone has no proven survival benefit in women diagnosed as UCCC but may provide local control, therefore radiotherapy alone seems unreasonable.

A chemotherapy regimen specific to UCCC has not been studied; however, UCCCs are included in endometrial cancer clinical trials. GOG177 showed that combination of paclitaxel, doxorubicin, and cisplatin (TAP) regimen achieved an improvement in overall response rate, PFS, and OS when compared to doxorubicin and cisplatin (AP) regimen for endometrial cancer [80]. A recent report from GOG209, which compared TAP regimen with less-toxic regimen TC (paclitaxel and carboplatin), showed noninferiority for TC compared to the TAP regimen for endometrial cancer. Thus, paclitaxel and carboplatin is a reasonable first-line therapy for UCCCs.

Ansari et al. and Chan et al. reported that chemotherapy and radiotherapy may be useful in CCAC [81], but no prospective clinical trial exists to confirm or refute their data.

19.3.2.3 Metastatic Disease and Relapse

CCAC is refractory to chemotherapy and radiation therapy. Patients who could not complete the optimal resection have extremely poor prognosis (3-year overall survival was 22%).

Patients with recurrent or metastatic disease not manageable with surgery or irradiation should receive chemotherapy. The most optimal chemotherapy has not been determined yet for recurrent UCCC. Today, options in first line are chemotherapy with cisplatin, taxol, and doxorubicin either in a doublet or triplet combination, which have demonstrated efficacy in UCCC1. Patients with recurrent or metastatic disease not manageable with surgery or irradiation should receive chemotherapy with the same regimens used for recurrent endometrioid carcinoma, i.e. CDDP + DOX, CDDP + DOX + TAX, or CBDCA + TAX [11].

McMeekin et al. assessed the relationship between histological type and clinical outcome in advanced and recurrent endometrial cancer patients who were enrolled in four GOG first-line chemotherapy. While there was a trend for a lower response rate for UCCC, histological type was not an independent predictor of response [82].

Phase II trials for temsirolimus or everolimus showed a response rate of around 25% for recurrent or metastatic endometrial cancer [83]. PTEN mutations might play an important role for PI3K-AKT-mTOR pathway when using mTOR inhibitors. Less than 20% of UCCCs have PTEN mutation or inactivation and the role of PIK3CA status in UCCC is unclear [84]. Bevacizumab has demonstrated the most promising efficacy in the treatment of recurrent endometrial cancer with a response rate of 13.5% and PFS at 6 months of 40.4%. VEGF expression was seen in nearly 60% endometrioid endometrial carcinomas, and was strongly correlated with angiogenesis and poor patient outcome. These molecular targets together with taxane and platinum-based backbone might improve the outcome, but thus far there is no evidence for the biological therapy in UCCC.

19.3.3 Carcinosarcoma

Carcinosarcomas (also known as "malignant mixed Mullerian tumors") are rare and highly aggressive epithelial malignancies that contain both malignant sarcomatous and carcinomatous elements. Uterine carcinosarcomas (UCSs) are uncommon with about 35% not confined to the uterus at diagnosis. Prognosis remains poor with high risk of recurrences (50%), either local or distant, occurring within 1 year. The survival of women with advanced uterine carcinosarcoma is poor with a pattern of failure indicating greater likelihood of upper abdominal and distant metastatic recurrence [85–88].

19.3.3.1 Initial Treatment
Optimal treatment remains uncertain. Ovarian and uterine carcinosarcomas are routinely excluded from upfront clinical trials. Treatment recommendations are mainly based upon retrospective studies with small patient populations especially for OCs [85].

Surgery
The primary treatment for UCS is surgery. Surgical treatment should comprise total abdominal hysterectomy, bilateral salpingo-oophorectomy, omentectomy, peritoneal cytology and biopsies, pelvic and para-aortic lymph node dissection, and tumor debulking. However, the necessity of omentectomy and/or lymphadenectomy is a matter of current debate. Lymph node dissection is indicated for UCS given their relatively high incidence of lymph node involvement (14–38% in early stage). Regarding its impact on survival, the majority of studies confirm a significant survival benefit [89, 90]. The possible mechanisms for the improvement of survival from lymphadenectomy include removal of micro metastatic foci and reduction of locoregional recurrence risk. The number of lymph nodes collected (pelvic and/or Para aortic) in early stages has also been correlated with recurrence and death. So, adequate lymphadenectomy is needed for both staging and therapeutic reasons. In advanced disease, primary cytoreduction surgery is recommended despite no clear evidence.

Adjuvant Treatment for Early Stage

Due to the high rate of local and distant recurrence, even for the early-stage disease, most patients need adjuvant treatments. There is still no clear consensus on the best adjuvant therapy for patients with UCS due to the fact that many studies are retrospective, with a small number of patients and various treatment regimens.

Pelvic failure is common, even in early stages. Thus pelvic radiotherapy (with or without brachytherapy) is commonly used and contributes to the reduction in the incidence of local pelvic recurrence. However, its impact on patient survival is not proven and it remains a subject of controversy [91].

The only phase III study comparing pelvic radiotherapy and observation is the EORTC study from Reed [24]. 224 uterine sarcomas including 91 stages I–II UCSs were randomized. This trial shows no difference in both overall and disease-free survival but radiation was associated with a significant improved local control. Local recurrences were 18, 8% for patients with radiotherapy and 35, 9% for patients with observation only. A phase III trial from GOG [92] compared whole abdominal radiotherapy (WART) to three cycles of combination chemotherapy (ifosfamide-cisplatin). 206 patients with stage I–IV resected ECs were included. The local and distance recurrence rates were 44, 7% and 25, 7% respectively, with WART and 42.5% and 23.3% respectively with chemotherapy. Although there was no statistically significant difference in survival, after adjusting for age and stage, a nonstatistically significant advantage in recurrence rate and survival was noted in the chemotherapy group (21% lower recurrence and 29% lower death). Less toxicity was also noted with chemotherapy [92].

Three large observational studies using the SEER database were published. The SEER database from Wright registered 1819 patients with stage I–II ECs, and demonstrated a significant 21% reduction of death for women who underwent radiotherapy in a multivariate model [93]. The benefit was exclusively observed for women who did not undergo lymph node dissection. In another SEER database from Clayton Smith of 2461 women with UCS, 5 year overall survival rates were 41.5% and 33.2% ($p < 0.001$) for women receiving or not receiving radiotherapy respectively [91]. The limitations of such large databases need to be emphasized because of the lack of standardization procedures for surgery, radiotherapy, and chemotherapy; the lack of centralized pathological review; and the potential impact of patient's and physician's preference on adjuvant choice of adjuvant treatment.

The role of adjuvant chemotherapy in UCS is still being debated. Only one trial has prospectively addressed the question of adjuvant chemotherapy (three cycles of ifosfamide-cisplatin) for UCS in comparison with radiotherapy (WART) [92]. This study was not able to demonstrate a significant difference in relapse rate or OS, but a slight advantage favors the use of chemotherapy. Another trial, which included other types of gynecologic sarcomas, failed to show a significant advantage on PFS and OS with adjuvant chemotherapy. To note, a significant trend to a better PFS but not OS was observed in the French study [26]. In a prospective phase II GOG study, 65 stage I–II completely resected ECs received three cycles of ifosfamide-cisplatin chemotherapy. PFS and OS at 7 years were 54% and 52% respectively [94]. The Cochrane database concluded that in advanced stage uterine carcinosarcoma as well as in recurrent disease, adjuvant combination chemotherapy with ifosfamide should be considered. Combination chemotherapy with ifosfamide and paclitaxel is associated with lower risk of death compared to ifosfamide alone [95].

Several retrospective studies have shown favorable survival outcomes with sequential multimodality therapy, including pelvic radiotherapy and polychemotherapy with cisplatin–ifosfamide or paclitaxel–paraplatine. These studies suggest a better outcome with combined treatment compared to radiotherapy alone. In the Makker study where 49 stage I–IV patients received platinum-based chemotherapy after surgery (mainly paraplatine–paclitaxel) with or without radiation therapy or radiotherapy alone, the 3-year PFS for the chemotherapy group was 35% versus 9% for radiotherapy group (NS) and 3-year OS rates were 66% and 34% respectively (NS) [96]. The 2010 NCCN guidelines recommend treatment for all stages of uterine carcinosarcoma except for IA. For stage IB–IV disease, treatment recommendations include chemotherapy with or without radiation or whole abdominal radiation with or without brachytherapy (https://www.nccn.org).

19.3.3.2 Advanced/Metastatic Phase and Relapse

Patients with advanced, unresectable, or recurrent UCSs have a poor prognosis with a median survival rate of less than 1 year.

The main cytotoxic agents studied in ECs are ifosfamide (32% response), cisplatin (19% response) and paclitaxel (18% response as first- or second-line therapy). In contrast to other gynecologic sarcomas, doxorubicine is only minimally active (10% response). Responses are usually partial and brief in duration.

Two prospective randomized trials had compared mono- and poly-chemotherapy with ifosfamide. Sutton et al. reported on 194 evaluable patients who received ifosfamide with or without cisplatin [94]. Although response rates were higher with the combination (54% versus 36%) and PFS slightly but significantly higher (6 months versus 4 months), no overall survival improvement was observed and toxicity of the combination was notable. The other GOG study included 179 patients treated with ifosfamide with or without paclitaxel. Significant differences in objective response (45% versus 29%), PFS (5.8 months versus 3.6 months) and even overall survival (13.5 months versus 8.4 months) were noted [97]. Thus, the ifosfamide–paclitaxel combination is currently the standard arm treatment in US.

The paclitaxel–paraplatine combination is a well-tolerated, outpatient regimen. Several phase II trials reported high response rates (54–69%), including complete response, a median PFS of 7.6 months and an OS of 14.7 months [98]. The GOG 261 ongoing phase III noninferiority trial is comparing ifosfamide–paclitaxel and paraplatine–paclitaxel. Paraplatine–paclitaxel is commonly used as standard therapy due to easier administration schedules and a better tolerability profile.

Many biological anticancer treatments have been evaluated (sorafenib, imatinib, thalidomide VEGF-Trap, iniparib plus paclitaxel, and carboplatine) [99]. Response rates to targeted agents are poor in unselected populations (0–5%). Ongoing studies including UCSs evaluate BSI-202, paraplatine–paclitaxel and PARP inhibitor (GOG 232-C), bevacizumab and temsirolimus, sunitinib, temozolomide, trabectedin, liposomal doxorubicine, ixabepilone, etc.

19.4 Other Very Rare Tumors

19.4.1 Uterine Tumor Resembling Ovarian Sex-Cord Tumor (UTROSCT)

Uterine tumor resembling ovarian sex-cord tumor (UTROSCT) is a rare and relatively newly defined clinical entity. The original identification of UTROSCT, as a histopathological entity by Clement and Scully in 1976, included two distinct tumors of unclear origin hypothesized-originating cells including endometrial stromal cells, adenomyosis, stromal myosis, endometriosis, or multipotential cells within the myometrium [100]. Since then, the entity has been recently delineated into the two distinct subtypes. Type I tumors, known as endometrial stromal tumors with sex-cord-like elements (ESTSCLE), have been recognized to have more malignant potential than Type II, and the outcome of Type I disease is contingent upon type, grade, and stage of the underlying stromal neoplasm [101]. Type II tumors, comprising classic UTROSCTs, are considered to be of low-grade malignant potential, secondary to occasional recurrence, although they typically exhibit benign behavior [2].

While both ESTSCLE and UTROSCT most likely arise from pluripotential uterine mesenchymal cells, UTROSCT is predominantly differentiated into sex-cord components, unlike ESTSCLEs, which typically express only one sex-cord marker [101]. This classification of UTROSCT into two histologic subtypes is relatively new, and a large portion of literature refers to UTROSCT generally without subcategorization. Diagnosis of UTROSCT is primarily based upon morphologic features on hematoxylin/eosin staining with confirmation by immunohistochemically staining. Positive staining for at least two sex-cord markers is supportive, including calretinin and at least one other marker [102–104]. Other commonly expressed markers include inhibin, cluster of differentiation 99 (CD99), and Melan A [104].

Additionally, these tumors are variably immunoreactive for mesenchymal and epithelial elements as well. Frequently positive stains include vimentin, desmin, cytokeratin, epithelial membrane antigen (EMA), CD10, and estrogen or progesterone receptors (ER/PR) [102]. A review of immunohistochemical markers associated with UTROSCTs identified inhibin as the most specific marker and calretinin as the most sensitive marker of the tumor [102, 105]. Given its rarity, the diagnosis of UTROSCT is usually made postoperatively per histopathological analysis. In addition, current available literature mainly focuses on the diagnosis of UTROSCT, and there is scant information available to define the clinical characteristics and outcomes of UTROSCT.

19.4.1.1 Initial Treatment

Optimal treatment for the disease has yet to be defined. Stricter definitions of UTROSCT in recent literature requires immunohistochemical positivity for calretinin and at least one sex-cord marker [103]. As these tumors have become more widely recognized and diagnostic technology has improved, the definition has evolved, and Type I and Type II tumors have become more distinct. Index of suspicion is relatively low due to the extremely low incidence of this tumor, however awareness of this entity is important and clinicians should consider it especially in patients with a history of UTROSCT or tamoxifen use.

UTROSCT is a tumor of low malignant potential that has been shown to recur in rare cases, and, as such, the primary management strategy remains surgical. The majority of patients with UTROSCT had a total abdominal hysterectomy with bilateral salpingo-oophorectomy, and it is evident that the pure form of UTROSCT behaves like a benign neoplasm. However, fertility preservation in patients of childbearing age is an important consideration, and a risk factor model was recently published to guide clinical decision making [106]. In none of the 18 patients, for which follow-up data was available (mean follow-up time of 32 months; range 4–84 months), recurrence had been observed. It has been suggested that the aggressive potential of UTROSCT can be evaluated by using the criteria for endometrial stromal sarcomas, e.g. pushing versus infiltrative border, vascular invasion, and mitotic count [16]. Therefore, the pure form of UTROSCT seems not to have the same risk as low-grade endometrial sarcoma, but the mean follow-up time of these cases was only 25 months. Nevertheless, there are reports on distant metastases and recurrences. UTROSCT is a tumor of low malignant potential that has been shown to recur in rare cases, and, as such, the primary management strategy remains surgical. However, fertility preservation in patients of childbearing age is an important consideration, and we propose a risk factor model in this paper with which to guide clinical decision making. The data that is available can be used to determine management strategies despite the relative scarcity of documented cases of UTROSCTs. Although these neoplasms are less aggressive than ESTSCLE, they have been known to recur, and, as such, are defined as tumors of low malignant potential. Thus, surgery alone can remain the mainstay of treatment. The study published by Blake et al., did not show a statistical difference in DFS between those patients that received a total abdominal hysterectomy alone and combined with an adnexectomy [106]. The decision to remove adnexa should be made based on the clinical situation and discussions between the provider and their patients.

19.4.1.2 Metastatic Phase

Kantelip et al. described an UTROSCT with two omental metastases showing the same histology as the uterine tumor. Unfortunately, no follow-up information was given [107]. The case described by Malfetano and Hussein as recurrent UTROSCT probably was not of the pure type [106]. Interestingly, the majority of tumors screened for ER and PR expression were positive, 71.4% and 88.9%, respectively. Management of metastatic disease reported frequent surgery and reoperation as soon as possible in the literature. No clear data on chemotherapy sensitivity can be identified in the literature until now. So a pragmatic attitude is to consider these metastatic patients for chemotherapy only when surgery is not an option. One treatment option that has not yet been explored for UTROSCT is hormonal treatment, such as a progestin agent.

19.4.1.3 Trophoblastic Disease

Gestational trophoblastic disease (GTD) is a group of disorders that arise from the placenta encompassing the premalignant complete (CHM) and partial (PHM) hydatidiform moles, and the malignant invasive hydatidiform mole, choriocarcinoma, placental site trophoblastic tumor (PSTT), and epithelioid trophoblastic tumor (ETT) [108]. The malignant forms of GTD are also collectively known as gestational trophoblastic tumors (GTT) or neoplasia (GTN).

19.4.1.4 Management of Molar Pregnancies

The risk of developing GTN is 15–20% and 0.5–1% after CHM and PHM, respectively [108]. Factors associated with an increased risk of GTN after a CHM include a pre-evacuation hCG level >100,000 IU/L, excessive uterine volume (>20-week size), theca lutein cysts >6 cm in diameter, and age more than 40 years [109, 110].

Prophylactic chemotherapy with methotrexate or actinomycin D at the time of, or immediately after, evacuation of CHM reduces post-CHM GTN risk to 3–8%. However this exposes >80% of patients to unnecessary toxicity which does not eliminate the need for surveillance and may induce drug-resistant disease. Therefore its use should be limited to very special situations where adequate hCG and patient follow-up is not possible [111].

Follow-up after evacuation of CHM or PHM requires serial serum quantitative hCG measurements every 1–2 weeks until at least two consecutive tests will show normal levels. After which, hCG levels should be determined monthly for up to 6 months in patients with CHM. However this can be stopped in patients with PHM as the risk of subsequent GTN is less than 1:3000 (ISSTD 2013).

During hCG follow-up, patients should use contraception for at least 6 months. Oral contraceptives have the advantage of suppressing endogenous LH, which may interfere with the measurement of hCG [112]. Since most relapses occur in the first 12 months, avoiding pregnancy during this period seems sensible.

19.4.1.5 Indications for Chemotherapy

The most common FIGO criteria [113, 114] for commencing chemotherapy for post-mole GTN is a rising or plateau of hCG level. In some institutions criteria for chemotherapy treatment include a serum hCG level greater than 20,000 IU/L more than 4 weeks after evacuation because of the risk of uterine perforation [108] and histological diagnosis of choriocarcinoma.

19.4.1.6 Risk Stratification for Chemotherapy

Several scoring systems based on a variety of prognostic factors were developed to stratify GTN patients into low- and high-risk groups. Among these, the International Federation of Gynecology and Obstetric (FIGO 2000) scoring/staging system is the most commonly used and is summarized in Table 19.1 [12, 114]. A score of 0–6 indicates a disease that should be treated with single-agent chemotherapy (methotrexate (MTX) or dactinomycin (ActD)). Patients scoring >6 are at high risk of developing single-agent resistant disease and therefore should receive combination chemotherapies. In this system, patients are also assigned a stage (see Table 19.2).

Table 19.2 FIGO 2000 scoring system for GTN

Prognostic factor	Score			
	0	1	2	4
Age (years)	<40	≥40	–	–
Antecedent pregnancy (AP)	Mole	Abortion	Term	–
Interval (end of AP to chemotherapy in months)	<4	4–6	7–12	>12
hCG (IU/L)	$<10^3$	10^3–10^4	10^4–10^5	$>10^5$
Number of metastases	0	1–4	5–8	>8
Site of metastases	Lung	Spleen, kidney	GI tract	Brain, liver
Largest tumor mass	–	3–5 cm	>5 cm	
Prior chemotherapy	–	–	Single drug	≥2 drugs

This stratification system presents several limitations. In particular, while nearly all patients scoring 0–3 will be cured with single-agent therapy, 70% of those scoring 5–6 will require combination therapy [115].

19.4.1.7 Imaging and Staging of Low- and High-Risk GTN Post Molar Pregnancy

Staging and scoring of disease is based on serum hCG measurement, clinical history and examination, pelvic ultrasound, and chest X-Ray (CXR). If the CXR is suggestive of lung metastases, a confirmatory CT chest can be helpful; however, only visible lesions on CXR should be scored [116]. Patients with lung metastases are at increased risk of CNS involvement so a MRI of the brain is needed. For those patients with a histological diagnosis of choriocarcinoma or suspected GTN following a nonmolar pregnancy, much more intensive imaging is required including: a CT of chest and abdomen; MRI of brain and pelvis; and an ultrasound of the pelvis. FDG-PET-CT is most helpful in relapsed patients to identify the location of active disease prior to attempted curative surgical resection [117]. The value of a lumbar puncture to measure the CSF serum hCG ratio; which should be less than 1:60 [115], in the era of high resolution (3 Teslar) MRI imaging of the CNS, is unclear but is still practiced by some centers [108].

19.4.1.8 Treatment of Low- and High-Risk GTN

Low-risk GTN (evidence IB) is treated with either MTX with or without folinic acid (FA) or ActD. Many different schedules have been studied, all of which appear to have activity but comparison of results is hampered by several factors, in particular, differences in patient inclusion criteria. In Europe and in many international centers, MTX/FA (See Table 19.2) is the preferred regimen because of lower toxicity. On the contrary, ActD appears to be more manageable in the schedule of administration and some authors suggest it to be more effective. However, the only randomized trial comparing the two treatments used a low dose (30 mg/m^2) of MTX. All patients with low-risk disease can expect to be cured regardless of whether they need to switch to second- or even occasionally third-line treatments [118].

19 Management of Rare Uterine Malignant Tumors

Table 19.3 Most widely used treatment schedules of low-risk GTN

– MTX 8 day regimen (50 mg total dose IM days 1, 3, 5, 7 with FA rescue 15 mg given 24 or 30 h later on (days 2, 4, 6, 8) repeated every 14 days termed the MTX/FA regimen [10]. Some centers prefer to adjust the MTX dose by weight and give as 1 mg/kg
– Pulsed ActD 1.25 mg/m^2 biweekly [22]
– 5 days ActD (0.5 mg IV) repeated every 14 days [21]
– Low-dose MTX (30/50 mg/m^2 IM) repeated weekly [21] but 30 mg/m^2 can no longer be recommended [22]
– MTX IV 0.4 mg/kg days 1–5 (max 25 mg/day) repeated every 14 days [30]

Response to therapy is assessed by serial serum 1–2 weeks hCG measurements. Once the hCG is normal, three consolidation treatments over 6 weeks are required to minimize the risk of recurrence. Generally accepted criteria for the definition of resistance to first-line therapy are an hCG plateau over three consecutive samples or rising hCG value on two consecutive samples over more than 2 weeks.

For women who become refractory or resistant to first-line single-agent chemotherapy, poly-chemotherapy can be administered (evidence grade 2C). However, it is possible to identify a group of patients able to receive another single-agent therapy depending on the hCG level at the time of resistance. Thus, in the case of 8-day MTX/FA regimen resistance, with hCG values less than 100–300 IU/L, a 0.5 mg 5 days IV ActD treatment every 14 days is highly effective [115].

High-risk patients without brain or liver involvement can be managed with multi-agent chemotherapy. The most frequently used regimen comprises etoposide, MTX, and ActD (EMA) alternating weekly with cyclophosphamide and vincristine (Oncovin™) (CO) (grade 2C) [115]. After hCG normalization, 6 weeks of consolidation therapy equivalent to three additional cycles are usually administered. If the disease is refractory to EMA/CO (Table 19.3), many patients can still be salvaged with various alternative platinum-based regimens including: EMA (omitting day 2 etoposide and ActD) alternating weekly with etoposide and cisplatin (EP) [119, 120]; paclitaxel and etoposide (TE) alternating 2 weekly with paclitaxel and cisplatin (TP) [115]; etoposide (VP16), ifosfamide and cisplatin (VIP) given 3 weekly, bleomycin, etoposide, and cisplatin (BEP) given 3 weekly [12].

The two most frequently used salvage regimens are EMA/EP and TE/TP. The former is highly active but is very toxic, the latter may be equally effective and appears much less toxic so a randomized trial comparing these regimens has been proposed.

19.4.1.9 Management of Ultrahigh Risk Disease

For patients presenting with very advanced disease or who have poor prognostic factors (i.e. liver metastasis with or without central nervous system (CNS) involvement) commencing treatment with standard EMA/CO or other multi-agent chemotherapy, can cause severe hemorrhage or worsening organ failure resulting in early deaths [121]. This can be avoided by using gentle induction therapy with low-dose etoposide 100 mg/m^2 and cisplatin 20 mg/m^2 on days 1 and 2 repeated every week, up to three times, before commencing standard chemotherapy [121]. Patients with poor risk features may benefit from 8 weeks (instead of 6 weeks) of consolidation therapy after normalization of serum hCG [115].

19.4.1.10 Management of CNS Disease and Role of Radiotherapy
The main therapeutic options for CNS metastasis are escalated dose EMA/CO in which the MTX is increased to 1 g/m² and intrathecal MTX 12.5 mg is given; or whole brain radiotherapy (20–30 Gy in two daily fractions) concurrent with chemotherapy [122]. Neurosurgery can be employed to remove and/or control bleeding metastases and/or relieve increased intracranial pressure. The use of whole brain radiotherapy is controversial given the long-term toxicity. Less-toxic alternatives, such as stereotactic radiotherapy or gamma-knife treatment at the end of chemotherapy for any residual lesions unsuitable for resection, are suggested [115].

19.4.1.11 Role of Surgery
Surgery is indicated to manage bleeding complications and to remove chemoresistant residual disease. In this setting FDG-PET/CT imaging can help to identify active residual disease sites after chemotherapy suitable for resection [117]. In nonmetastatic patients who do not desire to preserve fertility, hysterectomy may also be useful.

19.4.1.12 Placenta Site Trophoblastic Tumor (PSTT) and Epithelioid Trophoblastic Tumors (ETT)
PSTT may be less responsive to chemotherapy than choriocarcinoma. The FIGO prognostic scoring system is not used for determining therapy in these patients. While several prognostic factors have been identified, the most important is the time interval from the last pregnancy and the diagnosis of the PSTT. In a UK study, 98% of patients presenting the disease within 4 years from the previous pregnancy had a long-term survival, while all patients who were diagnosed PSTT beyond 4 years died [123]. In patients presenting PSTT within 4 years from their last pregnancy, hysterectomy alone is a sufficient treatment for localized disease while patients with metastatic tumor respond well to either EP/EMA or EMA/CO often followed by resection of residual disease and hysterectomy [123]. For patients presenting diagnosis of PSTT beyond 4 years from their last pregnancy, given the very poor outcomes, experimental therapies should be considered including the use of high-dose treatment even when the disease appears localized [123]. ETT is a relatively new entity and may or may not behave distinctly from PSTT. Currently most investigators manage ETT like PSTT until more data is available.

19.5 General Conclusion

The aim of this chapter is to provide a detailed summary based on contemporary views and international consensus on the management of patients with rare uterine tumors The information provided recognizes that there is limited evidence for many of the tumor subtypes. The challenge remains not only to accurately diagnose patients but also to design clinical trials for these rare cancers to develop a more robust evidence base. International efforts and investigator-led trials, with the support of the pharmaceutical industry, will help to narrow the current knowledge gap and lead to progress.

Unfortunately, sharing of data across institutions is challenging, but efforts are underway by GCIG, EORTC, IRCI, NCI, and other organizations to work together. In particular, sharing information regarding rare tumors will help increase knowledge and help retrospectively analyze study outcomes with the aim to better identify patients who can benefit from targeted treatment and be entered in clinical trials. Many organizations are creating biobanks of tissue and conducting molecular genetic analysis to identify patients for trials with targeted therapy. However, the registration needs to follow a standardized process to ensure homogeneity and must include an expert pathology review and have the support of national organizations. The French model, supported by the national cancer institute (Inca) for rare gynecologic cancer has been very effective. It has improved patient management and has been able to facilitate new clinical trials. More than 5000 patients with rare tumors have been included in the French rare tumor database over 5 years, and all patients have had their histological diagnosis systematically reviewed. In view of this success, the GINECO group (leader of the project) has been able to design a randomized clinical trial in SCT which has recruited more than 39 patients in 2 years (ALIENOR). Similarly, the Scottish group has designed the NiCCC trial which is recruiting patients with recurrent CCC of the uterus and ovary.

It is sobering that 37% of patients with rare gynecological cancers are misdiagnosed on initial pathological review, underscoring the importance of having all patients being reviewed by an expert pathologist in gynecological cancers [18]. This alone will enable the identification of potential patients suitable for clinical trial from a database. The French model of a national organization supported by national cooperative groups needs to be duplicated and broadly developed to an international level. Subsequently, sharing and merging data and biological results will be possible. With the new data reported by the TCGA for endometrioid carcinoma for subgroups as POLE or MSI, and the probable specific interest of such subgroups for immune checkpoint inhibitors [64]; the tendency to include molecular biology in the classification of cancers will improve. It is possible that more new rare subgroups of cancer will emerge for uterine localization, and thus prompt us to work and organize management for many subgroups of rare disease with specific treatment.

The key messages are the same as previously published for other rare cancer:

- Almost 50% of gynecological cancers meet the definition of rare cancers.
- A multidisciplinary approach is important for the diagnosis and treatment of these rare cancers.
- Research and drug development for these cancers is lacking due to their rarity.
- More resources dedicated to the education of the public, primary care physicians and general oncologists are required to ensure appropriate diagnosis and treatment.
- International consortia is important to develop studies dedicated to these rare cancers.

References

1. Gatta G, van der Zwan JM, Casali PG, Siesling S, Dei Tos AP, Kunkler I, et al. Rare cancers are not so rare: the rare cancer burden in Europe. Eur J Cancer. 2011;47(17):2493–511.
2. Sankaranarayanan R, Ferlay J. Worldwide burden of gynaecological cancer: the size of the problem. Best Pract Res Clin Obstet Gynaecol. 2006;20(2):207–25.
3. Bogaerts J, Sydes MR, Keat N, McConnell A, Benson A, Ho A, et al. Clinical trial designs for rare diseases: studies developed and discussed by the International Rare Cancers Initiative. Eur J Cancer. 2015;51(3):271–81.
4. Ray-Coquard I, Weber B, Lotz JP, Tournigand C, Provencal J, Mayeur D, et al. Management of rare ovarian cancers: the experience of the French website "observatory for rare malignant tumours of the ovaries" by the GINECO group: interim analysis of the first 100 patients. Gynecol Oncol. 2010;119(1):53–9.
5. Kurman RJ, Shih I. The dualistic model of ovarian carcinogenesis: revisited, revised, and expanded. Am J Pathol. 2016;186(4):733–47.
6. Hensley ML, Barrette BA, Baumann K, Gaffney D, Hamilton AL, Kim JW, et al. Gynecologic Cancer InterGroup (GCIG) consensus review: uterine and ovarian leiomyosarcomas. Int J Gynecol Cancer. 2014;24(9 Suppl 3):S61–6.
7. Amant F, Floquet A, Friedlander M, Kristensen G, Mahner S, Nam EJ, et al. Gynecologic Cancer InterGroup (GCIG) consensus review for endometrial stromal sarcoma. Int J Gynecol Cancer. 2014;24(9 Suppl 3):S67–72.
8. Satoh T, Takei Y, Treilleux I, Vouassoux-Shisheboran M, Ledermann J, Viswanathan AN, et al. Gynecologic Cancer InterGroup (GCIG) consensus review for small cell carcinoma of the cervix. Int J Gynecol Cancer. 2014;24(9 Suppl 3):S102–8.
9. Pautier P, Nam EJ, Provencher DM, Hamilton AL, Mangili G, Siddiqui NA, et al. Gynecologic Cancer InterGroup (GCIG) consensus review for high-grade undifferentiated sarcomas of the uterus. Int J Gynecol Cancer. 2014;24(9 Suppl 3):S73–7.
10. Friedlander ML, Covens A, Glasspool RM, Hilpert F, Kristensen G, Kwon S, et al. Gynecologic Cancer InterGroup (GCIG) consensus review for mullerian adenosarcoma of the female genital tract. Int J Gynecol Cancer. 2014;24(9 Suppl 3):S78–82.
11. Hasegawa K, Nagao S, Yasuda M, Millan D, Viswanathan AN, Glasspool RM, et al. Gynecologic Cancer InterGroup (GCIG) consensus review for clear cell carcinoma of the uterine corpus and cervix. Int J Gynecol Cancer. 2014;24(9 Suppl 3):S90–5.
12. Mangili G, Lorusso D, Brown J, Pfisterer J, Massuger L, Vaughan M, et al. Trophoblastic disease review for diagnosis and management: a joint report from the International Society for the Study of Trophoblastic Disease, European Organisation for the Treatment of Trophoblastic Disease, and the Gynecologic Cancer InterGroup. Int J Gynecol Cancer. 2014;24(9 Suppl 3):S109–16.
13. Ducimetiere F, Lurkin A, Ranchere-Vince D, Decouvelaere AV, Peoc'h M, Istier L, et al. Incidence of sarcoma histotypes and molecular subtypes in a prospective epidemiological study with central pathology review and molecular testing. PLoS One. 2011;6(8):e20294.
14. Park JY, Park SK, Kim DY, Kim JH, Kim YM, Kim YT, et al. The impact of tumor morcellation during surgery on the prognosis of patients with apparently early uterine leiomyosarcoma. Gynecol Oncol. 2011;122(2):255–9.
15. Pelmus M, Penault-Llorca F, Guillou L, Collin F, Bertrand G, Trassard M, et al. Prognostic factors in early-stage leiomyosarcoma of the uterus. Int J Gynecol Cancer. 2009;19(3):385–90.
16. Zivanovic O, Jacks LM, Iasonos A, Leitao MM Jr, Soslow RA, Veras E, et al. A nomogram to predict postresection 5-year overall survival for patients with uterine leiomyosarcoma. Cancer. 2012;118(3):660–9.
17. Einstein MH, Barakat RR, Chi DS, Sonoda Y, Alektiar KM, Hensley ML, et al. Management of uterine malignancy found incidentally after supracervical hysterectomy or uterine morcellation for presumed benign disease. Int J Gynecol Cancer. 2008;18(5):1065–70.

18. Leitao MM, Sonoda Y, Brennan MF, Barakat RR, Chi DS. Incidence of lymph node and ovarian metastases in leiomyosarcoma of the uterus. Gynecol Oncol. 2003;91(1):209–12.
19. Goff BA, Rice LW, Fleischhacker D, Muntz HG, Falkenberry SS, Nikrui N, et al. Uterine leiomyosarcoma and endometrial stromal sarcoma: lymph node metastases and sites of recurrence. Gynecol Oncol. 1993;50(1):105–9.
20. Leitao MM Jr, Hensley ML, Barakat RR, Aghajanian C, Gardner GJ, Jewell EL, et al. Immunohistochemical expression of estrogen and progesterone receptors and outcomes in patients with newly diagnosed uterine leiomyosarcoma. Gynecol Oncol. 2012;124(3):558–62.
21. Kapp DS, Shin JY, Chan JK. Prognostic factors and survival in 1396 patients with uterine leiomyosarcomas: emphasis on impact of lymphadenectomy and oophorectomy. Cancer. 2008;112(4):820–30.
22. Leitao MM Jr, Zivanovic O, Chi DS, Hensley ML, O'Cearbhaill R, Soslow RA, et al. Surgical cytoreduction in patients with metastatic uterine leiomyosarcoma at the time of initial diagnosis. Gynecol Oncol. 2012;125(2):409–13.
23. Dinh TA, Oliva EA, Fuller AF Jr, Lee H, Goodman A. The treatment of uterine leiomyosarcoma. Results from a 10-year experience (1990-1999) at the Massachusetts General Hospital. Gynecol Oncol. 2004;92(2):648–52.
24. Reed NS, Mangioni C, Malmstrom H, Scarfone G, Poveda A, Pecorelli S, et al. Phase III randomised study to evaluate the role of adjuvant pelvic radiotherapy in the treatment of uterine sarcomas stages I and II: an European Organisation for Research and Treatment of Cancer Gynaecological Cancer Group study (protocol 55874). Eur J Cancer. 2008;44(6):808–18.
25. Hensley ML, Miller A, O'Malley DM, Mannel RS, Behbakht K, Bakkum-Gamez JN, et al. Randomized phase III trial of gemcitabine plus docetaxel plus bevacizumab or placebo as first-line treatment for metastatic uterine leiomyosarcoma: an NRG Oncology/Gynecologic Oncology Group study. J Clin Oncol. 2015;33(10):1180–5.
26. Pautier P, Floquet A, Gladieff L, Bompas E, Ray-Coquard I, Piperno-Neumann S, et al. A randomized clinical trial of adjuvant chemotherapy with doxorubicin, ifosfamide, and cisplatin followed by radiotherapy versus radiotherapy alone in patients with localized uterine sarcomas (SARCGYN study). A study of the French Sarcoma Group. Ann Oncol. 2013;24(4):1099–104.
27. Burt BM, Ocejo S, Mery CM, Dasilva M, Bueno R, Sugarbaker DJ, et al. Repeated and aggressive pulmonary resections for leiomyosarcoma metastases extends survival. Ann Thorac Surg. 2011;92(4):1202–7.
28. Muss HB, Bundy B, Disaia PJ, Homesley HD, Fowler WC Jr, Creasman W, et al. Treatment of recurrent or advanced uterine sarcoma. A randomized trial of doxorubicin versus doxorubicin and cyclophosphamide (a phase III trial of the Gynecologic Oncology Group). Cancer. 1985;55(8):1648–53.
29. Sutton G, Blessing JA, Malfetano JH. Ifosfamide and doxorubicin in the treatment of advanced leiomyosarcomas of the uterus: a Gynecologic Oncology Group study. Gynecol Oncol. 1996;62(2):226–9.
30. Look KY, Sandler A, Blessing JA, Lucci JA III, Rose PG. Phase II trial of gemcitabine as second-line chemotherapy of uterine leiomyosarcoma: a gynecologic oncology group (GOG) study. Gynecol Oncol. 2004;92(2):644–7.
31. Hensley ML, Blessing JA, DeGeest K, Abulafia O, Rose PG, Homesley HD. Fixed-dose rate gemcitabine plus docetaxel as second-line therapy for metastatic uterine leiomyosarcoma: a Gynecologic Oncology Group phase II study. Gynecol Oncol. 2008;109(3):323–8.
32. Hensley ML, Blessing JA, Mannel R, Rose PG. Fixed-dose rate gemcitabine plus docetaxel as first-line therapy for metastatic uterine leiomyosarcoma: a Gynecologic Oncology Group phase II trial. Gynecol Oncol. 2008;109(3):329–34.
33. Maki RG. Gemcitabine and docetaxel in metastatic sarcoma: past, present, and future. Oncologist. 2007;12(8):999–1006.
34. Pautier P, Floquet A, Penel N, Piperno-Neumann S, Isambert N, Rey A, et al. Randomized multicenter and stratified phase II study of gemcitabine alone versus gemcitabine and docetaxel in patients with metastatic or relapsed leiomyosarcomas: a Federation Nationale

des Centres de Lutte Contre le Cancer (FNCLCC) French Sarcoma Group study (TAXOGEM study). Oncologist. 2012;17(9):1213–20.
35. van der Graaf WT, Blay JY, Chawla SP, Kim DW, Bui-Nguyen B, Casali PG, et al. Pazopanib for metastatic soft-tissue sarcoma (PALETTE): a randomised, double-blind, placebo-controlled phase 3 trial. Lancet. 2012;379(9829):1879–86.
36. Monk BJ, Blessing JA, Street DG, Muller CY, Burke JJ, Hensley ML. A phase II evaluation of trabectedin in the treatment of advanced, persistent, or recurrent uterine leiomyosarcoma: a Gynecologic Oncology Group study. Gynecol Oncol. 2012;124(1):48–52.
37. Sanfilippo R, Grosso F, Jones RL, Banerjee S, Pilotti S, D'Incalci M, et al. Trabectedin in advanced uterine leiomyosarcomas: a retrospective case series analysis from two reference centers. Gynecol Oncol. 2011;123(3):553–6.
38. Pautier P, Floquet A, Chevreau C, Penel N, Guillemet C, Delcambre C, et al. Trabectedin in combination with doxorubicin for first-line treatment of advanced uterine or soft-tissue leiomyosarcoma (LMS-02): a non-randomised, multicentre, phase 2 trial. Lancet Oncol. 2015;16(4):457–64.
39. Demetri GD, von Mehren M, Jones RL, Hensley ML, Schuetze SM, Staddon A, et al. Efficacy and safety of trabectedin or dacarbazine for metastatic liposarcoma or leiomyosarcoma after failure of conventional chemotherapy: results of a phase III randomized multicenter clinical trial. J Clin Oncol. 2016;34(8):786–93.
40. Garcia-Del-Muro X, Lopez-Pousa A, Maurel J, Martin J, Martinez-Trufero J, Casado A, et al. Randomized phase II study comparing gemcitabine plus dacarbazine versus dacarbazine alone in patients with previously treated soft tissue sarcoma: a Spanish Group for Research on Sarcomas study. J Clin Oncol. 2011;29(18):2528–33.
41. Schoffski P, Chawla S, Maki RG, Italiano A, Gelderblom H, Choy E, et al. Eribulin versus dacarbazine in previously treated patients with advanced liposarcoma or leiomyosarcoma: a randomised, open-label, multicentre, phase 3 trial. Lancet. 2016;387(10028):1629–37.
42. George S, Feng Y, Manola J, Nucci MR, Butrynski JE, Morgan JA, et al. Phase 2 trial of aromatase inhibition with letrozole in patients with uterine leiomyosarcomas expressing estrogen and/or progesterone receptors. Cancer. 2014;120(5):738–43.
43. FIGO Committee on Gynecologic Oncology. FIGO staging for carcinoma of the vulva, cervix, and corpus uteri. Int J Gynaecol Obstet. 2014;125(2):97–8.
44. Amant F, Coosemans A, Biec-Rychter M, Timmerman D, Vergote I. Clinical management of uterine sarcomas. Lancet Oncol. 2009;10(12):1188–98.
45. Shah JP, Bryant CS, Kumar S, Li-Fehmi R, Malone JM Jr, Morris RT. Lymphadenectomy and ovarian preservation in low-grade endometrial stromal sarcoma. Obstet Gynecol. 2008;112(5):1102–8.
46. Amant F, De Knijf A, Van Calster B, Leunen K, Neven P, Berteloot P, et al. Clinical study investigating the role of lymphadenectomy, surgical castration and adjuvant hormonal treatment in endometrial stromal sarcoma. Br J Cancer. 2007;97(9):1194–9.
47. Li AJ, Giuntoli RL, Drake R, Byun SY, Rojas F, Barbuto D, et al. Ovarian preservation in stage I low-grade endometrial stromal sarcomas. Obstet Gynecol. 2005;106(6):1304–8.
48. Altman AD, Nelson GS, Chu P, Nation J, Ghatage P. Uterine sarcoma and aromatase inhibitors: Tom Baker Cancer Centre experience and review of the literature. Int J Gynecol Cancer. 2012;22(6):1006–12.
49. Leath CA III, Huh WK, Hyde J Jr, Cohn DE, Resnick KE, Taylor NP, et al. A multi-institutional review of outcomes of endometrial stromal sarcoma. Gynecol Oncol. 2007;105(3):630–4.
50. Piver MS, Rose PG. Advanced uterine sarcoma; response to chemotherapy. Eur J Gynaecol Oncol. 1988;9(2):124–9.
51. Chan JK, Kawar NM, Shin JY, Osann K, Chen LM, Powell CB, et al. Endometrial stromal sarcoma: a population-based analysis. Br J Cancer. 2008;99(8):1210–5.
52. Malouf GG, Lhomme C, Duvillard P, Morice P, Haie-Meder C, Pautier P. Prognostic factors and outcome of undifferentiated endometrial sarcoma treated by multimodal therapy. Int J Gynaecol Obstet. 2013;122(1):57–61.

53. Tanner EJ, Garg K, Leitao MM Jr, Soslow RA, Hensley ML. High grade undifferentiated uterine sarcoma: surgery, treatment, and survival outcomes. Gynecol Oncol. 2012;127(1):27–31.
54. Gadducci A, Cosio S, Genazzani AR. Old and new perspectives in the pharmacological treatment of advanced or recurrent endometrial cancer: hormonal therapy, chemotherapy and molecularly targeted therapies. Crit Rev Oncol Hematol. 2006;58(3):242–56.
55. Vergote IB, Jimeno A, Joly F, Katsaros D, Coens C, Despierre E, et al. Randomized phase III study of erlotinib versus observation in patients with no evidence of disease progression after first-line platin-based chemotherapy for ovarian carcinoma: a european organisation for research and treatment of Cancer-Gynaecological Cancer Group, and Gynecologic Cancer Intergroup study. J Clin Oncol. 2014;32:320–6.
56. McCluggage WG. Mullerian adenosarcoma of the female genital tract. Adv Anat Pathol. 2010;17(2):122–9.
57. D'Angelo E, Prat J. Uterine sarcomas: a review. Gynecol Oncol. 2010;116(1):131–9.
58. Clement PB, Scully RE. Mullerian adenosarcoma of the uterus: a clinicopathologic analysis of 100 cases with a review of the literature. Hum Pathol. 1990;21(4):363–81.
59. Clement PB, Scully RE. Uterine tumors with mixed epithelial and mesenchymal elements. Semin Diagn Pathol. 1988;5(2):199–222.
60. Michener CM, Simon NL. Ovarian conservation in a woman of reproductive age with mullerian adenosarcoma. Gynecol Oncol. 2001;83(2):424–7.
61. Schroeder BA, Rodler ET, Loggers ET, Pollack SM, Jones RL. Clinical benefit of trabectedin in uterine adenosarcoma. Med Oncol. 2013;30(2):501.
62. Maeda M, Mabuchi S, Matsumoto Y, Hisamatsu T, Ohashi H, Kimura T. Activity of pegylated liposomal doxorubicin for extragenital mullerian adenosarcoma with sarcomatous overgrowth: a case report and a review of the literature. Eur J Gynaecol Oncol. 2011;32(5):542–6.
63. Tanner EJ, Toussaint T, Leitao MM Jr, Hensley ML, Soslow RA, Gardner GJ, et al. Management of uterine adenosarcomas with and without sarcomatous overgrowth. Gynecol Oncol. 2013;129(1):140–4.
64. Kandoth C, Schultz N, Cherniack AD, Akbani R, Liu Y, Shen H, et al. Integrated genomic characterization of endometrial carcinoma. Nature. 2013;497(7447):67–73.
65. Hendrickson M, Ross J, Eifel P, Martinez A, Kempson R. Uterine papillary serous carcinoma: a highly malignant form of endometrial adenocarcinoma. Am J Surg Pathol. 1982;6(2):93–108.
66. Naumann RW. Uterine papillary serous carcinoma: state of the state. Curr Oncol Rep. 2008;10(6):505–11.
67. Sagae S, Susumu N, Viswanathan AN, Aoki D, Backes FJ, Provencher DM, et al. Gynecologic Cancer InterGroup (GCIG) consensus review for uterine serous carcinoma. Int J Gynecol Cancer. 2014;24(9 Suppl 3):S83–9.
68. Growdon WB, Rauh-Hain JJ, Cordon A, Garrett L, Schorge JO, Goodman A, et al. Prognostic determinants in patients with stage I uterine papillary serous carcinoma: a 15-year multi-institutional review. Int J Gynecol Cancer. 2012;22(3):417–24.
69. Fader AN, Boruta D, Olawaiye AB, Gehrig PA. Uterine papillary serous carcinoma: epidemiology, pathogenesis and management. Curr Opin Obstet Gynecol. 2010;22(1):21–9.
70. Kelly MG, O'Malley DM, Hui P, McAlpine J, Yu H, Rutherford TJ, et al. Improved survival in surgical stage I patients with uterine papillary serous carcinoma (UPSC) treated with adjuvant platinum-based chemotherapy. Gynecol Oncol. 2005;98(3):353–9.
71. Fader AN, Nagel C, Axtell AE, Zanotti KM, Kelley JL, Moore KN, et al. Stage II uterine papillary serous carcinoma: carboplatin/paclitaxel chemotherapy improves recurrence and survival outcomes. Gynecol Oncol. 2009;112(3):558–62.
72. Viswanathan AN, Macklin EA, Berkowitz R, Matulonis U. The importance of chemotherapy and radiation in uterine papillary serous carcinoma. Gynecol Oncol. 2011;123(3):542–7.
73. Sutton G, Axelrod JH, Bundy BN, Roy T, Homesley HD, Malfetano JH, et al. Whole abdominal radiotherapy in the adjuvant treatment of patients with stage III and IV endometrial cancer: a Gynecologic Oncology Group study. Gynecol Oncol. 2005;97(3):755–63.

74. Randall ME, Filiaci VL, Muss H, Spirtos NM, Mannel RS, Fowler J, et al. Randomized phase III trial of whole-abdominal irradiation versus doxorubicin and cisplatin chemotherapy in advanced endometrial carcinoma: a Gynecologic Oncology Group study. J Clin Oncol. 2006;24(1):36–44.
75. Slomovitz BM, Broaddus RR, Burke TW, Sneige N, Soliman PT, Wu W, et al. Her-2/neu overexpression and amplification in uterine papillary serous carcinoma. J Clin Oncol. 2004;22(15):3126–32.
76. Aghajanian C, Sill MW, Darcy KM, Greer B, McMeekin DS, Rose PG, et al. Phase II trial of bevacizumab in recurrent or persistent endometrial cancer: a Gynecologic Oncology Group study. J Clin Oncol. 2011;29(16):2259–65.
77. Zhao S, Choi M, Overton JD, Bellone S, Roque DM, Cocco E, et al. Landscape of somatic single-nucleotide and copy-number mutations in uterine serous carcinoma. Proc Natl Acad Sci U S A. 2013;110(8):2916–21.
78. Thomas M, Mariani A, Wright JD, Madarek EO, Powell MA, Mutch DG, et al. Surgical management and adjuvant therapy for patients with uterine clear cell carcinoma: a multi-institutional review. Gynecol Oncol. 2008;108(2):293–7.
79. Hogberg T, Signorelli M, de Oliveira CF, Fossati R, Lissoni AA, Sorbe B, et al. Sequential adjuvant chemotherapy and radiotherapy in endometrial cancer—results from two randomised studies. Eur J Cancer. 2010;46(13):2422–31.
80. Fleming GF, Filiaci VL, Bentley RC, Herzog T, Sorosky J, Vaccarello L, et al. Phase III randomized trial of doxorubicin + cisplatin versus doxorubicin + 24-h paclitaxel + filgrastim in endometrial carcinoma: a Gynecologic Oncology Group study. Ann Oncol. 2004;15(8):1173–8.
81. Chan KK, Ip P, Kwong P, Tam KF, Ngan HY. A combination of chemoirradiation and chemotherapy for treatment of advanced clear cell adenocarcinoma of the cervix. Int J Gynecol Cancer. 2008;18(3):559–63.
82. McMeekin DS, Filiaci VL, Thigpen JT, Gallion HH, Fleming GF, Rodgers WH. The relationship between histology and outcome in advanced and recurrent endometrial cancer patients participating in first-line chemotherapy trials: a Gynecologic Oncology Group study. Gynecol Oncol. 2007;106(1):16–22.
83. Slomovitz BM, Lu KH, Johnston T, Coleman RL, Munsell M, Broaddus RR, et al. A phase 2 study of the oral mammalian target of rapamycin inhibitor, everolimus, in patients with recurrent endometrial carcinoma. Cancer. 2010;116(23):5415–9.
84. Tredan O, Treilleux I, Wang Q, Gane N, Pissaloux D, Bonnin N, et al. Predicting everolimus treatment efficacy in patients with advanced endometrial carcinoma: a GINECO Group study. Target Oncol. 2013;8(4):243–51.
85. Berton-Rigaud D, Vouassoux-Shisheboran M, Ledermann JA, Leitao MM, Powell MA, Poveda A, et al. Gynecologic Cancer InterGroup (GCIG) consensus review for uterine and ovarian carcinosarcoma. Int J Gynecol Cancer. 2014;24(9 Suppl 3):S55–60.
86. Murray S, Linardou H, Mountzios G, Manoloukos M, Markaki S, Eleutherakis-Papaiakovou E, et al. Low frequency of somatic mutations in uterine sarcomas: a molecular analysis and review of the literature. Mutat Res. 2010;686(1–2):68–73.
87. de Jong RA, Nijman HW, Wijbrandi TF, Reyners AK, Boezen HM, Hollema H. Molecular markers and clinical behavior of uterine carcinosarcomas: focus on the epithelial tumor component. Mod Pathol. 2011;24(10):1368–79.
88. Garg G, Shah JP, Kumar S, Bryant CS, Munkarah A, Morris RT. Ovarian and uterine carcinosarcomas: a comparative analysis of prognostic variables and survival outcomes. Int J Gynecol Cancer. 2010;20(5):888–94.
89. Nemani D, Mitra N, Guo M, Lin L. Assessing the effects of lymphadenectomy and radiation therapy in patients with uterine carcinosarcoma: a SEER analysis. Gynecol Oncol. 2008;111(1):82–8.
90. Vorgias G, Fotiou S. The role of lymphadenectomy in uterine carcinosarcomas (malignant mixed mullerian tumours): a critical literature review. Arch Gynecol Obstet. 2010;282(6):659–64.

91. Clayton SD, Kenneth MO, Gaffney DK. The impact of adjuvant radiation therapy on survival in women with uterine carcinosarcoma. Radiother Oncol. 2008;88(2):227–32.
92. Wolfson AH, Brady MF, Rocereto T, Mannel RS, Lee YC, Futoran RJ, et al. A gynecologic oncology group randomized phase III trial of whole abdominal irradiation (WAI) vs. cisplatin-ifosfamide and mesna (CIM) as post-surgical therapy in stage I-IV carcinosarcoma (CS) of the uterus. Gynecol Oncol. 2007;107(2):177–85.
93. Wright JD, Seshan VE, Shah M, Schiff PB, Burke WM, Cohen CJ, et al. The role of radiation in improving survival for early-stage carcinosarcoma and leiomyosarcoma. Am J Obstet Gynecol. 2008;199(5):536–8.
94. Sutton G, Kauderer J, Carson LF, Lentz SS, Whitney CW, Gallion H. Adjuvant ifosfamide and cisplatin in patients with completely resected stage I or II carcinosarcomas (mixed mesodermal tumors) of the uterus: a Gynecologic Oncology Group study. Gynecol Oncol. 2005;96(3):630–4.
95. Shylasree TS, Bryant A, Athavale R. Chemotherapy and/or radiotherapy in combination with surgery for ovarian carcinosarcoma. Cochrane Database Syst Rev. 2013;2:CD006246.
96. Makker V, Bu-Rustum NR, Alektiar KM, Aghajanian CA, Zhou Q, Iasonos A, et al. A retrospective assessment of outcomes of chemotherapy-based versus radiation-only adjuvant treatment for completely resected stage I-IV uterine carcinosarcoma. Gynecol Oncol. 2008;111(2):249–54.
97. Homesley HD, Filiaci V, Markman M, Bitterman P, Eaton L, Kilgore LC, et al. Phase III trial of ifosfamide with or without paclitaxel in advanced uterine carcinosarcoma: a Gynecologic Oncology Group study. J Clin Oncol. 2007;25(5):526–31.
98. Hoskins PJ, Le N, Ellard S, Lee U, Martin LA, Swenerton KD, et al. Carboplatin plus paclitaxel for advanced or recurrent uterine malignant mixed mullerian tumors. The British Columbia Cancer Agency experience. Gynecol Oncol. 2008;108(1):58–62.
99. Huh WK, Sill MW, Darcy KM, Elias KM, Hoffman JS, Boggess JF, et al. Efficacy and safety of imatinib mesylate (Gleevec) and immunohistochemical expression of c-kit and PDGFR-beta in a Gynecologic Oncology Group phase II trial in women with recurrent or persistent carcinosarcomas of the uterus. Gynecol Oncol. 2010;117(2):248–54.
100. Clement PB, Scully RE. Uterine tumors resembling ovarian sex-cord tumors. A clinicopathologic analysis of fourteen cases. Am J Clin Pathol. 1976;66(3):512–25.
101. Czernobilsky B, Mamet Y, David MB, Atlas I, Gitstein G, Lifschitz-Mercer B. Uterine retiform sertoli-leydig cell tumor: report of a case providing additional evidence that uterine tumors resembling ovarian sex cord tumors have a histologic and immunohistochemical phenotype of genuine sex cord tumors. Int J Gynecol Pathol. 2005;24(4):335–40.
102. Carta G, Crisman G, Margiotta G, Mastrocola N, Di FA, Coletti G. Uterine tumors resembling ovarian sex cord tumors. A case report. Eur J Gynaecol Oncol. 2010;31(4):456–8.
103. Pradhan D, Mohanty SK. Uterine tumors resembling ovarian sex cord tumors. Arch Pathol Lab Med. 2013;137(12):1832–6.
104. Irving JA, Carinelli S, Prat J. Uterine tumors resembling ovarian sex cord tumors are polyphenotypic neoplasms with true sex cord differentiation. Mod Pathol. 2006;19(1):17–24.
105. Movahedi-Lankarani S, Kurman RJ. Calretinin, a more sensitive but less specific marker than alpha-inhibin for ovarian sex cord-stromal neoplasms: an immunohistochemical study of 215 cases. Am J Surg Pathol. 2002;26(11):1477–83.
106. Blake EA, Sheridan TB, Wang KL, Takiuchi T, Kodama M, Sawada K, et al. Clinical characteristics and outcomes of uterine tumors resembling ovarian sex-cord tumors (UTROSCT): a systematic review of literature. Eur J Obstet Gynecol Reprod Biol. 2014;181:163–70.
107. Kantelip B, Cloup N, Dechelotte P. Uterine tumor resembling ovarian sex cord tumors: report of a case with ultrastructural study. Hum Pathol. 1986;17(1):91–4.
108. Seckl MJ, Sebire NJ, Berkowitz RS. Gestational trophoblastic disease. Lancet. 2010;376(9742):717–29.
109. Berkowitz RS, Goldstein DP. Clinical practice. Molar pregnancy. N Engl J Med. 2009;360(16):1639–45.

110. Savage PM, Sita-Lumsden A, Dickson S, Iyer R, Everard J, Coleman R, et al. The relationship of maternal age to molar pregnancy incidence, risks for chemotherapy and subsequent pregnancy outcome. J Obstet Gynaecol. 2013;33(4):406–11.
111. Fu J, Fang F, Xie L, Chen H, He F, Wu T, et al. Prophylactic chemotherapy for hydatidiform mole to prevent gestational trophoblastic neoplasia. Cochrane Database Syst Rev. 2012;10:CD007289.
112. Deicas RE, Miller DS, Rademaker AW, Lurain JR. The role of contraception in the development of postmolar gestational trophoblastic tumor. Obstet Gynecol. 1991;78(2):221–6.
113. Kohorn EI. Negotiating a staging and risk factor scoring system for gestational trophoblastic neoplasia. A progress report. J Reprod Med. 2002;47(6):445–50.
114. Ngan HY, Bender H, Benedet JL, Jones H, Montruccoli GC, Pecorelli S. Gestational trophoblastic neoplasia, FIGO 2000 staging and classification. Int J Gynaecol Obstet. 2003;83(Suppl 1):175–7.
115. Seckl MJ, Sebire NJ, Fisher RA, Golfier F, Massuger L, Sessa C. Gestational trophoblastic disease: ESMO clinical practice guidelines for diagnosis, treatment and follow-up. Ann Oncol. 2013;24(Suppl 6):vi39–50.
116. Ngan HY, Chan FL, Au VW, Cheng DK, Ng TY, Wong LC. Clinical outcome of micrometastasis in the lung in stage IA persistent gestational trophoblastic disease. Gynecol Oncol. 1998;70(2):192–4.
117. Mapelli P, Mangili G, Picchio M, Gentile C, Rabaiotti E, Giorgione V, et al. Role of 18F-FDG PET in the management of gestational trophoblastic neoplasia. Eur J Nucl Med Mol Imaging. 2013;40(4):505–13.
118. Brown J, Friedlander M, Backes FJ, Harter P, O'Connor DM, de la Motte RT, et al. Gynecologic Cancer Intergroup (GCIG) consensus review for ovarian germ cell tumors. Int J Gynecol Cancer. 2014;24(9 Suppl 3):S48–54.
119. Newlands ES. Management of ovarian germ cell tumours. Forum (Genova). 2000;10(4):368–80.
120. Newlands ES, Mulholland PJ, Holden L, Seckl MJ, Rustin GJ. Etoposide and cisplatin/etoposide, methotrexate, and actinomycin D (EMA) chemotherapy for patients with high-risk gestational trophoblastic tumors refractory to EMA/cyclophosphamide and vincristine chemotherapy and patients presenting with metastatic placental site trophoblastic tumors. J Clin Oncol. 2000;18(4):854–9.
121. Alifrangis C, Agarwal R, Short D, Fisher RA, Sebire NJ, Harvey R, et al. EMA/CO for high-risk gestational trophoblastic neoplasia: good outcomes with induction low-dose etoposide-cisplatin and genetic analysis. J Clin Oncol. 2013;31(2):280–6.
122. Neubauer NL, Latif N, Kalakota K, Marymont M, Small W Jr, Schink JC, et al. Brain metastasis in gestational trophoblastic neoplasia: an update. J Reprod Med. 2012;57(7–8):288–92.
123. Schmid P, Nagai Y, Agarwal R, Hancock B, Savage PM, Sebire NJ, et al. Prognostic markers and long-term outcome of placental-site trophoblastic tumours: a retrospective observational study. Lancet. 2009;374(9683):48–55.

Index

A
Abdominal hysterectomy, 155
Aberrations in endometrial hormonal milieu, 69
Adjuvant chemotherapy, 232
Adjuvant treatment, indication for
 endometrioid tumors, 144
 non-endometrioid tumors, 145
Advanced endometrial cancer, 52, 55, 138, 243
Advanced/recurrent endometrial cancer hormone therapy, 244
Aflibercept, vascular endothelial growth factor, 256
Age independent hypermethylation of ESR1 promoter, 83
Age Standardized Incidence Rates of Endometrial Cancer, 62
AKT inhibitor, 266
AKT mutation, 261
Altered cell differentiation, 9
Alternative splicing of ESR1 and ESR2 pre-mRNA, 77
American Association of Gynecologic Laparoscopists (AAGL), 158
AMP-activated protein kinase (AMPK), 261
Amsterdam criteria, 105
Androgen intracrinology, 76
Androgen receptors (AR), 78
Androgens in women, 71
Androstenedione, 71
Ang-2, 257
Angiogenesis, 239, 254, 255
Anovulation with unperturbed estrogen production, 83
Antiangiogenic agents, 40, 41, 239, 240, 255, 266
Antiangiogenic inhibitors, 251
Anti-estrogenic therapy, 27
Anti-HER2 therapies, 220
Antitumor activity, 41
Anti-tumour effect of melatonin, 87
Aortic bifurcation, 168
Apoptosis, endometrial cancer cells to, 83
Apparent diffusion coefficient (ADC), 50, 52
ARID1A, 26, 27
Aromatase inhibitors (AI), 252
A Study in the Treatment of Endometrial Cancer (ASTEC) trial, 183, 187, 225
Atypical hyperplasia (AH), 24
Atypical hyperplasia/endometrioid intraepithelial neoplasia (AH/EIN), 8

B
Base-pair mismatch in the microsatellite regions, 103
Basket trials, 129
β-catenin stabilization, 27
11β-hydroxy dehydrogenase type 1 (11βHSD1), 79
Bevacizumab, 254, 256
Bilateral common iliac lymphadenectomy, 168, 169
Bilateral salpingo-oophorectomy (BSO), 141, 155
Biological treatments, 238
Biphasic tumor, 14
Bladder and ureter base terminal, 165
Bladder lesion, 166
Bleeding complications, surgery, 304
Bowel handling, 166
Brachytherapy, 145
Breast cancer, 34
 tamoxifen use of, 64
Broad ligament, posterior leaflet, 160

C

Cabozantinib, 257
Cancer Genome Atlas project, 217
Cancer Registries, 65
Cancer staging system, 3
Carcinogenesis effect of androgens, 85
Carcinogenic catechol estrogens, 83
Carcinomatosis, 159
Carcinosarcomas, 5, 13–15, 279, 296
    adjuvant chemotherapy, 297, 298
    advanced/metastatic phase and relapse, 298
    pelvic failure, 297
    SEER database, 297
    sequential multimodality therapy, 298
    treatment, 296
Cardinal-uterosacral ligament complex, 159
Cediranib, 256
Cell biology, 251
Cell cycle, 251
Cellular control, 102
Cellular signalling of estrogen, 77
Central nervous system (CNS) metastasis, 304
Cervical invasion, 52
Cervical involvement, 153
Cervical stromal invasion, 178
Cervical stromal involvement, 51
Cervical uterine cancer, 53
Chemoprevention against endometrial cancer, 109, 110
Chemotherapy, endometrial cancer
    cisplatin-based chemoradiation, 237
    distant metastasis, 232
    histological classification, 231
    recurrence rates, 237
    survival, 231
Circumflex iliac nodes distal to the external iliac nodes (CINDEIN), 180
Clear cell carcinoma (CCC), 12, 62
    glycogen, 12
    immunohistochemistry, 12
    molecular studies, 12
    of uterine corpus and cervix, 293
        adjuvant treatment, 294, 295
        biological therapy, 296
        laparoscopic radical trachelectomy, 294
        lymphatic involvement, 294
        metastatic disease and relapse, 295, 296
        surgical staging, 294
Clinical effect, 120
Clinical trials, 130, 147
Clinical/epidemiological classification, 24
    type I, 24
    type II, 24

Cluster of differentiation 99 (CD99), 299
Clustering based on mRNA, 33
Cochrane Consumer Network (CCN), 120, 121
Cochrane meta-analysis of randomized trials, 225
Colorectal cancer (CRC), 102
Colpotomy, 164
Combination targeted therapy agents, 264–265
Combination therapy trials, 42
Comparative trials, 129
Computational models, 107
Consensus and expert opinion, 112
Copy-number high (serous-like), 250
Copy-number low (endometrioid) and microsatellite stable (MSS), 250
Corpus uteri, 4
Corticosteroids, 71, 72
Cowden syndrome, 110
Cox-2 inhibitors, 110
Cross clustering, 33
CTNNB1 mutations, 27, 266
    and endometrioid histology, 37
Cyclin A expression, 254
Cyclin-dependent kinases (CDKs), 254
Cytological atypia, 89
Cytoreductive surgery, 292
Cytotoxic chemotherapy/endocrine therapy, 243

D

Dalantercept, anti-angiogenic, 256
Dedifferentiated carcinomas, 13
Deep myometrial invasion, 51, 53
Deforolimus, 36
Dehydroepiandrosterone (DHEA), 71
Dehydroepiandrosterone sulphate (DHEAS), 71
Deiodinase 2 (DIO2), 73
Deregulated pathways in EC, 25, 26
Diabetes and obesity, 88
Dilation and curettage (D&C), 201
Direct antiproliferative action of progesterone, 83
Direct digestive wounds, 170
Disease characterization, targeted therapy, 251
Disease specific survival (DSS), 128
Disseminated metastases, 145, 146
Division of Cancer Prevention and Control, 101

Index

DNA damage, 83
DNA methylation, 251
  in estrogen signalling, 83
DNA ploidy, 178
DNA polymerase epsilon (POLE), 250
DNA repair pathways, 251
Double-blind, placebo-controlled randomized trial, 254
Douglas cul-de-sac and pararectal fossa, 166
Dovitinib, 256
Dual PI3K/mTOR inhibitor, 261
Dynamic contrast-enhanced (DCE)-MRI, 50

E

Early stage endometrial cancer, 155
  molecular factors, 220
  risk factors
    aneuploidy, 219
    FIGO classification, 213
    5-year survival rate, 214
    histologic differentiation, 214
    positive peritoneal cytology, 219–220
    recurrence-free survival, 219
    surgical stage, 213
    tumor differentiation, 214
    tumor size, 219
Embryo implantations, 73
Endocrine therapy resistance, 28
Endocrine treatment, 243
Endogenous hormones, 88, 89
Endometrial hyperplasia, 24
Endometrial sampling, 143
Endometrial stromal sarcoma (ESS)
  adjuvant hormonal therapy, 285
  adjuvant pelvic radiotherapy, 285
  chemotherapy regimens, 286
  gonadotrophin-releasing hormone agonists, 286
  HGUS, 287
  hormone-sensitive nature, 283
  lymphatic system, 283
  metastatic disease and relapse, 285–286
  treatment strategy, 283, 284
Endometrial stromal tumors with sex cord-like elements (ESTSCLE), 299
Endometrial tissue, 27
Endometrial tumour initiation, 83
Endometrioid adenocarcinoma, histotypes in, 24
Endometrioid and serous histotype, mutations between, 25
Endometrioid histology, 143
Endometrioid intraepithelial neoplasia (EIN), 8
Endometrioid/mucinous subtype, 220
ENGOT-EN1/FANDANGO trial, 240
ENGOT-EN 2 trial, 237
Epidermal growth factor receptor (EGFR), 35, 263
Epigenetic modification of progesterone, 85
Epithelial cell adhesion molecule (EPCAM) mutation carriers, 104
Epithelioid trophoblastic tumors (ETT), 304
ERBB2-amplified serous-like tumors, 35
ERBB2 gene alteration, 35
Estradiol (E2), 71
Estrogen, 71
  associated genotoxicity, 83
  independent pathway in EC, 249
  induced carcinogenesis, 82
  interaction alteration in EC, 27
  intracrinology, 76
  on proliferation and growth of reproductive tissues, 82
  receptors, 77, 244
Estrogen-dependent endometrial cancer, 243
Estrogenic stimulation, 24
Estrogen-producing ovarian tumors, 64
Estrone (E1), 71
European Society for Medical Oncology (ESMO), 133
  bilateral salpingo-oophorectomy, 135
  endometrial biopsy, 134
  follow-up, 138
  geriatric assessment, 134
  immunohistochemistry, 135
  levels of evidence and grades, 147–148
  pre-surgery evaluation, 134
  risk groups, 137
  surgical staging, 138
  surveillance for women, cancer risk, 134
  total hysterectomy, 135
European Society for Radiotherapy and Oncology (ESTRO), 133
  bilateral salpingo-oophorectomy, 135
  endometrial biopsy, 134
  follow-up, 138
  geriatric assessment, 134
  immunohistochemistry, 135
  pre-surgery evaluation, 134
  risk groups, 137
  surgical staging, 138
  surveillance for women, cancer risk, 134
  total hysterectomy, 135

European Society of Gynecological Oncology (ESGO), 133
  bilateral salpingo-oophorectomy, 135
  endometrial biopsy, 134
  follow-up, 138
  geriatric assessment, 134
  immunohistochemistry, 135
  pre-surgery evaluation, 134
  risk groups, 137
  surgical staging, 138
  surveillance for women, cancer risk, 134
  total hysterectomy, 135
European Society of Urogenital Radiology (ESUR) Endometrial Cancer Staging guidelines, 50, 51
Everolimus, 36
Evidence guidelines, 120
Evidence-based guidelines, 133
Evidence-based medicine (EBM), 119, 130
Evidence-based recommendations, 146
Evolution of endometrial cancer characterization, 250
Exogenous hormones, 89
Expanded Accordion Classification, 183
External beam radiotherapy (EBRT) treatment, 226, 227
  vs. brachiterpy, 233
  cochrane analysis of, 225
  pelvic, 232
  postoperative, 224–228
Extracellular signal-related kinase (Erk) 1/2 signalling pathway, 83
Extra-uterine disease spread, 53, 54

F
Familial syndromes, 102
Fédération Internationale de Gynécologie et d'Obstétrique (FIGO) staging system, 4, 5, 10, 176, 178
  for endometrial stromal sarcoma, 284
  for uterine sarcoma, 5
Fertility preserving treatment for grade 1 endometrioid tumors, 136
Fertility-sparing treatment, 137, 143
  close surveillance, 203
  conservative management, 202
  decision making process, 207
  definitive surgery, 204
  disease recurrence, 207
  early-stage G1 disease, 207
  HR and progestin therapy, 204
  hysteroscopic resection and progestin therapy, 205
  hysteroscopic surgical excision, 204
  imaging techniques, 202
  LNG-IUD, 203
  oral progestin therapy, 203
  outcomes of, 202
  patient selection, 201
  pregnancy outcome, 207
  progestin, 206
  progestin-containing IUD, 204
  randomised trial, 204
  recurrence rates, 203
  serum CA125, 202
  TAH-BSO, 204
Fibroblast growth factor-1 (FGF-1) expression, 256
Fibroblast growth factor receptor (FGFR), 256
Fibroblastic growth factor 2 (FGFR2), 36
Field-specific association resources, 120
FIGO staging system, Fédération Internationale de Gynécologie et d'Obstétrique (FIGO) staging system, see
Finnish trial, 233
Follicle stimulating hormone (FSH), 63, 71, 72, 80
Freeing pelvic ureter, 164
Functional decline (FD), 128

G
GDC-980, 40
Gene alterations, 25
Gene mutations, 26
Genetic Information Non-discrimination Act (GINA), 108
Genetic risk assessment, 111
Genito-femoral nerve injury, 170
Genome wide analyses, 27
Genomic pathway, 81
Geographical differences, 61
Germline DNA mutation, 108
  in DNA mismatch repair (MMR) genes, 202
  exonuclease domain of DNA polymerase POLE, 217
Gestational trophoblastic disease (GTD), 279, 301
  chemotherapy, 301, 302
  FIGO 2000 scoring system, 302
  staging and scoring of disease, 302
  treatment, 302, 303
  ultrahigh risk disease, 303, 304
Glucocorticoid production, 71
Glucocorticoid receptor (GR), 79, 87, 88

Index

Glucocorticoids, 72, 88
Glucose metabolism, 261–263
Gonadotropin-releasing hormone (GnRH) inhibitors, 72, 86, 252
Gonadotropin-releasing hormone (GnRH) receptor (GnRHR), 80
G protein-coupled receptor 30 (GPR30), 83
Grade 1 intramucous endometrial adenocarcinoma, 155
Grades of evidence, 120, 121
    CCN, 121
    OCEBM, 121
Grading of endometrioid carcinomas, 10
Granulosa and theca cell tumors, 64
Gs/adenylyl cyclase/cAMP/PKA pathways, 80
G3 tumors/deep myometrial invasion, 143
Gynecologic Cancer Inter-Group (GCIG) project, 207, 279
Gynecologic Oncology Group (GOG) trial, 41, 246, 292
    GOG 81 trial, 244
    GOG 86P, 239
    GOG-99 study, 225
    GOG 119 (Whitney) trial, 244, 246
    GOG 177 study, 237
    GOG 209 trial, 238
    GOG 258 phase III study, 233, 293
    phase II trial, 41
Gynecologic sarcomas, 297

H

Harmonization of research activities, medical practice and education, 278
Hazard ratios (HRs), 226, 227
Hemorrhagic urine, 166
Hepatic sex hormone-binding globulin (SHBG), 85
HER2 gene, 216, 263, 293
Hereditary breast and ovarian cancer syndrome (HBOCS), 102, 111
Hereditary cancers, screening, 108, 109
Hereditary non-polyposis colorectal cancer (HNPCC) syndrome, 101
High grade (grade 3) endometrioid EC, 34, 245
High-grade neuroendocrine tumors, 14
High grade serous carcinoma, 279
High grade undifferentiated sarcoma (HGUS), 286, 287
High grade uterine serous carcinoma (USC), 289–291
High-risk endometrial cancer, 136, 228
Histopathologic grades (G), 4–5

Homologous recombination deficiency (HRD) score, 268
Homologous recombination DNA repair pathway, 268
Hormonal aberrations, 88
Hormonal and metabolic pathways, steroid hormones homeostasis, 84
Hormonal blockade, 283
Hormonal therapy, 65
    with Tamoxifen (GOG-81F), 244
    toxicity profile, 245
Hormone dependent tissue, 27
Hormone induced carcinogenesis, 82
Hormone receptor
    in endometrium cells, 75
    expression, 27, 28, 251
    status, 245, 247
Hormone regulators of endometrium
    non-steroidal hormones, 72, 73
    steroid hormones, 70–72
Human chorionic gonadotropin (hCG), 80, 86
Human chorionic gonadotropin receptors, 86
Human endometrium, 69
Human epidermal growth factor receptor 2 (Her2) alteration, 35
Human epididymis protein 4 (HE4), 178, 217, 218
Human nuclear TRs, 79
Hyperandrogenism, 85, 86
Hyperinsulinism, 85
Hypothalamic-pituitary regulation of circulating steroid horemones, 70
Hysterectomy, 143, 155, 158, 166
    bilateral salpingo-oophorectomy, 187
Hysteroscopic biopsy, 202
Hysteroscopic intra-operative submucosal injection, 157
Hysteroscopic tumor resection, 207

I

Iatrogenic risk factors, 64
Iliac arterial bifurcation, 167
Immune checkpoint inhibitors, 305
Immune microenvironment in EC tumor, 267
Immunohistochemistry (IHC) analysis, 107, 135
    defective DNA mismatch repair, 140
    tissue markers of proliferation, 262
Immuno-profiling, 130
Immunotherapy, 267
Incidence of endometrial cancer, 61
Inferior mesenteric artery, 168
Infertility, 63

Infrarenal lymphadenectomy, 180
Infundibulopelvic ligament, 160
Infundibulopelvic ligament, 160
Inoperable metastasis, 243
Insulin, 73
   receptors, 79, 80
   resistance, 63
   signalling, 85
Insulin-like growth factor 1 (IGF-1), 85
Inter-aorto-caval lymph nodes, 168
Intermediate-risk endometrial cancer, 136, 223
International Collaborative Group on Hereditary Non-polyposis Colorectal Cancer, 105
International Federation of Gynecology and Obstetrics, 3
Interventional radiology techniques, 281
Intra-abdominal metastasis, 243
Intracrinology process, 73, 75
Irreversible steroid sulphatase (STS) inhibitor, 252
Isolated metastases, 145
Isolated para aortic recurrences, 171
Isolated tumor cells in pelvic and para-aortic lymph nodes, 196
Isolated vaginal recurrences of endometrial cancer, 171

J
Juxtavesical ureter, 164

K
KEYNOTE-028 study, 267
Kocher forceps, 161
Kocher maneuver, 167
Korean Gynecologic Oncology Group (KGOG), 178
KRAS mutation, 41

L
Laparoscopic hysterectomy, 158
Laparoscopically assisted vaginal hysterectomy, 155
Laparoscopic-directed preparation for vaginal hysterectomy, 158
Laparoscopy, 142
L1-cell adhesion molecule (L1CAM), 218, 219
Leg lymphedema, 187
Lenvatanib, 257
Lethal bleeding, 169

Levonorgestrel-releasing intrauterine device (LNG-IUD), 65
Ligand-induced signalling pathways, 81
Limited or inconsistent scientific evidence, 111
Local staging, 49, 50
Loco-regional relapse, 145
Low-grade endometrial cancers, 244
Low-grade neuoendocrine tumors of the endometrium, 14
Low-risk endometrial cancer, 136, 223
Low risk gestational trophoblastic neoplasia, 302
Low stage endometrioid histotype endometrial cancer, 24
Luteinizing hormone, 72, 86
Luteinizing hormone receptors (LH-R), 80, 86
Luteinizing hormone-releasing hormone (LHRH), 269
Lymph node dissection, 187
Lymph node dissemination, 176, 178, 180
Lymph node enlargement, 153
Lymph node involvement, 4
   prevalence, 177
Lymph node metastasis, 176, 178
   imaging modalities, 177
   in paraaortic area, 181
   molecular and serum biomarkers, 178
   pattern, 179, 180
Lymph node status, 187
Lymphadenectomy, 53, 135, 136, 141, 142, 156, 157, 167–170, 183, 187
   adjuvant therapy, 183
   assessment of, 182
   clinical trial, 183
   diagnostic and therapeutic benefits, 175
   morbidity, 182
   surgical staging, 180
   therapeutic role, 181, 182
Lymphatic circulation, 179
Lymphatic dissemination, 178, 180
Lymphatic drainage pathways of myometrium, 157
Lymphatic space involvement (LVSI), 214, 215
   age, 215
   estrogen and progesterone receptors, 216
   HER2/neu, 216
   hormonal therapy, 216
   molecular analysis, 215
   molecular markers, 216
   p53 alterations, 216
   progestins, 216
   PTEN mutation, 216

race, 215
tumor growth and disease spreading, 215
Lymphatic spread, 188
Lymphatic tissue, 168
Lymphedema, 183
Lymphocele, 170
Lymphocyst formation, 187
Lymphonodectomy (LNE), 215
Lymphorrhoea, 170
Lymphostasis, 168, 170
Lymphovascular space invasion (LVSI), 10, 137, 143, 178
Lynch syndrome (LS), 62, 102, 103
    families, 62
    genetic risk assessment, 104
    germline mutations in mismatch repair genes, 103
    histologic subtypes, 104
    incidence, 104
    lower uterine segment, 104
    lymph-vascular invasion, 104
    MLH1 promoter methylation, 104

M

Macroscopic lymph node metastasis, 243
Maggi's italian trial, 232
Maintenance therapy, 268
Malignant mixed Müllerian tumor (MMMT), 14
Mammalian target of rapamycin (mTOR), 238, 239
MAP kinase-dependent phosphorylation, 87
Matrix metalloproteinase-2 (MMP-2), 83
Matrix metalloproteinase-9 (MMP-9), 83
Medical insurance coverage, 108
Medium-high-risk endometrial cancer, 228
MEK/ERK MAPK pathway, 83
Melatonin, 73
    administration, 87
    levels, 87
    receptors, 80, 81
Membrane located ER, 82
Memorial Sloan-Kettering Cancer Center's pathologic ultrastaging algorithm for sentinel lymph nodes, 195
Mesenchymal tumors, 279
    LMS, 279, 280
Metabolic syndrome, 63
Metabolism pathway, 263
Metastatic disease, 237, 238, 281
    biological anticancer treatments, 298
    HER2/neu, 293
    paclitaxel-paraplatine combination, 298
    platinum/taxane-based regimens with trastuzumab, 293
Metastatic high grade sarcomas, 289
Metformin, 261, 262
Microarray mRNA expression, 33
Microcystic, elongated and fragmented (MELF) growth pattern, 10
Micrometastasis, 196
Microscopic lymph node metastasis, 243
Micropapillary growth, 11
Microsatellite instability (MSI), 26, 103, 107, 140, 217, 250
Microsatellite mismatch repair (MMR) status, 266
Mineralocorticoid, 71
    production, 72
Mineralocorticoid receptor (MR), 79
Minimal invasive surgery, 135, 172
Mismatch repair (MMR), 103
    deficiency, 103
    mutations, 109
    predict model, 107
Mismatch repair-related protein expression and clinicopathologic features in EC, 267
MITO END 2 trial, 41, 239
Mixed carcinomas, 14
MMRpro model, 107
Molecular aberrations, endometrioid carcinomas, 10
Molecular analysis, 129
Molecular classification of EC-TCGA, 28
    mutational status, 29–30
Molecular methods of drug delivery, 42
Monoclonal antibodies to small molecule inhibitors, 35
MRI protocol, 50
mTOR inhibitors, 36, 37, 258, 266
    and anti-angiogenic agent, 266
    mTORC1/2 inhibitor, 266
Muir-Torre Syndrome, 110
Mullerian adenosarcoma of female genital tract, 288
Multitargeted anti-angiogenic agents, 257
Mutated PI3Kinase and PI3K pathway aberrations, 216–217
Mutation and copy number alteration spectra, 32
Mutational alteration, 34
Mutation-based trial design, 42
Myometrial invasion, 49, 51, 53, 153, 178, 214

N

N-acetyle-5-methoxy-tryptamine, 73
National Comprehensive Cancer Network (NCCN) guidelines, 140, 147, 245
 primary treatment, 140, 141
Near infrared (NIR) fluorescence imaging system using ICG, 189
NEU gene, 293
Neuroendocrine tumors, 14
Neurovascular injury, 187
Next generation sequencing (NGS), 42, 129, 130
Nodal staging, 53
Non-endometrioid histology, 142, 143
Non-endometrioid tumors, adjuvant chemotherapy, 138
Non genomic estrogen signalling, 82
Non genomic pathway, 81
Non-genomic transcription independent effects, 79
Non-sentinel lymph nodes, 188
Nonsteroidal anti-inflammatory drugs (NSAIDs), 110
Non-steroidal hormones, 69
 FSH and LH, 72
 GnRH, 72
 insulin, 73
 melatonin, 73
 TH, 72, 73
Non-transcriptional response to estrogen, 82
NORDCAN database, 65
NSGO9501/EORTC 55991 trial, 233
Nuclear DNA replication and repair, 250

O

Obesity, 155
Observational studies, 120
Occult ovarian malignancy, 202
Olaparib, 268
Onapristone, 252
Oncological safety of the laparoscopic approach, 155
Open label trials, 129
Open-technique laparoscopy, 159
Oslo trial, 224, 225
Ovarian cancer (OC), 34, 102
Ovarian preservation, 136, 155
Ovarian steroid hormones, 69
Ovarian theca cells, 71
Overall treatment utility (OTU), 128
Oxford Centre for Evidence-based Medicine (OCEBM), 121

P

Palbociclib, 254
PALETTE trial, 288
Para-aortic lymph node dissemination, 180, 181
Para-aortic lymph nodes, 141
Para-aortic lymphadenectomy, 142, 167, 180
PARAGON study, 252
Paravesical fossa, 165
PARP inhibitor, 266
Pathologic ultrastaging, 196
Patient-derived tumour xenograft models, 251
PD-1 targeted immunotherapies, 267
Pelvic and para-aortic lymph node dissection, 180
Pelvic and para-aortic lymph node involvement, 4
Pelvic and para-aortic lymph node metastasis, 176, 179
Pelvic and para-aortic lymphadenectomy, 183
Pelvic and para-aortic nodal disease, 176
Pelvic external beam radiotherapy, 232
Pelvic lymphadenectomy, 156, 167
Pelvic nodal dissection, 141
Pelvic radiation, 256
Peritoneal incision, 167
Peritoneum vesicouterine cul-de-sac, 166
Personalized medicine, 19, 129
Pfannenstiehl laparotomy, 167
Pharmacogenomics, 129
Pharmacological measures, risk reduction, 65
Phase I clinical trials, 129
Phase II clinical trial, 130
Phase II study KEYNOTE-158, 267
Phase II target agents trials in advanced/recurrent endometrial cancer, 38–39
Phase III clinical trials, 130
Phase 3 randomized placebo-controled trial, ENGOT-EN5/ SIENDO, 268
Phase IV clinical trial, 130
Phosphatidylinositol 3-kinase pathway, 216, 217
PI3K inhibitors, 37, 40, 258, 268
PI3K/AKT/mTOR pathway, 25, 28, 35–37, 40, 41, 217, 251, 257–261
PI3Kinase/mTOR inhibitors, 217
PIK3CA mutation, 41
Pilaralisib, 37
Placebo-controlled randomized trial, 257
Placenta site trophoblastic tumor (PSTT), 304
Platelet-derived growth factor receptor (PDGFR), 256
Platinum-based therapy, 238

POLE-mutated cancers polymerase
    proofreading, 217
POLE proofreading mutation, 217
POLE ultramutated subgroup, 250
Poly(ADP-ribose) polymerase (PARP)
    inhibitors, 40
Polycystic ovarian syndrome (PCOS), 63,
    85, 88
Polycystic ovary (PCO), 64
PORTEC system, 19
    PORTEC-1, 15, 224
    PORTEC-2, 228
    Portec 3 trial, 237
    PORTEC-4 study, 19
Posterior dissection and vesico-uterine
    dissection, 160
Posterior dissection, Douglas cul de sac,
    161, 162
Postmenopausal (PM) endometrium, 82
Postmenopausal vaginal bleeding, 134
Postoperative vaginal brachy therapy
    (VBT), 228
Post transcriptional deactivation of PR
    isoforms, 85
PPP2R1A, 26
PR knockout (PRKO) mice, 85
Pre- and post-test counseling, 108
Precancers of endometrioid carcinoma, 8
Precision medicine, 129
Premenopausal endometrium, 81, 82
PREMM$_{1,2,6}$ model, 107
Preoperative endometrial carcinoma
    biopsies, 178
Preoperative hysteroscopy, 202
Proactive molecular risk classifier for
    endometrial cancer (ProMisE), 17
Progesterone, 71
    insufficiency, 85
    interaction alteration in EC, 27
    intracrinology, 75, 76
    tumour suppressive role, 83, 85
Progesterone-based treatment, 143
Progesterone receptors (PR), 28, 77,
    78, 244
Progestin and antiestrogenic therapy, 28
Progestin-based contraception, 110, 112
Prognosis, 3
Prognostic factors, 153
Progression free survival (PFS), 128
Prohormones, 71
Prophylactic surgery, 109
PTEN mutation, 216
p53-tumor-suppressor gene, 216
Pulmonary metastasis, 243

Q
Querleu classification, 162–164

R
Radiation therapy, 292
Radical hysterectomy, 162, 166
    lateral peritoneum, 163
    pararectal fossa, 163
    paravesical fossa, 163
    pelvic ureter, 163
Radioactive tracers, 189
Randomized clinical trials (RCTs), 120,
    122–128
Randomized phase II study, 255
Randomized phase III trials, 232, 234–236
Rare gynecologic tumors (RGT), 278
RAS pathway, 41
RAS/MEK/ERK pathway, 41
RAS-RAF-MEK-ERK pathway mediators, 26
Rat endometrial stromal cells, 81
Receptor tyrosine kinases (RTK), 216
Rectovaginal space, 164
Recurrent endometrial cancer, 171
Regional pelvic recurrence, 138
Relapsed/metastatic endometrioid tumors, 138
Renovascular azygo lumbar arch, 169
Reproductive and genetic counseling, 207
Retinoid X receptor (RXR), 79
Revised 2009 FIGO staging, EC, 154
Revised Amsterdam criteria and Bethesda
    guidelines, 105, 106
Ridaforolimus, 36
Right colon, 167
Right pedicle infundibulopelvic, 168
Risk scoring systems, 178
Robotic-assisted laparoscopy, 142
Robotic-assisted surgery, 155
Round ligament, 160

S
Second-line chemotherapy for endometrial
    carcinoma, 238
Selective estrogen receptor modulators
    (SERM), 252
Selective inhibitor of nuclear export (SINE)
    drug, 268
Selective lymphadenectomy, Mayo
    criteria, 177
Selective progesterone receptor modulators
    (SPRM), 89
SENTI-ENDO study, 197
Sentinel lymph node dissection (SLND), 136

Sentinel lymph node (SLN) mapping, 142, 183
  algorithm, 193
  algorithm-specific sensitivity, 194
  blue dyes, 189
  blue SLNs, 192
  clinical care, 188
  colorimetric blue dye, 189
  detection rate, 192
  diagnostic accuracy, 193–194
  dye positive lymph nodes, 193
  fallopian tubes, 189
  fluorescent indocyanine green dye, 189
  ICG dye, 189
  image-guided procedure, 188
  location in pelvis, 191
  lymph node dissection, 193
  lymph node metastases, 194
  lymphatic anatomy, 190, 191
  lymphatic channels, 188
  lymphatic mapping, 188
  lymphatic pathway, 191
  pathologic ultrastaging, 194
  peritumoral injection, 188
  precaval and paraaortal lymph node dissection, 193
  radioactive isotopes, 189
  SLN algorithm, 192
  tracers detection, 190
  uterine corpus (subserosal/myometrial), 188
Sentinel lymph nodes, 158, 170
Serous adenocarcinoma, histotypes in, 24
Serous carcinomas, 10–12, 62
Serous endometrial intraepithelial carcinoma (SEIC), 8
Sex steroid hormone receptors, 81
Simple hysterectomy, 160–162
Single agent anti-tumour activity of selinexor, 268
Society of Gynecologic Oncology (SGO), 106, 110, 140, 246
Society of Gynecologic Oncology education committee, inherited gynecologic cancer predispositions, 106
Somatic copy number alterations (SCNA), 217
Somatic copy numbers (SCN), 217
Sporadic mutations, 25
Sporadic POLE mutations, 217
Stage I endometrial carcinoma, 176
Stage-I endometrioid uterine tumors ploidy, 219
Stage IVA cancer, 244

Staging of gynecological cancers, 3
Stathmin overexpression, 178
Steroid hormones
  androgens, 71
  corticosteroids, 70–72
  cortisol binding globulin, 71
  endometrial response to, 81
  estrogens, 71
  Hypothalamic-Pituitary regulation, 70
  intracrinology, 74
  progesterone, 71
  receptors, 77
  sex steroids, 70
  sex-hormone binding globulin, 71
Steroid hormones intracrinology of endometrium
  androgen intracrinology, 76
  estrogen intracrinology, 76
  progesterone intracrinology, 75
Steroid receptor signalling, 81
Stratification system, 177
Stratified medicine, 129
Stromal decidualisation in endometrium, 71
Subserosal injection, 189
Subserosal intraoperative injection, 157
Sunitinib, 256
Surgery, uterus cancer, 154
Surgical management, 135
Surgical-pathological patterns of spread, 4
Surgical restaging with lymph node dissection, 142
Surveillance, Epidemiology, and End Results (SEER) database, 3, 182
Survival effect of para-aortic lymphadenectomy in endometrial cancer (SEPAL) study, 182

T
Targeted chemotherapy, 269
Targeted medicine, 129
Targeted therapy in EC management, 238, 251, 263–266
  clinico-pathological characteristics, 249
  estrogen and progesterone receptors
  clinical trials, 253
  low grade endometrioid histology, 251
  oestrogen antagonist, 252
  response rates, 252
  tamoxifen and megestrol, 252
  target-specific therapy, 251
Temsirolimus, 37
Testosterone, 71

The Cancer Genome Atlas consortium
      (TCGA), 250
Thyroid-binding globulins (TBGs), 72
Thyroid hormone receptor (TR), 79
Thyroid hormones (TH), 72, 73, 87
Thyroid stimulating hormone (TSH), 87
Tibolone, 89
Tissue microstructure, 53
Tissue recombination studies, 83
Total abdominal hysterectomy and bilateral
      salpingo-oophorectomy (TAH-
      BSO), 202
Total extrafascial non conservative
      hysterectomy, 160–162
Total hysterectomy, 141
Total laparoscopic hysterectomy, 155
TP53 master regulator gene suppression, 26
TP53 mutations, 12
Translational clinical trials, 251
Translational research activities, 129
Transperitoneal approach, 170
Transperitoneal laparoscopy, 167
Transtubal dissemination, 159
Transvaginal ultrasonography (TVS), 202
Tumor Cancer Genome Atlas (TCGA), 15
    copy-number high serous-like
      group, 16, 17
    copy-number low endometrioid-like
      group, 16
    endometrial carcinoma analysis, 15
    histologies distribution, 31
    genomic subtypes, 18
    hypermutated/microsatellite-unstable
      group, 31
    hypermutated POLE group, 16
    ultramutated POLE group, 15, 16, 31
Tumor cell migration and invasion, 87
Tumor diameter, 178
Tumor testing, 107, 108
Tumoral metabolical properties, 52
Tumor-infiltrating lymphocytes (TILs), 267
Tumor-volume-directed radiation
      therapy, 292
Tumour microenvironment, 69
Tumour progression, 69
Tumour suppressive role of progesterone,
      83, 85
Tumour suppressor proteins and growth
      regulatory proteins, 268
Type I endometrial cancer, 62, 63, 214
    risk factors, 63, 64
Type II cancer, 62, 63, 214
Type II diabetes mellitus (T2DM), 63
Tyrosine kinase inhibitor (TKI), 256

U
Ultrastaging, 158
    protocols, 195
    sensitivity and specificity, 195, 196
Umbrella trials, 129
Undifferentiated carcinomas, 13
Univariate disease-free survival analyses for
      FIGO stage, 218
Unopposed estrogen therapy, 65
Unresectable metastatic disease, systemic
      treatment, 281
    dacarbazine and temozolomide, 283
    doxorubicin, 282
    Eribulin, 283
    fixed dose-rate gemcitabine plus
      docetaxel, 282
    gemcitabine, 282
    ifosfamide, 282
    pazopanib, 282
    Trabectedin, 282, 283
Ureteral damage, 170
Uterine adenosarcomas, 288, 289
Uterine arterys, 158, 159, 163
Uterine carcinosarcomas (UCs), 296
Uterine corpus, 62, 188
Uterine extraction and vaginal closure, 161
Uterine fundus, 164
Uterine malignant tumors
    histological diagnosis, 278
    level 1 evidence, 278
    patient management, 278
Uterine manipulator, 158, 159
Uterine mobilisation, 158
Uterine neoplasm, 140
Uterine perforation, 159
Uterine resection, 155
Uterine sarcomas, 287
Uterine serous carcinoma, 27
Uterine tumor resembling ovarian sex-cord
      tumor (UTROSCT), 299
    metastatic phase, 300
    treatment, 299, 300
Uterine vessels dissection, 160
Uterine vessels ligation, 162
Uterosacral ligaments, 160, 164

V
Vagina, circular colpotomy, 161
Vaginal approach, 142
Vaginal bank, 161
Vaginal brachytherapy, 225
Vaginal cuff, 165
Vaginal hysterectomy, 135

Vaginal recurrence, 138
Vaginal suture, 164
Vaginal vault, 166
Vascular endothelial growth factor receptor (VEGFR), 256
Vascular surgery, 169
Vesico vaginal dissection, 161
Vesicouterine peritoneal reflection, 160
Vesicovaginal dissection, 165

W
Whole abdominal pelvis irradiation (WAPI), 293
WNT and RAS dependent pathway alteration, 27
WNT-βcatenin signaling pathway, 26
Wnt inhibitory proteins, 83
Women with black ethnicity, 61